CLINICAL
ONCOLOGY

CLINICAL ONCOLOGY

Basic principles and practice

Fourth Edition

ANTHONY J NEAL MD MRCP FRCR
Consultant in Clinical Oncology
at St Luke's Cancer Centre
Guildford, Surrey, UK

PETER J HOSKIN MD FRCP FRCR
Professor in Clinical Oncology
at University College London, and
Consultant in Clinical Oncology
at Mount Vernon Hospital
Northwood, Middlesex, UK

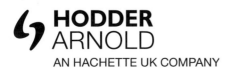

HODDER
ARNOLD
AN HACHETTE UK COMPANY

First published in Great Britain in 1997
Third edition 2003; reprinted 2005 by
Arnold, a member of the Hodder Headline Group,
This fourth edition published in Great Britain in 2009 by
Hodder Arnold, an imprint of Hodder Education, an Hachette UK Company,
338 Euston Road, London NW1 3BH
http://www.hoddereducation.com

Hachette UK's policy is to use papers that are natural, renewable and recyclable products and made from wood grown in sustainable forests. The logging and manufacturing processes are expected to conform to the environmental regulations of the country of origin.

Whilst the advice and information in this book are believed to be true and accurate at the date of going to press, neither the authors nor the publisher can accept any legal responsibility or liability for any errors or omissions that may be made. In particular (but without limiting the generality of the preceding disclaimer) every effort has been made to check drug dosages; however, it is still possible that errors have been missed. Furthermore, dosage schedules are constantly being revised and new side-effects recognized. For these reasons the reader is strongly urged to consult the drug companies' printed instructions before administering any of the drugs recommended in this book.

British Library Cataloguing in Publication Data
A catalogue record for this book is available from the British Library

Library of Congress Cataloging-in-Publication Data
A catalog record for this book is available from the Library of Congress

ISBN 978 0 340 972 939

1 2 3 4 5 6 7 8 9 10

Commissioning Editor: Sara Purdy
Project Editor: Jane Tod and Amy Mulick
Production Controller: Karen Tate
Cover Designer: Amina Dudhia
Copy-editor: Michèle Clarke
Indexer: Laurence Errington

Typeset in 10/12 pt Berling by Phoenix Photosetting, Chatham, Kent
Printed and bound in Italy

What do you think about this book? Or any other Hodder Arnold title?
Please visit our website: www.hoddereducation.com

CONTENTS

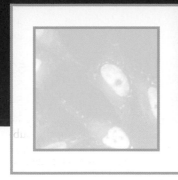

Preface ix

Acknowledgements x

List of abbreviations xi

1 PATHOGENESIS OF CANCER 1
Genetic factors 1
Chemical factors 3
Physical factors 4
Viral factors 5
Immune factors 7
Endocrine factors 7
Understanding the cause of cancer – the contribution to patient care 8

2 PRINCIPLES OF CANCER DIAGNOSIS AND STAGING 10
Securing a tissue diagnosis 10
Principles of cancer staging 11
The TNM staging system 19
Use of pathological information 20

3 DECISION-MAKING AND COMMUNICATION 22
Treatment options 23
Quality of life 25
Communication 26
Conclusion 28
Clinical evidence and clinical trials 28
Conclusion 35

4 PRINCIPLES OF SURGICAL ONCOLOGY 36
Management of the primary tumour 36
Combined surgery and radiotherapy 37
Management of regional lymph nodes 37
Palliative surgery 38

5 PRINCIPLES OF RADIOTHERAPY 42
Types of radiotherapy 42
Other forms of radiation 44

Biological actions of ionizing radiation   44
Clinical use of radiotherapy   45
Side-effects of radiotherapy   48
Radiation protection   49

6 PRINCIPLES OF SYSTEMIC TREATMENT   52
Chemotherapy agents   52
Efficacy and toxicity of chemotherapy   54
Clinical use of chemotherapy   56
Drug resistance   56
Administration of chemotherapy   57
Hormone therapy   61
Biological therapy   63
Growth factors   64
Experimental chemotherapy   65

7 LUNG CANCER AND MESOTHELIOMA   67
Lung cancer   67
Mesothelioma   84

8 BREAST CANCER   89
Epidemiology   89
Aetiology   90
Pathology   91
Natural history   92
Symptoms   95
Signs   95
Differential diagnosis   96
Investigations   97
Staging   100
Treatment   100
Prognosis   113
Screening   114
Prevention   115

9 GASTROINTESTINAL CANCER   118
Carcinoma of the oesophagus   118
Carcinoma of the stomach   124
Carcinoma of the pancreas   130
Hepatocellular cancer   135
Cholangiocarcinoma   139
Carcinoma of the gallbladder   141
Carcinoma of the colon and rectum   142
Carcinoma of the anus   152
Tumours of the peritoneum   156

10 UROLOGICAL CANCER   160
Renal cell carcinoma   160
Prostate cancer   163

Bladder cancer 172
Cancer of the testis 177
Cancer of the penis 180

11 GYNAECOLOGICAL CANCER 185
Cervical cancer 185
Endometrial cancer 191
Ovarian cancer 194
Cancer of the vagina 198
Cancer of the vulva 200
Choriocarcinoma 202

12 CNS TUMOURS 207
Astrocytoma 211
Oligodendroglioma 213
Meningioma 213
Pituitary tumours 214
Craniopharyngioma 216
Pineal tumours 216
Germ cell tumours 216
Ependymomas 217
Medulloblastoma 217
Chordoma 218
Haemangioblastoma 218
Lymphoma 218
Metastases 219
Carcinomatous meningitis 221

13 HEAD AND NECK CANCER 225
Carcinoma of the oral cavity 225
Carcinoma of the oropharynx 232
Carcinoma of the larynx 232
Carcinoma of the hypopharynx 233
Carcinoma of the nasopharynx 234
Carcinoma of the paranasal sinuses 235
Salivary gland tumours 235
Orbital tumours 237

14 ENDOCRINE TUMOURS 239
Thyroid cancer 239
Tumours of the parathyroid gland 246
Tumours of the adrenal glands 246
Carcinoid tumours 248
Multiple endocrine neoplasia (MEN) 251

15 SARCOMAS 254
Soft tissue sarcomas 254
Osteosarcoma 259
Ewing's sarcoma 263
Other bone tumours 265

16 LYMPHOMA   268
Hodgkin's lymphoma   268
Non-Hodgkin's lymphoma (NHL)   275

17 HAEMATOLOGICAL MALIGNANCY   288
Leukaemia   288
Multiple myeloma   299

18 PAEDIATRIC CANCER   310
Leukaemia   310
Central nervous system tumours   310
Bone and soft tissue tumours   313
Lymphoma   315
Neuroblastoma   316
Nephroblastoma (Wilms' tumour)   318
Other tumours   321

19 SKIN CANCER   325
Squamous and basal cell carcinoma   325
Melanoma   331
Metastases   338
Rare tumours   338

20 AIDS-RELATED CANCER   341
Management problems   341
Kaposi's sarcoma (KS)   342
Primary cerebral lymphoma   343
Non-Hodgkin's lymphoma   344
Hodgkin's disease (HD)   345
Other tumours   345

21 CARCINOMA OF UNKNOWN PRIMARY   347
Differential diagnosis   347
Investigations   348
Management   350
Prognosis   351

22 ONCOLOGICAL EMERGENCIES   354
Hypercalcaemia   354
Spinal cord and cauda equina compression   355
Superior vena cava obstruction   357
Neutropenic sepsis   359
Tumour lysis syndrome   360

23 PALLIATIVE CARE   363
Pain control   363
Other symptoms   368
The dying patient   371

Appendices   375
Index   380

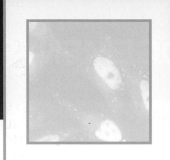

PREFACE

Approximately 1 million people in the European Union die from malignant disease each year, representing one in four of deaths from all causes. Over the last 30 years, the overall incidence of cancer has increased by 25%, with a 15% increase in men and double that for women, although during the last decade, the overall incidence has started to reach a plateau. Over the last 20 years, the diagnosis of cancer at an earlier stage and advances in treatment and supportive care have led to an ongoing fall in age-standardized mortality.

The management of cancer patients forms a significant part of the daily practice of doctors in clinical specialities and general practice. This concise textbook has been written to give an insight into the basic principles and practice of clinical oncology. With both general and site-specific chapters, it provides a readily available source of information on the epidemiology, aetiology, pathology, presentation, staging, management and prognosis of malignant disease. Recent advances and topical issues are covered. This book will be of interest and relevance to undergraduates in medicine, junior doctors, nurses with an interest in oncology and other healthcare professionals who wish to acquire a core of basic knowledge in this field. Case studies and MCQs will be used to reinforce key points. The text of this fourth edition has been fully revised to reflect recent advances and changes in practice in this field, the statistics updated and many new figures added to illustrate key points.

Anthony J Neal & Peter J Hoskin

2009

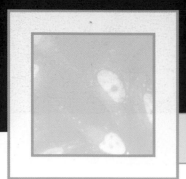

ACKNOWLEDGEMENTS

The authors acknowledge with thanks the support of various colleagues in producing this edition. In particular Dr A Padhani (Figures 11.5 and 17.4), Dr RJ Chambers (Figure 16.5) and Varian Medical Systems (Figures 5.1 and 5.2).

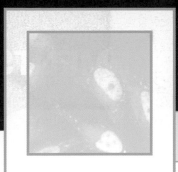

LIST OF ABBREVIATIONS

ABVD	chemotherapy schedule comprising Adriamycin, bleomycin, vincristine and dacarbazine
AFP	α-fetoprotein
AIDS	acquired immune deficiency syndrome
AIN	anal intraepithelial neoplasia
ALL	acute lymphoblastic leukaemia
AML	acute myeloid/myeloblastic leukaemia
AP	anteroposterior
APR	abdominoperineal resection
APUD	amine precursor uptake and decarboxylation
ATRA	all-transretinoic acid
AUC	area under the serum concentration vs time curve
BBB	blood–brain barrier
BCC	basal cell carcinoma
BEACOPP	chemotherapy schedule comprising bleomycin, etoposide, Adriamycin, cyclophosphamide, vincristine (Oncovin), procarbazine and prednisone
BEAM	chemotherapy schedule comprising BCNU, etoposide, cytosine arabinoside and melphelan
BEP	chemotherapy schedule comprising bleomycin, etoposide and cisplatin
BEV	beam's eye view
BOPP	chemotherapy schedule comprising bleomycin, vincristine, cisplatin and prednisolone
BSE	breast self-examination
CAP	chemotherapy schedule comprising cyclophosphamide, Adriamycin, cisplatin
CDT	chemotherapy schedule comprising cyclophosphamide, dexamethasone and thalidomide
CEA	carcinoembryonic antigen
CGL	chronic granulocytic leukaemia
CHART	continuous, hyperfractionated, accelerated radiotherapy
ChlVPP	chemotherapy schedule comprising chlorambucil, vinblastine, procarbazine and prednisolone
CHOP	chemotherapy schedule comprising cyclophosphamide, hydroxydaunorubicin (Adriamycin), oncovin and prednisolone

CHRPE	congenital hypertrophy of the retinal pigment epithelium
CIN	cervical intraepithelial neoplasia
CIS	cell carcinoma in situ
CNS	central nervous system
CRM	circumferential resection margin
CRT	chemoradiotherapy
CSF	colony-stimulating factors
CT	computed tomography
CVAD	chemotherapy schedule comprising cyclophosphamide, vincristine, doxorubicin (Adriamycin) and dexamethasone
DCIS	ductal carcinoma in situ
DMC	data monitoring committee
DNA	deoxyribonucleic acid
DRE	digital rectal examination
EBV	Epstein–Barr virus
ECF	chemotherapy schedule comprising epirubicin, cisplatin and 5FU
ECX	chemotherapy schedule comprising epirubicin, cisplatin and capecitabine (xeloda)
EDTA	ethylene diamine tetra-acetic acid
EGFR	epithelial growth factor receptor
EMA-CO	chemotherapy schedule comprising etoposide, actinomycin D, methotrexate, vincristine and cyclophosphamide
EORTC	European Organization for Research and Treatment of Cancer
EPID	electronic portal imaging device
ER	oestrogen receptor
ERCP	endoscopic retrograde cholepancreaticogram
ESR	erythrocyte sedimentation rate
EUA	examination under anaesthetic
FACT	Functional Assessment of Cancer Therapy questionnaire
FAD	chemotherapy comprising fludarabine in combination with Adriamycin and dexamethasone
FDG	fluorodeoxyglucose
FDPs	fibrin degradation products
FISH	fluoresence in situ hybridization
FMD	chemotherapy schedule comprising fludarabine in combination with mitozantrone and dexamethasone
FNA	fine needle aspiration
FOBT	faecal occult blood testing
5FU	5-fluorouracil
GC	chemotherapy schedule comprising gemcitabine with cisplatin
G-CSF	granulocyte colony-stimulating factor
GEP	gastroenterohepatic peptide
GIST	gastrointestinal stromal tumour
GnRH	gonadotrophin-releasing hormone
GST	glutathione S-transferase
HAART	highly active antiretroviral therapy
HAD	Hospital Anxiety Depression
HCG	human chorionic gonadotrophin
HHV	human herpes virus
5-HIAA	5-hydroxyindoleacetic acid
HIV	human immunodeficiency virus

HNPCC	hereditary non-polyposis colon or colorectal cancer
HPOA	hypertrophic pulmonary osteoarthropathy
HPV	human papilloma virus
HTLV-1	human T-cell lymphotrophic virus type 1
HVA	homovanillylmandelic acid
IDL	indirect laryngoscopy
IJV	internal jugular vein
IL	interleukin
IMRT	intensity-modulated radiotherapy
INR	international normalized ratio
IPI	International Prognostic Index
IVC	inferior vena cava
IVU	intravenous urography
KS	Kaposi's sarcoma
LCA	leukocyte common antigen
LCIS	lobular carcinoma in situ
LD	latissimus dorsi
LDH	lactate dehydrogenase
LET	linear energy transfer
LOPP	chemotherapy schedule comprising chlorambucil (Leukeran), vinblastine, procarbazine and prednisolone (same as ChlVPP)
MAB	maximal androgen blockade
MAB	monoclonal antibodies
MALT	mucosal associated lymphoid tissue
MDR	multidrug resistance
MDT	chemotherapy schedule comprising melphalan, dexamethasone and thalidomide
MEN	multiple endocrine neoplasia
mIBG	meta-iodobenzyl guanidine
MIP	maximum intensity projection
MOPP	chemotherapy schedule comprising mustine, vincristine, procarbazine and prednisolone
MRA	magnetic resonance angiography
MRI	magnetic resonance imaging
MTD	maximum tolerated dose
MTIC	monomethyl triazenoimidazole carboxamide
MVAC	chemotherapy schedule comprising methotrexate, vinblastine and Adriamycin plus cisplatin
MVC	chemotherapy schedule comprising methotrexate, vinblastine and cisplatin
NAT2	N-acetyl transferase 2
NHL	non-Hodgkin's lymphoma
NLPHL	nodular lymphocyte-predominant Hodgkin's lymphoma
NMDA	N-methyl-D-aspartate
NSAID	non-steroidal anti-inflammatory drug
NSE	neurone-specific enolase
OAF	osteoclast-activating factor
OEPA	chemotherapy schedule comprising vincristine, etoposide, prednisolone and Adriamycin
OPPA	chemotherapy schedule comprising vincristine, procarbazine, prednisolone and Adriamycin
PBPC	peripheral blood progenitor cell

PCI	prophylactic cranial irradiation
PDGF	platelet derived growth factor
PDGFRB	platelet derived growth factor receptor B
PET	positron emission tomography
PICC	peripherally inserted central catheter
PIN	prostate intraepithelial neoplasia
PLAP	placental alkaline phosphatase
PNET	primitive neuroectodermal tumours
POMBACE	chemotherapy schedule comprising cisplatin, vincristine, methotrexate, bleomycin, actinomycin D, cyclophosphamide and etoposide
PSA	prostate-specific antigen
PTC	percutaneous transhepatic cholangiography
PUVA	psoralens and ultraviolet A
PVI	protracted venous infusion
RCHOP	chemotherapy schedule comprising rituximab, cyclophosphamide, hydroxydaunorubicin (Adriamycin), vincristine and prednisolone
RCVP	chemotherapy schedule comprising rituximab, cyclophospamide, vincristine and prednisolone
REAL	Revised European American Lymphoma classification
RECIST	Response Evaluation Criteria in Solid Tumours
RMI	Risk of Malignancy index
RR	relative risk
SCC	squamous cell carcinoma
SCLC	small cell lung cancer
SIADH	syndrome of inappropriate antidiuretic hormone secretion
SRT	stereotactic radiotherapy
STD	sexually transmitted disease
SUV	glucose uptake rates (standardized uptake value)
SVC	superior vena cava
SVCO	superior vena cava obstruction
TCT	transitional cell tumours
TME	total mesorectal excision
TNM	tumour, nodes, metastases
TP	thymidine phosphorylase
TSH	thyroid stimulating hormone
TURBT	transurethral resection of bladder tumour
TURP	transurethral resection of the prostate
VAC	chemotherapy schedule comprising vincristine, actinomycin D and cyclophosphamide
VAIN	vaginal intraepithelial neoplasia
VAS	visual analogue scale
VDA	vascular disrupting agents
VEGF	vascular endothelial growth factor
VHL	von Hippel–Lindau
VMA	vanillylmandelic acid
Z-DEX	chemotherapy schedule comprising idarubicin and high-dose dexamethasone

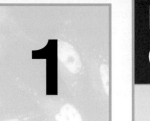

1 PATHOGENESIS OF CANCER

- Genetic factors   1
- Chemical factors   3
- Physical factors   4
- Viral factors   5
- Immune factors   7

- Endocrine factors   7
- Understanding the cause of cancer –
  the contribution to patient care   8
- Further reading   8
- Self-assessment questions   9

Pathogenesis is defined as 'the manner of development of a disease'. An understanding of the causes of a given cancer is an integral part of formulating strategies for successful treatment, screening and prevention. We owe much of our current understanding to epidemiologists who have discovered associations between different cancers and a number of genetic and environmental factors. In many cases, these lead directly to malignancy, e.g. smoking and lung cancer. The causative factors can be divided into genetic, chemical, physical and viral. It is becoming increasingly clear that changes in the host genome are the final common pathway in the process of carcinogenesis whatever the initial aetiology. However, for most patients with cancer it is still not possible to identify why that particular person developed cancer. Some of the examples cited are for historical interest only.

GENETIC FACTORS

The 23 pairs of human chromosomes contain the genetic material of the cell made up of unique sequences of deoxyribonucleic acid (DNA) base pairs, which code for the amino acid building blocks of proteins responsible for all the basic metabolic processes that enable the individual cells to survive, reproduce and express properties characteristic of their tissue of origin. Subtle changes in the genes comprising the chromosome may lead to a malignant tumour characterized by loss of the normal cellular mechanisms responsible for control of proliferation, cell differentiation, programmed cell death (apoptosis), cellular organization and cellular adhesion. The uncoupling of the usual balance between cell loss and multiplication leads to growth of the tumour and its subsequent invasion both locally and at distant sites.

Over the last two decades, the field of molecular biology has made great progress in elucidating the likely mechanisms of carcinogenesis. Much of this is due to the development of techniques for the isolation and identification of genetic material, such as the polymerase chain reaction and gel electrophoresis. It is becoming apparent that genetic aberrations can be found in the majority of human cancers. The site of the responsible genes can be inferred by 'linkage studies' on individual members of families in which there is an inherited pattern of cancer incidence. The known positions of marker genes are used to deduce where the cancer gene lies along a given chromosome. The gene can then be sequenced, cloned and used to test patients thought to harbour the gene.

Factors suggesting a genetic predisposition to cancer include:

- family clustering of a specific type(s) of cancer
- cases occurring in very young individuals relative to the age distribution of that cancer within the rest of the population
- associations noted between different tumour types
- multiplicity of cancers, e.g. bilaterality.

The genetic aberrations associated with cancer can be classified according to whether they are associated with activated oncogenes or tumour-suppressor genes.

Activated oncogenes

These are genes which, when expressed, code for a protein that in some way is related to the proliferative cycle of cells or cell differentiation. These products may be growth factors, growth factor receptors on the cell surface or the chemicals that transmit the receptor signals from the cytoplasm to the nucleus. These oncogenes are well preserved throughout the evolutionary scale, remaining very similar right down to primitive organisms such as yeasts. Their over-expression or amplification leads to uncoupling of the usual cell loss/gain equilibrium in favour of cell multiplication, resulting in an increase in cell numbers and ultimately a clinically apparent tumour. They are activated during the intense cell proliferation and differentiation of embryogenesis but, in the mature cells, are suppressed by regulating genes at other points along the chromosome. DNA strand breaks (e.g. from ionizing radiation or chemical carcinogens) with aberrant repair or translocations of genetic material might lead to loss of the genes responsible for regulation of a given oncogene. This may in turn lead to its activation.

The best characterized example is that of the Philadelphia chromosome of chronic myeloid leukaemia, which is confined to the malignant clone and can be identified in 95 per cent of patients with the disease. There is a translocation of part of chromosome 9 to chromosome 22 and vice versa, placing the *abl* oncogene from chromosome 9 adjacent to the breakpoint cluster region (*bcr*) on chromosome 22. The fusion of these genes leads to the transcription of a protein with tyrosine kinase activity, which leads to leukaemic transformation by increasing lymphocyte proliferation.

Tumour-suppressor genes

Each cell has one of a pair of tumour-suppressor genes on each homologous chromosome, and both must be inactivated for the cancer to develop. This means that individuals from a 'cancer family' with only a single gene inherited owing to a 'germ line' mutation have a normal phenotype, act as a carriers, but will develop cancer if the second gene is lost owing to a somatic mutation or other form of genetic miscoding. Normal individuals must lose both genes by a somatic mutation for a sporadic cancer to develop. Thus tumour-suppressor genes cause cancer not by amplification or overexpression (as with oncogenes) but by loss of their function.

The best known example of a tumour-suppressor gene is the *P53* gene, which has been called 'the guardian of the genome' and is found to be mutated in the majority of sporadic cancers. It is also mutated in Li–Fraumeni syndrome, characterized by cancers of the breast, adrenal glands, leukaemia, gliomas and soft tissue sarcomas. This gene is involved in inducing cell cycle arrest, which allows cells with DNA damage to repair these mutations before entering mitosis. Mutation of *P53* therefore makes the cell susceptible to carcinogenic mutations. Other examples include the retinoblastoma gene which is located on chromosome 13, breast cancer susceptibility genes *BRCA1* (chromosome 17) and *BRCA2* (chromosome 13), the Wilms' tumour gene on chromosome 11, and the familial polyposis coli gene on chromosome 5.

Some examples of inherited diseases associated with the development of cancer are listed in Table 1.1.

TABLE 1.1 Inherited diseases associated with the development of cancer

Disease	Type of cancer
Autosomal dominant	
Familial adenomatous polyposis	Adenoma/carcinoma of the colon/rectum
Peutz–Jeghers syndrome	Adenoma/carcinoma of the colon/rectum
Gardener's syndrome	Adenoma/carcinoma of the colon/rectum
Multiple endocrine neoplasia types 1 and 2 (see Chapter 14)	Endocrinologically active adenomata
von Recklinghausen's disease	Neurofibromas, schwannoma, phaeochromocytoma
Palmar/plantar tylosis	Carcinoma of the oesophagus
Cowden's disease	Colorectal cancer, breast cancer
Gorlin's syndrome	Basal cell carcinoma of skin, medulloblastoma
von Hippel–Lindau disease	Cerebellar haemangioblastoma, hypernephroma
Autosomal recessive	
Albinism	Melanoma, basal cell and squamous cell carcinomas of the skin
Xeroderma pigmentosum	Melanoma, basal cell and squamous cell carcinomas of the skin
Ataxia telangiectasia	Acute leukaemia
Fanconi anaemia	Acute leukaemia
Wiskott–Aldrich syndrome	Acute leukaemia
Bloom's syndrome	Acute leukaemia
Chromosomal disorders	
Down's syndrome (trisomy 21)	Acute leukaemia
Turner's syndrome (X0)	Dysgerminoma

CHEMICAL FACTORS

Cigarette smoking

Cigarette smoking is the single most important cause of preventable death in the UK. It accounts for around a quarter of all deaths from cancer, and 90 per cent of deaths from lung cancer. Polycyclic aromatic hydrocarbons in the tar (e.g. benzpyrene) rather than the nicotine are carcinogenic. Smoking is strongly associated with carcinomas of the lung (squamous and small cell variants), oral cavity, larynx, bladder and pancreas.

Asbestos

A history of asbestos exposure is usually elicited from dockers, plumbers, builders and engineers, and is associated with carcinomas of the lung, and mesotheliomas of the pleura and peritoneum. The blue variant is particularly carcinogenic.

Products of the rubber and aniline dye industry

Both beta naphthylamine and azo dyes are carcinogenic. These substances and their products are excreted in the urine, and cause cancers of the renal pelves, ureters and bladder.

Wood dust

Inhalation of hardwood dusts has been associated with adenocarcinoma of the nasal sinuses, first described in workers in the furniture factories of High Wycombe.

Soot

Before the advent of vacuum machines for cleaning chimneys, there was an increased risk of carcinoma of the scrotum in chimney sweeps from trapping of soot in the rugosity of the scrotal skin and poor personal hygiene.

Tar/bitumen

As with cigarette smoke, polycyclic aromatic hydrocarbons may lead to cancer of exposed skin.

Mineral oils

An increased risk of skin cancer was noted in workers using spinning mules from exposure to lubricating oils.

Chromates, nickel

These are associated with the development of lung cancer.

Arsenic

Its use as a 'tonic' during the early twentieth century led to multiple basal and squamous cell carcinomas of the skin. It has also been associated with lung cancer.

Aflatoxin

This is a product of the fungus *Aspergillus flavus*, which is a contaminant of poorly stored cereals and nuts, and causes hepatocellular carcinoma.

Nitrosamines

These are products of the action of intestinal bacteria on nitrogenous compounds in ingested food and have been implicated in stomach cancer.

Vinyl chloride monomer

Industrial exposure has led to angiosarcomas of the liver and cerebral gliomas.

Alkylating chemotherapy agents

The addition of alkyl groups to the DNA double helix drastically changes its configuration and leads to difficulty when the cell undergoes mitosis or meiosis, ultimately leading to loss and distortion of the genome. Prior use of these agents in the chemotherapy of lymphoma has led to an increased risk of acute myeloid leukaemia in long-term survivors.

PHYSICAL FACTORS

Physical factors can cause direct damage of the genome, such as DNA strand breaks or point mutations, both of which may lead to an aberration either of the gene sequence or of the genes themselves. This is a phenomenon of everyday life and the changes are either repaired by cellular protection mechanisms or are so severe that the cell perishes and does not multiply. However, if the effects are such that these mechanisms for repair are overloaded, the cell may divide and the genetic error expresses itself, possibly leading to a cell with a malignant phenotype. As the skin and mucosal surfaces are exposed to the external environment, it is these that are most prone to physical carcinogenic influences.

Solar radiation

Excessive ultraviolet exposure in normal individuals or minimal amounts in susceptible individuals (e.g. albinos, xeroderma pigmentosum) can lead to melanoma, basal cell carcinoma and squamous carcinoma (Fig. 1.1).

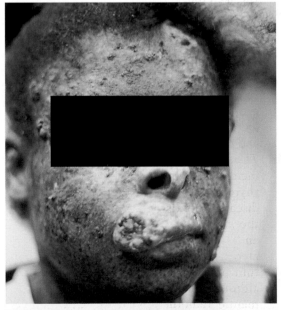

Figure 1.1 This young girl has xeroderma pigmentosum. She has developed multiple facial solar keratoses and both pigmented and non-pigmented skin cancers owing to ultraviolet radiation.

Ionizing radiation

Several categories of exposure can be identified and implicated in carcinogenesis:

- *Excessive background radiation* Radon gas is colourless and odourless, being a daughter product from the radioactive decay of uranium in the Earth's crust, particularly in granite-rich areas. It seeps into homes and reaches its highest level during winter when ventilation of dwellings is at its minimum. When inhaled, solid (α particle emitting) daughter products can be deposited on the bronchial epithelium leading eventually to lung cancer. Uranium miners are at particular risk, and many have died of lung cancer in Eastern Europe and Germany. Japanese atomic bomb survivors have an increased incidence of a number of solid tumours, particularly breast cancer, and radioiodine exposure from atomic bomb test fallout has caused thyroid cancer. Radium ingested by watch dial painters has led to bone sarcomas owing to concentration of the element in the skeleton.
- *Excessive diagnostic radiology exposure* There was an increased risk of carcinoma of the breast in a cohort of women who had many chest fluoroscopies to monitor iatrogenic pneumothoraces. The use of thorotrast (containing thorium, which has similar properties to radium) as a contrast agent led to tumours of the hepatobiliary tract and nasal sinuses.
- *Therapeutic radiation* There is an increased incidence of papillary carcinoma of the thyroid after thyroid irradiation for benign disease. Soft tissue sarcomas may arise at the edge of a previously irradiated area and skin carcinomas in previously irradiated skin. Breast irradiation for postpartum mastitis has caused breast cancer, although in the modern era the use of mantle radiotherapy in the treatment of Hodgkin's lymphoma during young adult life has led to a substantial ongoing risk of breast cancer.

Heat

Carcinomas of the skin have been described in chronic burn scars and the skin of Indians who wear heating lamps against their skin for warmth. Clay pipe smokers are at risk of carcinoma of the lip.

Chronic trauma/inflammation

Carcinomas can arise at sites of chronic skin/mucosal damage (e.g. the tongue adjacent to sharp teeth or a syphilitic lesion), at the site of a sinus from chronic osteomyelitis or inflammatory bowel disease, chronic venous (Marjolin's) ulcer on the lower limb (Fig. 1.2), or colonic carcinoma after chronic ulcerative colitis. Calculi and the associated infection may predispose to carcinomas of the urinary and hepatobiliary tracts. Skin cancers can arise in scarring from a previous burn (Fig. 1.3), and lung scars from previous tuberculosis may lead to adenocarcinoma.

VIRAL FACTORS

Viruses reproduce by integrating their own genes with those of the infected host, and in doing so the gene sequence of host chromosomes is adjusted. This may in turn lead to deregulation of oncogenes or inactivation of tumour-suppressor genes, ultimately resulting in malignant transformation. Evidence suggesting that a viral infection might have led to a tumour includes:

- geographical and community case clustering
- serological evidence of infection
- visualization of viral particles in the tumour cells, or
- identification of viral genome in the tumour DNA.

General observations include the following:

- The prevalence of infection is always much higher than the incidence of the associated tumour.
- Additional factors (e.g. genetic, immune) must be operative for malignant transformation.

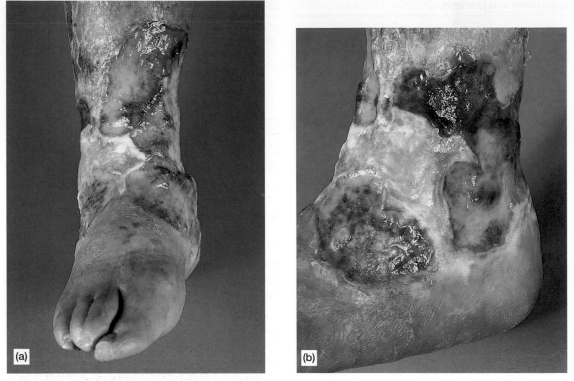

Figure 1.2 A large venous skin ulcer had been present for many years on the medial malleolus of the ankle. More recently it had enlarged and become irregular in shape with everted margins. Biopsy confirmed the clinical diagnosis of squamous carcinoma. (a) Frontal view. (b) Lateral view.

■ There is usually a long latent period between infection and presentation with cancer.

Some specific viruses related to cancer include the following:

Hepatitis B virus

There is a high lifetime incidence (up to 100 times) of hepatoma in parts of Africa where hepatitis B is endemic and there are many chronic carriers of the virus.

Epstein–Barr virus (EBV)

There is very strong evidence that this is the causative agent of undifferentiated nasopharyngeal carcinoma in South-East Asia, B-cell lymphomas in the immunosuppressed and Burkitt's lymphoma in Africa. There is also evidence linking it with Hodgkin's disease.

Human papilloma virus (HPV)

The potential for HPV to cause cancer is most frequently expressed as the development of benign papillomas (warts) on the genitalia. It is generally considered to be sexually transmitted, infection risk being related to the number of sexual partners and sexual practices such as oral sex. HPV types 6 and 11 are low risk for malignant change. HPV types 16 and 18 are higher risk and account for 70 per cent of cervical cancers. HPV infection is also implicated in the genesis of cancers of the oral cavity, oropharynx, and cancers of the vulva and anal canal. It is believed that the virus produces two oncoproteins, E6 and E7, and these inactivate the *P53* tumour-suppressor gene leading to cancer induction. Routine vaccination against HPV will undoubtedly impact on the incidence of such cancers in the future.

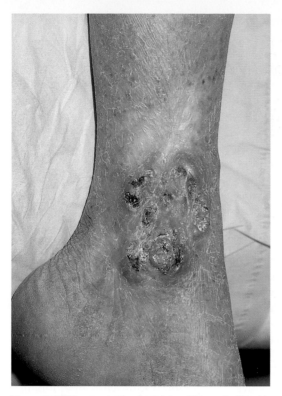

Figure 1.3 This woman had sustained burns to the skin above the lateral malleolus of the ankle 10 years earlier. She then developed nodularity and ulceration within the scar. Biopsy confirmed squamous carcinoma.

Human T-cell lymphotrophic virus type 1 (HTLV-1)

This is a retrovirus related to the human immunodeficiency virus (HIV, HTLV-3). It causes adult T-cell leukaemia–lymphoma in the endemic regions of Japan and the Caribbean where more than 95 per cent of cases have positive viral serology.

Human herpes virus type 8

This is the causative agent in HIV-associated Kaposi's sarcoma, primary effusion lymphoma and variants of multicentric Castleman's disease.

IMMUNE FACTORS

There is evidence that the body's immunosurveillance system mediated by T cells is capable of mounting an immune response to tumour cells. This is manifested as a lymphocytic infiltrate in tumours such as seminoma and melanoma, which correlates with a favourable prognosis, the phenomenon of spontaneous regression in hypernephroma and melanoma, and the objective responses seen when the T-cell population is boosted by cytokines such as interleukin 2 and interferon. There is evidence that immunosuppression leads to development of some forms of cancer, some of which are mediated by viruses.

Acquired immune deficiency syndrome (AIDS)

Up to 40 per cent of patients with AIDS will ultimately develop some form of malignant disease (see Chapter 20).

Drug induced immunosuppression

Transplant recipients receiving steroids and azathioprine or cyclosporin have an increased incidence of Kaposi's sarcoma, non-Hodgkin's lymphoma and skin cancer.

ENDOCRINE FACTORS

Many cells have receptors for hormones on their surface, within their cytoplasm and nucleus. Overstimulation of these receptors by endogenous or exogenous hormones can lead to excessive cell proliferation, usually resulting in an adenomatous change but sometimes malignancy.

Excessive endogenous steroids (e.g. from a granulosa cell tumour of the ovary) or long-term exogenous oestrogens (e.g. high-dose oestrogen-only oral contraceptive or hormone replacement therapy) can predispose to hyperplasia of the endometrium, which may progress to a well-differentiated adenocarcinoma. Similarly, excess physiological secretion of hormones can lead to hyperplasia, adenomatous change and eventually malignant transformation. For example, chronic severe iodine deficiency leads to a rise in thyroid-stimulating hormone (TSH), leading to goitre and in some cases follicular carcinoma.

UNDERSTANDING THE CAUSE OF CANCER – THE CONTRIBUTION TO PATIENT CARE

Identification of the aetiological agents responsible for cancers is vital for identifying individuals at high risk. Avoiding exposure of employees to industrial carcinogens either by the issue of protective clothing or restricted access is a vital part of health and safety practice to prevent cancers. Similarly, screening of high-risk asymptomatic individuals might be indicated, e.g. regular urine cytology in rubber workers at risk of bladder cancer. Identification of cancer patients in whom industrial exposure to a carcinogen is implicated will entitle the patient to industrial injuries compensation.

Understanding the cause of cancer also forms the backbone of more general health education programmes aimed at reducing tobacco consumption and exposure to excessive ultraviolet irradiation.

Molecular biology has already given us a particularly valuable insight into the mechanisms of carcinogenesis. Specific applications include:

- risk factor determination
- genetic counselling
- therapy
- screening
- prevention.

The ultimate goal of such research must be to give a greater understanding of cancer and ultimately facilitate more effective cancer therapies. The identification of precise genetic abnormalities may in turn make it possible to insert the appropriate genetic code into the genome (e.g. to replace a missing tumour-suppressor gene) or inactivate/downregulate an overexpressed oncogene, thereby reversing the cellular processes underlying the malignant phenotype.

Examples of such translational research include the development of the monoclonal antibodies such as trastuzumab (Herceptin®), which is a very active treatment in women with breast cancer who overexpress a receptor of the epidermal growth factor family, HER2 (see Chapter 8).

The antibody imatinib (Glivec®) is another example of rational drug design. It is highly active for blast-phase chronic myeloid leukaemia, as the tyrosine kinase protein it targets is BCR-ABL, produced by the Philadelphia chromosome (see above). Similarly, the recognition of gastrointestinal stromal tumours (GISTs) and their overexpression of *c-kit* has led to an effective therapeutic option with imatinib, in a tumour that was previously unresponsive to conventional treatments (see Chapter 9).

FURTHER READING

Eeles RA, Easton D. *Genetic Predisposition to Cancer.* Arnold, London, 2004.

Mendelsohn J, Howley PM, Israel MA *et al. The Molecular Basis of Cancer.* Saunders, London, 2008.

Ruddon RW. *Cancer Biology.* Oxford University Press, Oxford, 2007.

SELF-ASSESSMENT QUESTIONS

1. Which three of the following suggest a familial cancer?
   a. Other affected first degree relatives
   b. Cancer of the female genital tract
   c. Young age at diagnosis
   d. Cytogenetic abnormalities in the tumour
   e. Follicular carcinoma of the thyroid
   f. Presentation with metastatic disease
   g. Bilaterality

2. Which one of the following statements is not true about tumour suppressor genes?
   a. They prevent the development of cancer
   b. Mutations can be identified in most cases of cancer
   c. *P53* is a tumour-suppressor gene
   d. *BRCA1* is a tumour-suppressor gene
   e. Mutation analysis is clinically useful even if cancer has already developed

3. Which three of the following are cancers that can be caused by exposure to ionizing radiation?
   a. Pancreatic cancer
   b. Breast cancer
   c. Gallbladder cancer
   d. Parathyroid cancer
   e. Papillary carcinoma of the thyroid
   f. Kidney cancer
   g. Lung cancer

4. Which one of the following is not a form of cancer associated with viral infection?
   a. Nasopharyngeal cancer
   b. Hepatocellular cancer
   c. Adult T-cell leukaemia–lymphoma
   d. Non-Hodgkin's lymphoma
   e. Kidney cancer

2

PRINCIPLES OF CANCER DIAGNOSIS AND STAGING

■ Securing a tissue diagnosis 10
■ Principles of cancer staging 11
■ The TNM staging system 19
■ Use of pathological information 20
■ Further reading 20
■ Self-assessment questions 21

Diagnosis and staging are vital for determining the optimum management of a patient with cancer.

SECURING A TISSUE DIAGNOSIS

Cancer treatment usually involves major procedures with significant toxicity and the diagnosis of cancer has profound psychological, social and physical consequences for the patient. It is therefore mandatory to be certain of the diagnosis before informing the patient or starting therapy. This may entail a simple biopsy or a more invasive procedure such as a laparotomy or craniotomy. As a rule of thumb, the least invasive means of obtaining tissue should be employed. However, occasionally, several attempts at obtaining tissue from an ill-defined and poorly accessible tumour prove unsuccessful or the patient may be unfit to undergo an essential procedure by virtue of age or general condition. Under these circumstances, clinical judgement and common sense must prevail. Clearly it would be inappropriate to investigate exhaustively an elderly and infirm person with an extensive asymptomatic brain tumour or widespread metastatic disease if no treatment

or change in management would be considered. Specific methods of obtaining tumour tissue include the following techniques.

Cytology of bodily fluids

A small specimen of body fluid (e.g. sputum, ascitic fluid, pleural fluid, urine, cerebrospinal fluid) may be spun down and the cells in it stained and examined under the microscope within minutes of its collection. An experienced cytologist can then give an immediate and accurate diagnosis. The false positive rate is very low, although false negatives occur owing to errors in interpretation or sampling. This analysis has the advantage that the specimen can often be collected as an outpatient procedure with minimal discomfort and it gives a result quickly so that treatment can start as soon as possible. Of course the cellular material obtained may be insufficient for immunohistochemical analysis unless a centrifuge is used to produce a cellular pellet, which can be fixed in wax and sectioned/stained in the usual way.

Cytology of tissue scrapings

Superficial cells are removed from a body surface (e.g. skin, vagina, cervix, bronchial mucosa, oesophageal mucosa) by scraping or brushing, before being stained and examined under the microscope. The advantages and limitations are the same as for fluid cytology.

Fine needle aspiration (FNA)

This entails the passage of a fine-gauge hypodermic needle into a suspected tumour. Ultrasound or CT guidance may be necessary for deep-seated tumours that cannot be palpated, such as those at the lung apex or retroperitoneum. Cells are aspirated, smeared onto a microscope slide and sent to a cytologist. This method is particularly useful for discriminating between reactive and malignant lymphadenopathy and for assessing breast lumps. The advantages and disadvantages are comparable to those cited above for fluid cytology. If the needle washings are very cellular, a centrifuge can be used to produce a pellet for fixation, sectioning and staining as for a piece of tissue.

Needle biopsy

This is more invasive than FNA. A core of tissue is taken with a biopsy needle (e.g. Trucut®) under local anaesthetic and the specimen is sectioned after mounting and fixing in wax, which means that the result will not be available for several days after collection. The larger specimen makes a false negative result less likely. Tumour grading and architectural subtyping will be possible within the constraints of the sample. This is particularly the case for lymphoma which is not diagnosed effectively by cytology alone, and indeed excision biopsy of a suspicious lymph node is preferable. It is also possible to distinguish in situ malignant change from invasive. More extensive immunohistochemical analysis will be possible from the larger specimen left after standard staining has been undertaken.

Incision biopsy

A small ellipse of tissue is taken from the edge of the tumour using a small scalpel under local anaesthetic. A punch biopsy instrument can be used instead of a scalpel to obtain a core of tissue, but this is more traumatic.

Excision biopsy

The tumour is excised in toto with a narrow margin of normal tissue. Unlike the other investigations, this has the advantage of removing the lesion, which may be curative for benign tumours and certain skin malignancies if the microscopic margins are clear. It can, however, make further management difficult if the original boundaries of the tumour are not apparent after excision.

PRINCIPLES OF CANCER STAGING

Once the diagnosis has been confirmed, the stage of the cancer, which defines the size and extent of the tumour, must be ascertained. Staging has several purposes:

- It defines the locoregional and distant extent of disease.
- It helps to determine the optimum treatment.
- It permits a baseline against which response to treatment can be assessed.
- It provides prognostic information.

Staging entails a detailed assessment as to the local extent of the tumour and whether there is evidence of spread elsewhere, e.g. regional lymphatics, distant metastases. This will in turn help the referring specialist and oncologist to decide on the most appropriate therapy. For example, a patient with distant metastases is unlikely to be a candidate for aggressive surgery to remove the primary tumour but may be a candidate for systemic treatment such as chemotherapy. Alternatively, the detection of lymph node metastases alone may indicate to the surgeon that excision of the primary tumour should be combined with a lymph node dissection and/or systemic adjuvant therapy. Detailed surgical staging is also valuable to the radiotherapist in deciding the volume of tissue to be irradiated.

Staging permits assessment of the response to treatment. A thorough assessment of the tumour dimensions prior to therapy will permit a critical evaluation of the response to treatment at a later date. Accurate measurements in two planes perpendicular to each other can be used as a crude measure of tumour size before, during and after therapy.

Staging provides a guide to the likely prognosis. In most cancers, the ultimate outcome and therefore life expectancy is related to the stage. Patients with metastatic disease at presentation will clearly fare worse than patients with disease localized to the site of origin. The only tumours that are potentially curable when distant metastases are present are seminoma, teratoma, choriocarcinoma, lymphoma and leukaemia.

Staging may be *clinical*, based on the clinician's history and examination; *non-clinical*, comprising blood tests and radiological studies; or *pathological*, based on the surgical specimen.

History

A thorough and systematic history can reveal symptoms that may suggest the need for specific staging investigations or a certain disease stage. For example, systemic symptoms such as weight loss, anorexia, malaise and fever raise the suspicion of metastatic disease. Specific symptoms at a site away from the primary tumour may also cause suspicion of distant metastases, e.g. skeletal pain, early morning headache, haemoptysis, hepatic pain.

Examination

A full physical examination should be performed in all cases. The primary tumour's size, shape, position and mobility should be recorded, preferably with a diagram. The regional lymph nodes should be carefully palpated – involved nodes are enlarged, usually non-tender and hard, and may be fixed to each other, the overlying skin or underlying tissues. The sclerae should be examined for jaundice and the abdomen palpated for hepatomegaly in which the liver is typically hard and knobbly.

The chest is examined for signs of collapse, consolidation or effusion. The skin should be surveyed for any abnormal appearances, which may be biopsied if suspicious. A detailed neurological examination should be performed to exclude focal or global neurological deficit, and the fundi examined to exclude papilloedema. Tenderness over sites of bone pain is suspicious and should be followed up by appropriate X-rays.

Investigations

A knowledge of the patterns of spread of tumours will aid the selection of staging investigations. All patients should have a full blood count, liver function tests, calcium and alkaline phosphatase levels taken. The interpretation of deranged values is outlined in Table 2.1. Measurement of the erythrocyte sedimentation rate (ESR) is useful in lymphoma and myeloma. A chest X-ray should be obtained in all cases to exclude obvious pulmonary metastases, with equivocal cases proceeding to a CT scan of the thorax. In the case of bone/soft tissue sarcomas, a CT scan of the thorax is justified at the outset, as this will be more sensitive and, if positive, may spare the patient major surgery. Other investigations may be indicated depending on site and nature of the malignant disease:

- plain X-rays
- liver ultrasound
- isotope bone scan
- CT/MRI
- positron emission tomography
- other specialized investigations, e.g. bone marrow trephine, lumbar puncture
- tumour marker assays.

Plain X-rays

Plain X-rays of the skeleton should be taken at sites of any unexplained bone pain, particularly if affecting a long bone as these are prone to pathological fracture (Fig. 2.1), which may be prevented if the metastasis is detected early. A skeletal survey comprising views of the skull, thoracic spine, lumbar spine and pelvis is indicated in suspected myeloma, as an isotope bone

TABLE 2.1 Interpretation of abnormal screening blood tests

Test result	Interpretation
Normochromic normocytic anaemia	Suggests possibility of advanced cancer
Leucoerythroblastic anaemia	Suggests heavy bone marrow infiltration
Thrombocytopenia	Suggests heavy bone marrow infiltration or DIC
Elevated alkaline phosphatase with normal γ-glutamyltransferase	Suggests possible bone metastases ± elevated calcium
Elevated alkaline phosphatase and γ-glutamyltransferase ± elevated bilirubin	Suggests possible liver metastases

scan may be insensitive for this condition owing to lack of an osteoblastic response in the involved and surrounding bone (see below).

Ultrasound

It is sensitive, specific, non-invasive and can be performed at short notice but is no substitute for high-quality cross-sectional imaging. It is to some extent subjective and the final hard copies can be difficult for the non-radiologist to inter-

pret and utilize. Liver ultrasonography can be used for rapid staging of cancer, particularly gastrointestinal malignancies, as these preferentially metastasize to the liver via the portal circulation. Transoesophageal ultrasonography can be of help in staging oesophageal cancers and tumours arising in the trachea and proximal bronchial tree. Transvaginal ultrasonography may be of value in staging malignancies of the lower female genital tract.

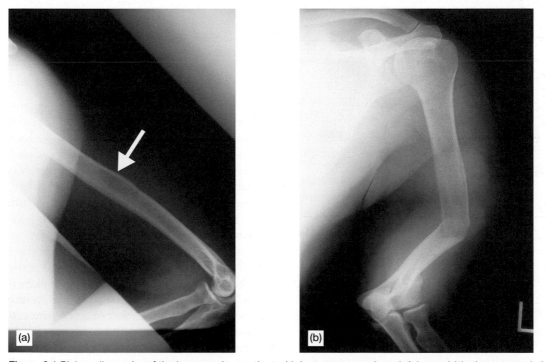

Figure 2.1 Plain radiographs of the humerus in a patient with lung cancer and a painful arm. (a) Lytic metastasis in the mid-shaft. This was noted by the radiologist but no prophylactic treatment was undertaken. (b) Subsequent pathological fracture at the same site.

Isotope bone scan

This is a useful way of imaging the whole skeleton. It is routinely performed as part of the staging of prostate cancer and breast cancer, which have a propensity for early dissemination to the skeleton, but is otherwise reserved for patients with widespread skeletal symptoms or when plain X-rays are equivocal for metastatic disease. A metastasis leads to an osteoblastic response, which in turn leads to increased accumulation of the bone-seeking radioisotope and therefore a hot spot (Fig. 2.2). Myeloma bone lesions are not particularly well visualized as they do not evoke a significant osteoblastic response. A very diffuse involvement of the skeleton may produce an intense uptake of isotope producing a 'superscan'. Benign disease such as degenerative changes in joints, vertebral collapse from osteoporosis or Paget's disease of bone can also lead to abnormal isotope uptake. Bone scans can be unreliable in assessing response to therapy in the short term, as activity may be increased at the sites of metastatic disease with regression of the metastasis and subsequent bone healing (Fig. 2.3).

Computed tomography (CT)

CT gives good soft tissue and bone contrast. A contrast-enhanced CT scan of the brain, thorax, abdomen and pelvis is indicated for potentially curable tumours with a propensity for widespread multiple metastases, and in all patients with metastatic disease as a baseline for assessing response to therapy. Abnormal lymph nodes on CT are defined as >1 cm in diameter, although CT cannot detect abnormal lymph node architecture and therefore cannot distinguish between benign and malignant enlargement. Localized CT imaging may be used to position a needle for biopsy of a mass. Care should be taken when interpreting images for treatment planning as occasional cases of situs inversus may lead to confusion (Fig. 2.4).

Magnetic resonance imaging (MRI)

This gives soft tissue contrast superior to that of CT and superb anatomical definition in transverse, sagittal and coronal views (Fig. 2.5). No

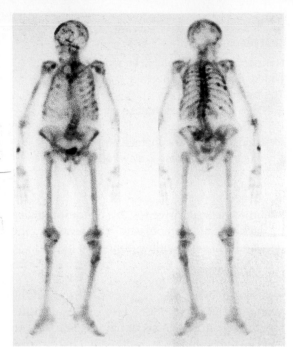

Figure 2.2 Isotope bone scan (anterior and posterior views) showing multiple skeletal metastases from breast cancer. Radioactive technetium has been injected and taken up by the skeleton, particularly in regions of increased bone metabolism. Note the uptake in the kidneys and bladder owing to urinary excretion of isotope. Metastases are seen in the skull, spine, pelvis and right proximal femur.

ionizing irradiation is involved and it is therefore better for investigating young children and pregnant women. Contraindications include cardiac pacemakers, metallic intracranial vessel ligation clips, previous metallic intraocular foreign bodies and claustrophobia. It is particularly sensitive for imaging the brain and spinal cord. MRI is useful for patients with apparently solitary cerebral metastases on CT as a means of excluding multiplicity, which may be important in determining optimal management, and is the investigation of choice for patients with primary CNS tumours. It also has a role in the delineation of the local extent of soft tissue sarcomas and primary liver tumours prior to definitive surgery where the tumour can be related to adjacent major blood vessels, and is the staging method of choice for pelvic tumours (e.g. carcinomas of the prostate, cervix, rectum).

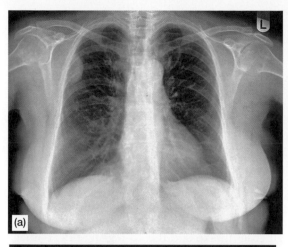

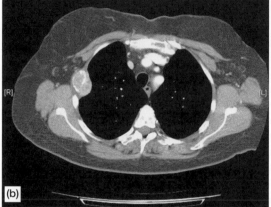

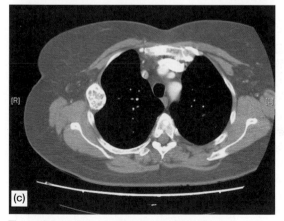

Figure 2.3 (a) Plain chest radiograph showing a peripheral opacity in the right upper zone.
(b) Corresponding CT image showing a large, destructive, soft tissue mass arising from a rib. (c) After appropriate systemic therapy, there has been a response showing as healing and sclerosis. Paradoxically, the isotope bone scan indicated increased isotope uptake at this site, which suggested disease progression.

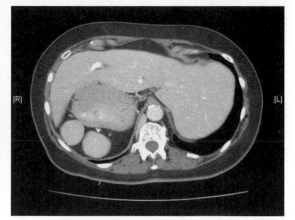

Figure 2.4 Situs inversus. Transverse CT image of the upper abdomen with the stomach and liver and spleen (abnormally developed into two splenunculi) transposed with respect to their usual left/right positions. Misplacement of CT films on a screen could lead to a significant error at the time of surgery.

MRI can be useful in determining the nature of persistent skeletal symptoms when plain X-rays and isotope bone scans are both normal (Fig. 2.6).

Positron emission tomography (PET)

This entails the systemic administration of positron-emitting molecules, which form part of the everyday metabolic processes of the living cell, e.g. fluorodeoxyglucose (FDG). These tracers are preferentially taken up by fast metabolizing tissues (e.g. tumours) and can then be detected and their uptake spatially localized. Patients fast beforehand to maximize glucose uptake, and have to be warm and relaxed to avoid shivering and brown fat metabolism, which can lead to spurious glucose uptake. These studies provide functional information entirely different to the structural information obtained from CT and MRI, and can provide a whole body snapshot of the likely sites of disease activity. CT imaging is often undertaken in the scanner at the same time as the PET study to facilitate anatomical appreciation of the sites of tracer uptake. PET is of particular value in the assessment of residual soft tissue masses after chemotherapy (e.g. lymph node masses in lymphoma and testicular

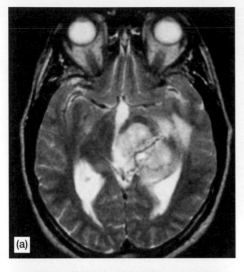

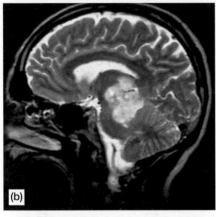

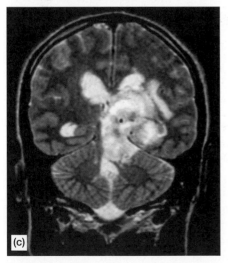

Figure 2.5 Brainstem glioma. MRI of the brain showing (a) transverse, (b) sagittal and (c) coronal views.

tumours) where the presence of viable tumour may be distinguished from fibrosis and/or necrosis. PET can also be used as part of a whole body staging procedure, particularly prior to radical surgery in diseases with an innately high risk of distant dissemination, e.g. lung cancer, pancreatic cancer (Fig 2.7). It can be of value in assessing response to therapy (Fig. 2.8). PET imaging is sensitive for detecting low-volume malignant lymphadenopathy (e.g. in the mediastinum, pelvis) that would otherwise be indeterminate by CT criteria (Fig. 2.9). PET is, however, not a good imaging modality for surveying the brain as this is an area of very avid glucose uptake and the co-registered CT imaging is usually of low resolution and without contrast enhancement.

Other specialized investigations

1. Bone marrow aspirate and trephine
This is a relatively non-invasive method for obtaining a sample of bone and bone marrow for microscopic examination. It is particularly useful in the diagnosis and staging of haematological malignancies (lymphoma, myeloma, leukaemia) and some solid tumours (small cell carcinoma of the lung, Ewing's tumour of bone).

2. Lumbar puncture
Some tumours have a particular propensity to spread to the central nervous system, particularly the meninges, and the CNS may act as a sanctuary allowing malignant cells to survive systemically administered chemotherapy. It is relatively easy to obtain a specimen of cerebrospinal fluid from the lumbar subarachnoid space, which can then be submitted for cytological examination. Lumbar puncture forms part of the routine staging of high-risk non-Hodgkin's lymphomas (e.g. primary testicular lymphomas, those with bone marrow involvement, lymphomas affecting the paranasal sinuses).

Tumour marker assays

Tumour markers are usually proteins associated with the malignant process. Common methods of detection include:

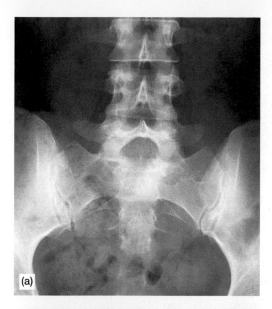

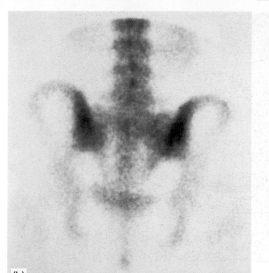

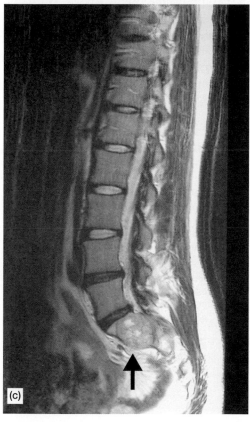

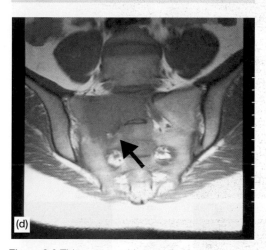

Figure 2.6 This woman with previously treated breast cancer presented with sciatica. (a) Normal plain radiograph of lower lumbar spine and adjacent pelvis. (b) Isotope bone scan of the same region showing normal, symmetrical uptake. (c) Sagittal MRI of the lumbar spine and sacrum showing a soft tissue mass at S1. (d) Transverse MRI showing a large metastasis in the superior aspect of the sacrum impinging on the ipsilateral S1 nerve root.

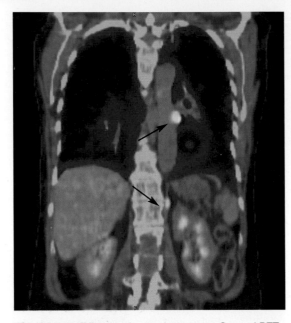

Figure 2.7 PET imaging for staging cancer. Coronal PET scan of the thorax and abdomen performed in a patient with lung cancer who was being considered for surgery. Although the staging CT scan was reported as normal, there is intense glucose metabolism in the left adrenal gland and a further focus just lateral to the thoracic aorta (arrows), both suggesting metastatic disease.

- immunohistochemistry
- fluoresence in situ hybridization (FISH).

Tumour markers in the serum, urine or cellular material are useful in many aspects of cancer management, and testicular tumours provide a number of examples (Table 2.2). The following are examples of tumour markers used for other tumour types:

- CA15-3 (blood) in breast cancer
- carcinoembryonic antigen (CEA – blood) in gastrointestinal cancer
- prostate-specific antigen (PSA – blood) in prostate cancer
- CA125 (blood) in ovarian cancer
- CA19-9 (blood) in pancreatic cancer
- α-fetoprotein (AFP – blood), β-human chorionic gonadotrophin (HCG – blood), placental alkaline phosphatase (PLAP – blood) and lactate dehydrogenase (LDH – blood) in testicular teratoma/seminoma
- thyroglobulin (blood) in follicular carcinoma of the thyroid
- calcitonin (blood) in medullary carcinoma of the thyroid
- 24-hour urinary vanillylmandelic acid (VMA) in phaeochromocytoma

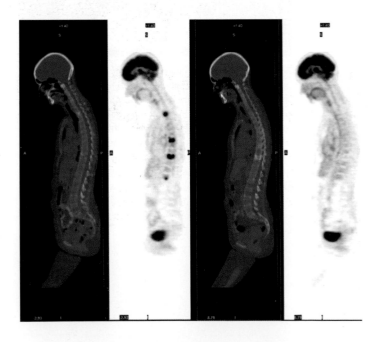

Figure 2.8 PET imaging to assess response to treatment. Sagittal whole body images of a patient with bone metastases. Left-hand panes represent the CT and PET images before treatment, the PET showing four areas of intense glucose uptake in the thoracic spine. The right-hand panes are the corresponding images after successful systemic therapy showing a metabolic response. Note the area of sclerosis that has appeared in the lower thoracic region to suggest a healing area of osteoblastic activity.

TABLE 2.2 Role of serum tumour markers in the management of patients with testicular tumours

Role	Example
Diagnosis	Elevation of AFP suggests yolk sac teratoma elements, elevation of HCG suggests trophoblastic teratoma elements, while elevated LDH is associated with seminoma
Staging	Failure of AFP/HCG/LDH to return to normal after orchidectomy suggests residual disease elsewhere
Prognosis	Very high levels of AFP/HCG are associated with poor prognosis in testicular teratoma
Indicator of response	Failure of AFP/HCG/LDH to fall with chemotherapy suggests drug-resistant disease
Detection of relapse	Sudden elevation of AFP/HCG/LDH while in clinical remission suggests subclinical relapse

- 24-hour urinary 5-hydroxyindoleacetic acid (5-HIAA) in carcinoid tumours
- urinary Bence–Jones protein, paraprotein/immunoglobulin levels (blood) and electrophoresis (blood) in myeloma.

THE TNM STAGING SYSTEM

The origins of this staging system go back to the 1940s. Since then it has evolved into a comprehensive system covering all types and stages of

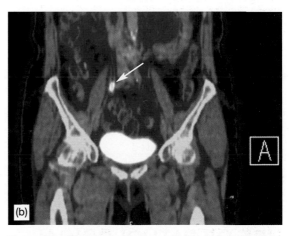

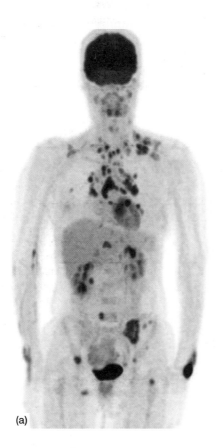

Figure 2.9 PET staging of cancer. (a) Coronal whole body PET image showing widespread metastatic disease. The mediastinal lymphadenopathy was not appreciated on an earlier CT scan. (b) Coronal PET image of the pelvis. Small but abnormal lymph node in the right iliac chain (arrow). Again, this had not been appreciated in an earlier CT survey.

cancer. It is accepted and contributed to by the most eminent cancer research groups such as the World Health Organization, International Union Against Cancer, and International Society of Paediatric Oncology. A formalized, universally applied staging scheme has several advantages. First, it aids the clinician in his or her appreciation of the extent of the cancer and gives a meaningful guide to likely prognosis. Secondly, it gives a consistency in the reporting of clinical trials and facilitates an exchange of meaningful information between clinicians without ambiguity, even if they do not speak the same language.

The system describes the anatomical extent of the disease by using three components:

- 'T' for the primary tumour
- 'N' for regional lymph nodes
- 'M' for distant metastases.

Each of these categories is assigned a number according to the extent of disease, which will vary according to anatomical site and type of malignancy. Other categories include:

- Tis – carcinoma in situ
- T0 – no evidence of primary
- Tx – primary cannot be assessed
- Nx – nodes cannot be assessed
- Mx – metastases cannot be assessed
- Gl – well differentiated
- G2 – moderately differentiated
- G3 – poorly differentiated
- G4 – undifferentiated
- pT/N/M – pathological staging.

The reader is referred to the site-specific chapters for more detailed staging descriptions.

USE OF PATHOLOGICAL INFORMATION

The pathologist plays a vital role in tumour diagnosis. The information on a pathology report is an integral part of the decision-making process for the clinician. Essential details include:

- tumour size and macroscopic appearance
- tissue of origin
- benign versus malignant
- if malignant, primary versus secondary
- tumour differentiation, i.e. grade
- degree of local invasion (blood vessels, lymphatic vessels, nerve fibres, organ capsule)
- number of regional lymph nodes retrieved and number involved
- host immune response
- tumour excised with an adequate margin of normal tissue
- immunocytochemical markers, e.g. HER2 in breast cancer.

Much of this information is of prognostic value and may assist in determining the optimal treatment of the patient. The recent advances in immunocytochemistry have allowed pathologists to identify the tissue of origin in very poorly differentiated tumours (see Chapter 21) which has improved the management of this small group of patients. As with the radiologist, it is not only courteous but essential that as much relevant clinical information as possible is put onto any form submitted to the pathologist.

FURTHER READING

Greene FL, Compton CC. *AJCC Cancer Staging Atlas*. Springer, New York, 2006.

Sobin LH, Wittekind C. *TNM Classification of Malignant Tumours*. Wiley-Liss, New York, 2002.

Wittekind C, Greene FL. *TNM Atlas*. Wiley-Liss, New York, 2008.

SELF-ASSESSMENT QUESTIONS

1. Which three of the following statements apply to cytology as a diagnostic tool?
   a. Can only be performed on specimens of body fluid
   b. Can provide a rapid diagnosis
   c. Allows precise characterization of the tumour
   d. Cannot distinguish in situ disease from invasive
   e. It has a low false positive rate
   f. A negative result makes cancer very unlikely
   g. Very useful for immediate diagnosis of lymphoma

2. Which of the following is the least important objective of staging cancer?
   a. Provides baseline of current disease status for assessing response to treatment
   b. Allows optimization of treatment
   c. Informs both patient and clinician
   d. Allows time for patient to come to terms with diagnosis
   e. Gives insight into likely prognosis

3. Which three of the following statements apply to an isotope bone scan?
   a. Images all the skeleton except the ribs
   b. Complements plain radiographs of painful areas of the skeleton
   c. Relies on isotope being taken up in areas of osteoclastic activity
   d. It is not good at imaging myeloma bone lesions
   e. Increased isotope uptake always suggests disease progression
   f. Benign disease can produce a hot spot
   g. Contraindicated in hypercalcaemia

4. Which three of the following are contra-indications to having a magnetic resonance scan?
   a. Previous hip replacement surgery
   b. Pregnancy
   c. Claustrophobia
   d. Raised intracranial pressure
   e. Cardiac pacemaker
   f. Spinal cord compression
   g. Intraocular metallic foreign body

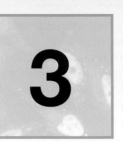

3

DECISION-MAKING AND COMMUNICATION

■ Treatment options   23
■ Quality of life   25
■ Communication   26
■ Conclusion   28

■ Clinical evidence and clinical trials 28
■ Conclusion   35
■ Further reading   35

The following chapters describe clear treatment policies for different types of malignant disease. These policies are based upon a knowledge of the natural history of the disease and, as detailed in the previous chapter, details of its extent – the clinical or pathological stage of the tumour.

However, the practice of clinical oncology demands more than simple application of these instructions in an uncritical fashion. The individualization of treatment for any given patient will be influenced by sociological, economic and psychological factors as well as oncological principles. The three levels of decision-making used when formulating a treatment policy for an individual are:

■ the decision to treat or not to treat
■ treatment intent, whether radical or palliative, and
■ specific aspects of treatment policy regarding local, systemic and supportive therapy.

Figure 3.1 illustrates the various options for treatment.

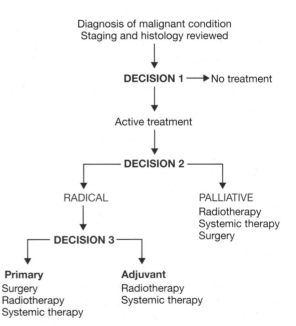

Figure 3.1 Treatment options.

TREATMENT OPTIONS

To treat or not to treat

Not every patient in whom a diagnosis of cancer is made will benefit from active treatment of their disease. There is, for example, good evidence to show that active local treatment in the form of radiotherapy for inoperable carcinoma of the bronchus in poor performance status patients will have no impact whatsoever on the survival of a patient. It follows therefore, that in asymptomatic patients diagnosed with this condition, treatment will only be meddlesome and indeed may detract from that patient's quality of life by invoking side-effects for no positive outcome. In contrast, treatment with radiotherapy or chemotherapy in good performance status patients may result in a 2-month gain in survival; it is then a judgement as to whether for an individual asymptomatic patient this is appropriate treatment, and it is important that those patients who develop symptoms from a bronchial carcinoma are not denied treatment by operating a blanket policy of no treatment for these patients. The actual decision to treat a patient will be based not only on their clinical state but also on the availability of treatment facilities and the emotional response of the patient and their relatives. It is often very difficult for a patient to accept that, having been told they have cancer, no treatment is proposed other than symptomatic measures, even though specific cancer treatment may have no proven benefit.

A more comfortable scenario in which a no-treatment decision may be taken is when the prognosis is so good and the risk of relapse so small that treatment for all patients will result in overtreatment with consequent side-effects for the majority. An example of this situation is the management of stage 1 testicular teratoma following orchidectomy where the probability of relapse is around 20 per cent and the use of tumour markers and scans enables early diagnosis of relapse in a tumour readily cured on exposure to appropriate chemotherapy. This is a much easier scenario for the patient, who will easily accept that they are almost certainly cured and require no further treatment other than close follow-up for a finite period.

Treatment should always have a positive benefit for the patient but treatment outcome for any individual is not predictable. The decision to treat or not then becomes a matter of balancing the probability of improving a patient's condition, whether by symptom control with palliative treatment or by cure with radical treatment, against the toxicity and disturbance to lifestyle that treatment will entail. Thus it is possible to justify an intensive course of chemotherapy with major side-effects when there is a high probability of cure but more difficult to do so in a patient with limited life expectancy in whom only minor symptom improvement can be anticipated. Wherever possible, the patient should be allowed to determine the level of input they wish to undergo; there is good evidence that, as a group, patients will often wish to undertake treatments with significant toxicity and very limited chances of possible benefit in contrast to the views of health professionals.

Radical or palliative treatment

Radical treatment is that which is given with the intent of long-term control or cure for the patient. Palliative treatment is that which is given to improve the quality of life for a patient with no implied impact upon their survival.

While this may seem to be a clear distinction, in practice it may be difficult to define treatment aims in these terms. For example, a patient presenting with small cell lung cancer may be offered a course of radical treatment comprising intensive chemotherapy and perhaps also chest radiotherapy. However, it is recognized that, while this treatment may prolong survival, the likelihood of cure is less than 15 per cent. Thus the treatment intent, although radical, will result for most patients in only very limited benefit. Conversely a patient with breast cancer relapsing with a single site of painful bone metastases may receive a low palliative dose of radiation for pain relief only, yet live, pain free, for several years.

In most cases, however, the decision of treatment intent if not outcome will be clear. Those patients who present with localized tumours accessible to local therapy and those with metastatic disease from chemosensitive tumours, such as germ cell tumour or lymphoma, will be offered radical treatment. Those who present with metastatic disease from other tumours and those who relapse after primary treatment will, with few exceptions, fall into the palliative group.

Palliative treatment has the aim of improving a patient's wellbeing usually through treatment for specific local symptoms such as pain, obstruction or haemorrhage. It follows therefore that patients in whom radical treatment is not appropriate and who have no symptoms do not require palliative treatment. The concept of prophylactic palliative treatment, in other words treatment to prevent symptoms emerging, is for most patients inappropriate and, in the asymptomatic patient, introduces treatment toxicity with little likelihood of benefit. There may be occasional exceptions to this concept, for example the prophylactic fixation of a bone damaged by extensive osteolytic metastases with impending pathological fracture. As always the probability of treatment benefit must be weighed against the natural history of the condition and probability of disease-related and treatment-related symptoms.

Local, regional or systemic treatment

As a general principle, a primary malignant tumour will require ablation with local treatment, which may be surgical excision and/or radiation treatment. Similarly, metastatic disease requires systemic treatment, which may be chemotherapy, hormone therapy or a biological agent.

Local treatment may involve simple excision of a tumour, removal of the entire organ or removal of the involved organ and regional tissues at risk of tumour involvement. In the past there have been advocates of extensive regional surgery around a tumour site in the hope of improving cure; however, such approaches are only rational where a tumour is known to spread in a predictable fashion. In practice most common tumours are thought to spread at an early stage in their evolution through blood and lymphatic dissemination of tumour cells. For this reason the use of radical regional surgery is usually inappropriate. This is well illustrated in the case of breast cancer where it is now clear that survival is largely independent of the type of local treatment for a given stage of disease. Thus radical mastectomy is no better at curing breast cancer than simple removal of the lump from the breast.

Although local control of a tumour is an important goal, most patients die from cancer because of metastatic disease. Where a cancer has been detected prior to the establishment of metastases, then radical local treatment can result in cure. However, the natural history of many cancers is such that even relatively early tumours will already be associated with distant micrometastases. In these cases improvements in survival are likely to come only from the use of adjuvant systemic treatment.

Adjuvant treatment

Adjuvant treatment is the prophylactic use of local or systemic treatment following primary treatment of a malignant tumour to prevent recurrence.

One of the most common adjuvant treatments given today is postoperative radiotherapy following excision of a malignant tumour, for example irradiation of the breast following local excision of an early carcinoma. Such adjuvant treatment may add significantly to patient morbidity and it is important therefore to consider the relative merits of treatment in these situations. For example, the risk of local relapse in the breast following simple excision with no radiotherapy is around 30–50 per cent depending upon tumour size. On this basis, if all patients are treated following lumpectomy, half may never have required treatment; the difficulty lies in predicting accurately those who will relapse. A further consideration is the fact that local relapse following lumpectomy may be treated successfully in many women and will still occur in 5–10 per cent even with radiotherapy. A small survival advantage with postoperative radiotherapy has also been shown. The decision to offer a woman breast radiotherapy following excision of a malignant breast lump therefore has to balance the potential benefits with the likely side-effects for each individual patient. The substantial reduction in local relapse in the breast from 50 to 5 per cent will be seen in most cases to justify a relatively simply, low morbidity treatment.

The use of adjuvant systemic therapy is also one in which the decision to offer a particular treatment must be balanced against the possible acute toxicity which, with chemotherapy, may be significant. There are, in fact, few sites of cancer where the use of adjuvant systemic therapy is of proven value. The area where there has been the greatest endeavour and the most reliable information is once again breast cancer. There is now little doubt that an overall survival benefit is achieved by offering women with early operable breast cancer some form of adjuvant systemic therapy. In postmenopausal women tamoxifen or anastrazole is recommended. This reduces the likelihood of dying from breast cancer by one-third and is a simple treatment involving the administration of a single tablet daily for a number of years with few, if any, associated side-effects. Therefore the decision in this case is reasonably straightforward. In contrast there is a less reliable effect of anti-oestrogen treatments in premenopausal women with an oestrogen receptor-negative tumour, but proven advantage with chemotherapy for those with high-risk tumours defined by high tumour grade or positive regional lymph nodes. However, this treatment involves 6 months of intravenous chemotherapy with attendant side-effects. The greatest efficacy is seen in those patients with positive axillary lymph nodes, but even so the difference in survival at 10 years between women who receive chemotherapy and those who do not in prospective randomized trials is only 6 per cent. Therefore the treatment decision for adjuvant chemotherapy in a premenopausal patient with negative lymph nodes in whom there may be only a small probability of survival gain for the individual becomes more difficult.

It can be difficult to translate clinical trial and population-based data to the individual patient. Breast cancer is a common cancer and therefore even a very small treatment effect of, say, an improvement in survival of 5 per cent over 10 years will result in many thousands of women worldwide living for longer after breast cancer. However, for the individual woman the odds that she will benefit from adjuvant treatment in that setting are small and it is possible that she will undergo a toxic treatment with no effect on her ultimate survival.

It is also difficult for those around the patient, be they family, friends or physicians, to evaluate and balance the risks of having a toxic treatment against the risk of relapse, particularly when there can never be the certainty of cure. There is evidence to suggest that patients have a much lower threshold for accepting treatment, even where there is significant associated toxicity, than would the nurses or doctors who look after them.

QUALITY OF LIFE

Whilst survival will always be the most important end-point of cancer treatment, the quality of life experienced and the impact of different treatment regimens upon this is an important further consideration. Measurement of quality of life has become increasingly sophisticated. Early attempts relied heavily upon assessments by a physician on a broad scale measuring physical performance status as illustrated in Chapter 6 (see Table 6.2, page 55). A true measure of the quality of life for an individual can, however, be acquired only from that individual, and a number of formal patient questionnaire-based scales have now been developed. These include the Rotterdam symptom checklist, the Hospital Anxiety Depression (HAD) score and the European Organization for Research and Treatment of Cancer (EORTC) standardized quality of life questionnaire (EORTC QLQ-C30), consisting of a core questionnaire to which can be added disease site-specific modules. The place for quality of life assessments in clinical trials will be discussed later in this chapter.

COMMUNICATION

Whilst the principles of communication in oncology should be no different to any other branch of medicine there are specific features that require consideration. In Western society the term 'cancer' remains one that is frequently surrounded by fear and dread for most of the population. In other cultures it may not even be mentioned in open discussion. Many patients passing through an oncology unit will have an incurable and ultimately fatal disease. This requires special skills in communication and support, which will span the entire range of oncological practice. Radical treatment might require lengthy discussion to consider the choice between different treatment options; at the other extreme, specific skills are required in imparting the news that a cancer may be incurable and death imminent.

Patients are increasingly well informed and wish to discuss the details of their disease and options for treatment. The diagnosis of cancer is often associated with many emotional responses, which will colour the consultation including anger, frustration, guilt and despair. These may present considerable barriers to open discussion particularly where there is a perception that earlier medical care has been inadequate or delayed the diagnosis of cancer.

Communication with a patient is affected by many factors relating to both the patient and the healthcare professional including environment, culture and content.

Environment

Wherever possible important discussions relaying news of a diagnosis of cancer, discussions relating to treatment options and the 'bad news interview' relaying news that the condition may be incurable and terminal should be carried out in an environment comfortable for the patient. Privacy is important but often difficult to achieve in a busy ward and wherever possible a dedicated side room or communication room should be available. The patient should be adequately clothed and not given important information during the process of physical examination or while still undressed.

If possible and provided this is desired by the patient they should have a relative or friend accompanying them or alternatively a health professional with whom they have empathy, for example their ward nurse. Despite inevitable pressures on the time available for such interviews the patient should not be aware of time pressures that may hinder their willingness to interact and ask questions.

Culture

There will be cultural differences in the way in which a diagnosis of cancer, a potentially fatal illness, and death are approached. Increasingly in Western civilization a direct approach is preferred. The word 'cancer' should not be avoided or hidden behind euphemisms. A clear and simple explanation of the disease relevant to that particular patient and the treatment options should be given. Patients may be unfamiliar with surgical procedures, and the processes of radiotherapy and chemotherapy; these will require additional explanation. It is unwise to assume that a patient has any background information unless confirmed. It is often helpful early in a consultation to ask the patient to give their understanding of their illness or the treatments being offered, against which background further discussion can proceed. A particular pitfall to avoid relates to fellow health professionals who may be disadvantaged by the assumption that they already are familiar with their condition and will have decided on the treatment they wish to receive; usually this is far from the case and they will welcome putting aside any background knowledge they may have acquired for a full and simple explanation of their position.

Content

Three common consultations can be identified in oncology that present specific challenges in communication; these are the choice between different radical or palliative treatments, the discussion of likely prognosis and discussion of matters related to the process of dying.

Treatment choices

Where there is a choice of treatment, this should be laid out for the patient and in each case the possible advantages and disadvantages discussed. It may be difficult to give a balanced view of treatment options particularly for specialists outside their own area of interest; this is the advantage of multidisciplinary discussions. Realistic estimates of success should be given with a clear explanation of the expected endpoint, whether 'cure', by which the patient will interpret a complete return to normal life and normal life expectancy; 'control' of the disease, which may be only temporary; or simply control of symptoms without any impact perhaps on survival. There is a recognized need to clearly highlight possible side-effects of treatment, in particular those that may result in a long-term alteration in lifestyle for the patient. Again realistic estimates of their likelihood and the balance between side-effects and positive benefit should be discussed.

It is well recognized that most patients do not retain information from their initial interview for long and that a significant amount of the information will be forgotten or misinterpreted. It is therefore important that written information is given to the patient to support the facts imparted in the interview and that this is followed up by an opportunity for the patient to return for further discussion. A readily available point of contact should be given to the patient and often it is helpful for another healthcare professional such as a specialist nurse to be available for them to discuss matters further.

Prognosis

Prediction of life expectancy is notoriously difficult and there is considerable evidence that estimates by healthcare professionals are often widely inaccurate. It is often difficult for patients and their relatives to accept that their medical advisers cannot give an accurate picture of the future. It is, however, usually possible to estimate survival in terms of days, weeks, months or years and, where lengthy survival is to be expected, a percentage likelihood of surviving, say, 5 years can be given. This should, however, be carefully interpreted since it is often difficult for patients to relate life-table curves giving a probability of survival at any point to their own individual survival.

The point at which patients wish to discuss such matters in detail will vary, some wishing to consider this in detail from the outset but many preferring to leave the matter unspoken for some time or on occasions throughout their illness. This should be respected and the issue dealt with sensitively, giving patients the opportunity to 'set the pace', by asking specific details of their outlook, rather than giving bald and alarming statements of a short prognosis. Open questions such as 'Is there anything else you would like to ask?' may give them the lead to pursue specific areas of concern when they wish to do so.

Dying

The mention of death and dying is often avoided by both carers and patients perhaps in an attempt to avoid facing the inevitability of this event. Meaningful discussions with a patient who has advanced incurable cancer can, however, only progress once the notion of dying has been accepted, if only to subsequently agree not to mention it further. Patients and their relatives will often hide behind euphemisms such as 'the end' or 'when it's all over', whilst healthcare professionals may use terms such as 'very serious' or 'incurable' to introduce the idea that an illness is fatal. Realistic expectations are important for practical issues to be faced such as where and by whom the patient wishes to be cared for in his or her last days, clarification of their wishes in the form of a will and, where dependent children are involved, arrangements for their future care. Patients and their relatives are often concerned over the process of dying rather than the event itself, and it is important to explore these fears with appropriate reassurance over the availability and efficacy of symptom control and nursing care. Above all, it is important not to avoid the issue when faced with direct questions from the patient but to reply honestly and with sensitivity.

Difficulties in communication

Expectations versus reality

For many patients the reality of a serious illness and the possibility of death is dealt with by unrealistic expectations from their treatment and their carers. This can be projected as anger and dissatisfaction when treatment failure is encountered. It is important that unrealistic expectations are not fuelled by unrealistic predictions of outcome from treatment and that such responses are met sympathetically but with clear and accurate information of realistic outcomes.

Lack of knowledge

Many patients may find it difficult to accept that their advisers do not understand all the details of their disease process and rarely can they attribute a cause to it. Patients often focus on events in their life and seek confirmation that this was the possible cause for their cancer, which it is not possible to confirm or refute. Similarly events may occur in their disease course that are unexpected and cannot necessarily be explained by previous experience. Healthcare professionals should not be reluctant to admit that they do not know or understand events and this is far better than fabrication of possible mechanisms which have no basis.

Identification

Patients who may be contemporaries of their carers and children are particularly likely to provoke strong emotional responses. This is a normal reaction to events and should be recognized as such but not be allowed to cloud objectivity. If this is found to be an overwhelming difficulty, healthcare professionals should have access to an another colleague who can take their place or support them through difficult events.

Conflict within families

The diagnosis of a life-threatening illness or impending death may unveil underlying conflicts between a patient and other family members. There is often guilt that the patient has not been given sufficient attention, symptoms have been missed and that more should have been done. This may be transferred to those looking after the patient as complaints relating to their diagnosis and care. Other more complex tensions may emerge with unmasking of relationship difficulties between partners or parents and children. There may be attempts to 'protect' the patient by asking professionals to withhold information, which relatives may see as distressing. Throughout the important principle is that the patient is pre-eminent and, while although you must deal with relatives sympathetically, the patient's wishes should at all times be respected.

CONCLUSION

Decision-making in oncology is not as straightforward as a simple knowledge of the disease process may imply. Relating the large body of knowledge regarding disease outcome, treatment outcome and treatment-related morbidity to an individual patient can be difficult. The probability of benefit from any treatment can be interpreted differently by each patient so that, while one might accept a 90 per cent probability of cure as very favourable, another will find a 10 per cent probability of relapse unacceptable. Treatment decisions rely on an accurate and realistic presentation of the facts but individual interpretations might come to very different conclusions from the same facts.

CLINICAL EVIDENCE AND CLINICAL TRIALS

Ultimately treatment decisions rely upon interpretation of the available data for a given clinical situation. Different sources of data, however, have different levels of reliability when applying them to a patient population. Perhaps the least reliable, but often most memorable, is that of the anecdote recalling the course of a similar patient treated in the past. The most reliable data will come from the results of a large randomized trial addressing a specific question. Clinical evidence is graded according to its level of reliability as follows:

- Level la – Meta-analysis of randomized controlled trials
- Level lb – Evidence from one or more randomized trial
- Level lla – Evidence from a non-randomized trial
- Level lll – Evidence from descriptive studies
- Level lV – Evidence from expert committee
- Reports or clinical experience.

A particular clinical question, whether in cancer treatment or any other speciality, can be addressed in a number of ways. Types of trial include:

- randomized controlled trials
- case–control studies
- cohort studies.

A clearly defined path for new treatment development in the clinical setting is defined as follows:

- Phase 1
  - First exposure in man
  - Low doses initially based on animal data
  - Dose escalation to maximum tolerated dose (MTD)
  - Measurement of pharmacokinetics in man
  - Definition of significant and limiting toxicities
- Phase 2
  - Testing for activity in a range of tumours
  - Define response rates
- Phase 3
  - Randomized controlled trial to compare with best current treatment or placebo
- Phase 4
  - Post marketing surveillance following successful phase 3 trial as use becomes widespread outside trial setting.

Randomized controlled trials

These are statistically the most reliable way of comparing two or more different treatments in a population of patients. The characteristics of the population are defined and patients fulfilling these criteria are allocated to one of the treatment options by a random process akin to tossing a coin, but more usually derived from a computer-generated list of random numbers. In this way fluctuations in the population that may affect the outcome of treatment are distributed evenly across the treatment groups allowing a true comparison of the treatment to be made.

End-points

It is important at the outset of a trial to *define* the end-points by which the results will be judged. This will also guide the assessments that will be required during the trial to provide the necessary information to answer the main questions posed. End-points are often defined as primary, reflecting the main question addressed by the trial, and secondary, which will include other important outcomes such as side-effects. Common end-points will include the following:

- survival
- disease-free survival
- response
- toxicity
- quality of life.

Survival is the commonest end-point for a large trial comparing two or more treatments for cancer. Whilst apparently straightforward in its definition time, cause of death may be difficult to trace, particularly in trials continuing for many years and where the condition has a long natural history, for example patients in trials of prostate and breast cancer. It is important to define the cause of death. This will allow a comparison of not only overall survival but also disease-specific survival, i.e. counting only those patients dying from the disease under investigation. It is always important, however, to analyse all causes of death, since this may on occasions reveal an excess of deaths from complications of the treatment. A typical example of this is the long-term analysis of the results of radiotherapy for breast cancer, where a reduction in breast cancer death rate is seen in patients receiving radiotherapy, but overall survival between those receiving radiotherapy and those who did not is no different. The explanation for this apparent anomaly was explained by an excess of non-cancer deaths, predominantly cardiovascular disease in the radiotherapy group which negated the reduction in breast cancer deaths.

Disease-free survival is defined by the period during which a patient remains in remission, without detectable disease, following treatment. It may be further subdefined as 'local disease-free survival' taking into account only relapse within a specified site, typically the primary site of the cancer, after local treatment such as surgery or radiotherapy, which would not be expected to directly influence other distant sites. 'Distant disease-free survival' may also be used to assess a treatment for metastatic disease. Where this is used as an end-point in a trial, it is important to account for the fact that relapse may only be defined by specific tests, which will be performed at specific time points. For example if a patient is most likely to relapse with lung metastases detected on a chest X-ray, where the trial design defines a chest X-ray to be performed once a year, relapse can only be defined once a year, assuming the patient did not become symptomatic and obtain a chest X-ray for their clinical management in the meantime. This would give only a very crude picture of the pattern of relapse, and a delay in appearance of metastases by less than 12 months would not be detected; a design, which called for a chest X-ray every 2 to 3 months during the period of risk, might be more suitable in such a scenario. It is also important to realize that patients can only be compared by disease-free interval if they become disease free; for example, it is a very common end-point for trials after local treatment of early breast cancer where virtually all patients are 'disease free' after treatment, but of little value in trials of treatment for metastatic disease where only modest response rates might be anticipated.

In these patients a similar concept may, however, be applied using progression or symptom response rather than tumour response and measuring '*progression-free survival*' or '*symptom-free survival*'.

Response may be an important end-point when testing new treatments to see whether they are effective. There are recognized formal definitions of response. The most commonly used are the RECIST response criteria as follows:

- *Complete response* (CR): complete disappearance of all detectable disease for a period of at least 1 month
- *Partial response* (PR): a 30 per cent reduction in measurable disease for at least 1 month
- *Stable disease* (SD): a reducing of <30 per cent in measurable disease or no increase in size for at least 1 month
- *Progressive disease* (PD): any increase in size of measurable disease during the assessment period.

Response may be quoted as overall reponse rates (OR or RR), which will usually include CR + PR, but it is important to check on precise definitions as some investigators will include stable disease in this category.

Toxicity is a vital component in assessing the outcome of any clinical trial since ultimately any benefit will be balanced with side-effects. Toxicity will include the immediate effects observed during the trial and may take the form of laboratory measures, such as full blood count or renal function, and symptom scores for expected side-effects of treatment. It is also important to consider later effects after treatment has been completed, and specific issues that might arise from cancer trials include the effects of treatment on fertility and the induction of second malignancies.

Quality of life measures will give a global view of the impact of the intervention to be tested taking into account the response of the disease, side-effects of treatment and also the more complex issues of the psychological and sociological consequences of the disease and its treatment.

Measurement of end-points is a very important component of the design of any trial and requires a knowledge of the natural history of the disease being studied together with a knowledge of the effects of the treatment interventions that will be available from preceding use of the agents in phase 1 and 2 trials (see below). There are two important considerations in deciding how measurements should be included in a trial.

Timing must be defined to give useful information but without burdening the patient or investigators with unnecessary measurements. In the early part of a trial more measures are likely than later on, the most intensive being during treatment. However, as illustrated by the example of annual chest X-rays in a disease that may relapse within a few months, appropriate time-points for assessment after treatment must also be incorporated. The nature of most cancer is for these to be most intensive over the first 2–3 years after treatment and then to become less intrusive as the high-risk period for relapse passes.

Measurement may require a range of methods to be applied:

- *Death* is a clear end-point but tracing patients after treatment to different centres and defining cause of death can be more troublesome. In some countries cancer registries might be able to supply the information independently.
- *Clinical* measurement of a tumour mass may appear straightforward but clear parameters will need to be defined, for example whether maximum diameter, minimum diameter or a calculated area or volume is to be used. Ideally measurements are made by independent observers or, if made by the investigators, then they should be blind to the treatment received. Trials that do not include these safeguards could be open to bias.
- *Radiological* measurements should similarly be carefully defined and ideally judged by an independent radiologist or preferably a central panel convened for the trial. This allows any variation between observers to be ironed out and greater uniformity in the observations will be achieved.
- *Laboratory* measures are in general more objective but validation of the laboratory methods used is important. It is preferable

to use a single reference laboratory distant from the treating centre with mechanisms in place to notify investigators of clinically relevant abnormal results.

- Measurement of *symptoms* is more complex. There are a number of accepted and validated measuring tools for common problems such as pain or vomiting and wherever possible these should be employed rather than individualized scales from a single trial or centre. These will typically take the form of categorical scales based on none, mild, moderate, severe format or visual analogue scales, using a 10 cm scale, on which patients mark the severity of a symptom. Critical to achieving good data is careful explanation and continued support during the data collection. Wherever possible it is important to have data completed by the patient themselves rather than a surrogate.
- *Quality of life* instruments are detailed questionnaires relating to the patients emotional and physical wellbeing. They can be general or have additional 'disease-specific modules' addressing issues that may be pertinent to a particular tumour site, for example urinary and sexual function in carcinoma of the prostate. Common examples used in cancer trials are the FACT and EORTC QLQ-C30 quality of life questionnaires.
- *Health economic* assessments are increasingly an integral component of randomized trials assessing new treatments as it becomes apparent that the resources allocated to health care in the developed world can no longer match the availability and demand for increasingly complex and expensive treatments. Demonstration of cost-effectiveness is therefore an important component of any clinical trial today evaluating new cancer treatments. The tools for evaluating this are also becoming more complex as it becomes clear that a simple balance sheet approach cannot address the issues that may arise. Attempts are made to relate the treatment effect with the length of time over which benefit may occur,

resulting in concepts such as the Quality Adjusted Life Year (QALY) to measure treatment outcome.

Placebo-controlled trials

Placebo-controlled trials will be appropriate when a new treatment is being tested in a situation where there is no recognized standard treatment with which to compare it. Although it may be possible to compare the new treatment with no treatment there is always the possibility that simply the process of delivering a treatment, whether a drug or other intervention, will have an unexpected beneficial or harmful effect. The use of a placebo, which will be made to resemble the active treatment as closely as possible, reduces this possibility. Placebos are most effective in trials that are blinded. This refers to a situation in which either the investigator or subject do not know the difference between the placebo and active drug (single blind design). The optimum design is a double blind trial in which neither the investigator nor the subject are aware whether a placebo or active drug is being used.

Where there is already a recognized treatment against which the new treatment is to be tested then placebo-controlled trials are inappropriate and the control arm will be the standard best available treatment. Alternatively, particularly in testing new treatment in advanced cancer, the control arm could be best supportive care. This is optimized symptomatic supportive care distinct from the use of 'anticancer' treatment and permits the test of a new treatment in the setting of symptomatic, advanced malignancy to evaluate the addition of an anticancer therapy where standard treatment is symptomatic care only.

Randomization

Randomization describes the method by which subjects in a trial are distributed into different treatment groups. Most trials have two 'arms': the standard arm, which should be the recognized best available treatment or, where there is none, then this will be a 'no treatment' or placebo arm and the experimental arm in which the new treatment will be tested. In most trials there will be balanced randomization, i.e. the trial will comprise equal numbers in each of the arms of the trial. Occasionally, however, a design can be used in which there is a weighted randomization, for example a 2:1 distribution of subjects, usually in favour of the experimental arm, i.e. twice as many subjects in the experimental arm as the control. Randomization should take place through an independent trials office totally separate from the facilities in which the trial will be undertaken; usually this will involve computer-generated blocks of random numbers, which will then allocate subjects to their arm of the trial. This may be accessed by researchers through a telephone call, fax or, increasingly, a voice-activated computer program.

Stratification

Stratification can be built into the design of a trial. This is to ensure that subgroups within the trial population, which may have different prognoses, are equally distributed. In oncology this might mean that trials are stratified by tumour stage or performance status. At randomization each tumour stage or performance status group will be independently randomized ensuring an equal distribution of stages or performance status across the arms of the trial. This precaution also aids later analysis using the stage or performance status subgroups without prejudice. Multicentre trials often stratify by treatment centre also.

Trial statistics

The major drawback of a randomized trial is that for a statistically robust result large numbers of patients are required. The total number required will be defined beforehand by the trial statistician who will be able to predict the number needed to give a defined level of statistical certainty for a given change in response rate from a known baseline. For example if a standard treatment has a known response rate of 70 per cent and 5-year survival of 45 per cent, the trial investigators must decide what improvement upon this they would expect, or wish to detect, in their trial. They will then need to define the power of the trial, i.e. how certain they wish to be of their result at the end. As an example, if a particular treatment has a survival rate of 50 per cent, in order to reliably detect an absolute improvement of 10–60 per cent from a new treatment, approximately 400 patients will be required to enter a randomized trial comparing the two. The precise number of patients will be affected by the degree of error in the trial results that will be accepted by those designing the trial. There are two types of error recognized:

- type I(α) error in which a difference may be observed which does not really exist; and
- type II(β) error in which a true difference may be missed.

These will commonly be set at an α error of 0.05 and a β error of 0.2 (often referred to as 80 per cent power). This means that it will be accepted that there is a 5 per cent chance of the result observed being false. As a general principle the more strict the statistical constraints, i.e. the smaller the α and β errors accepted and the smaller the difference to be detected between the arms of the trials, the larger the numbers required. As an example, for a trial in a condition where, with standard treatment, 5-year survival is 50 per cent, to detect a 10 per cent increase in survival with a new treatment in a two-arm randomized trial accepting an α error of 0.05 and β error of 0.2, then a total of 760 patients will be required. Trials designed to show equivalence, i.e. no difference between the treatment arms, require the highest numbers.

The 'p' value is often quoted alongside results of a clinical trial. This essentially relates to the α error accepted in the result. The conventional value required before a result is considered statistically significant is $p = 0.05$, which relates to an α error of 0.05 and means that there is a 5 per cent chance of the results not being a true reflection of the comparison in the trial, or in other words there can be a 95 per cent certainty that the result is a true result.

Trial infrastructure

Clinical trials demand an extensive infrastructure within a dedicated central clinical trials unit that will co-ordinate the trial and provide a central point for randomization, data collection and analysis. It should be independent from the investigators entering and treating patients in the trial who are usually based in many different centres all accruing relatively small numbers of patients. A randomized clinical trial may take several years before it is completed and analysed to give reliable results that will be translated into clinical practice. It is important during the running of such a trial that any new information from other trials that may affect the relevance of the outcome are considered and that any unexpected toxicity or difference in response is evaluated within the trial. For this reason most large trials will have associated with them a data monitoring committee (DMC) usually comprising a statistician and two or three clinicians or scientists who are not involved in that particular trial. They will review the results of the trial at defined time-points perhaps annually or after accrual of a predetermined number of subjects, e.g. after every 100 patients entered. They may recommend early closure of a trial if a large number of unexpected toxicities are found in one arm, or if a sufficiently large difference emerges between the arms of the trial early on that was unexpected and unlikely to be reversed by larger numbers. The data seen by the DMC must at all times remain confidential from the investigators involved in running the trial. In practice early closure is rare in a well-designed clinical trial but the DMC is an important component to ensure that patients are not given inappropriate treatment.

Ethics of clinical trials

It is a fundamental principle in designing and partaking in a clinical trial comparing two treatments that the patient should not be disadvantaged compared with other patients not taking part in the trial. For this to be satisfied the investigators must be confident that there is no proven advantage for the new treatment over the existing management and equally that there is no evidence of any greater toxicity that would disadvantage the patient. This will be based on information gained from earlier phase

I and phase II trials. In fact it has been shown that patients taking part in clinical trials have a better outcome than those who do not, possibly because of adherence to a rigid protocol and the greater clinical input that inevitably accompanies trial participation.

Meta-analysis

A meta-analysis is a means of overcoming the problem of patient numbers. This arises because most innovations in treatment have only a modest impact upon outcome; an improvement in survival of more than 10 per cent from any new intervention is very unusual. Other new treatments might not even be expected to improve survival but aimed at reducing toxicity or improving quality of life. Any clinical observation is inherently unreliable in statistical terms and will carry a range around which a repeat observation may be expected to fall – this is often quoted as the 95 per cent confidence interval within which 95 per cent of repeated observations might be expected. The smaller the number of observations the wider will be the confidence interval. To be certain that the observations in two groups of patients are truly different, there must be no overlap of the confidence intervals. Where there is a big difference, even relatively wide confidence limits will not overlap, but for a small true difference the confidence interval needs to be as small as possible to demonstrate the difference, and this will only be achieved with a large number of patients.

A meta-analysis therefore attempts to include as many patients as possible who have entered trials addressing a particular question. This approach has been used in several tumour sites of which breast cancer provides an excellent example. For a number of years a series of individual clinical trials across the world has addressed the question as to whether adding hormone therapy or chemotherapy to the primary treatment can prolong survival. The results of individual trials failed to give a clear answer, some showing benefit and others no benefit. A meta-analysis has therefore been performed combining the results of all known trials in this area and demonstrating in 30 000 women that adjuvant tamoxifen conveys a 6.2 per cent survival advantage after 10 years and in 10 000 women that polychemotherapy carries a 6.3 per cent survival advantage after 10 years. These figures illustrate the very small overall survival effect seen and explain why series of small trials gave conflicting results. With the large numbers in the meta-analysis, small differences can be found with a high level of statistical reliability as demonstrated by the very low 'p' value associated with these data; the tamoxifen result above has a p value of <0.00001, i.e. only a 1 in 10 000 chance that the observation is not real.

Case–control studies

In many situations, particularly in rare tumours where it is not possible to study large numbers of patients, randomized trials are not practical. The next best type of trial is the case–control trial in which a new treatment is given to a series of patients and then compared with previous patients treated for that condition. It is important in such a comparison to exclude any factors that might affect the result other than the treatment being tested. This is achieved by selecting matched controls, i.e. patients with otherwise identical characteristics to one of the new treatment group with whom they are matched. Parameters important to match for include age, sex, tumour stage and histological type, together with any other known prognostic factors. The comparison may be refined by selecting two matched controls for each patient receiving the new treatment.

The difference between the two groups is often quoted as an *odds ratio* comparing the probability of an event (e.g. death or tumour recurrence) occurring in the control group with that in the new treatment group.

Cohort studies

Cohort studies are not usually of value in comparing two different treatments but are used in particular to investigate aetiological factors. As their name suggests they are observational studies in which a group of patients (a cohort) is monitored over a period of time for a particular outcome, e.g. development of or death from cancer. This type of study is usually reported in terms of relative risk, comparing the incidence in the cohort with that of a control cohort. The value of this type of study is in defining the natural history of a particular tumour type and evaluating the impact of potential aetiological agents.

CONCLUSION

Subsequent chapters will describe for different tumour types their aetiology, natural history and various treatment options. The accuracy of this depends critically upon the data from which this information is derived. It can be seen that there are many pitfalls in obtaining and interpreting the results of clinical data sets. Any advances in cancer management depend critically upon rigorous evaluation with close attention to the design and interpretation of clinical trials to ensure that reliable outcome data are acquired to further advance knowledge. It also demands that clinicians and patients of the future are sufficiently informed to understand and partake in clinical trials.

FURTHER READING

Girling DJ, Parmar MKB, Stenning SP, Stephens RJ and Stewart LA. *Clinical Trials In Cancer: principles and practice*. Oxford University Press, Oxford, 2003

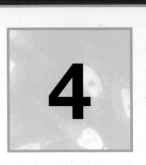

PRINCIPLES OF SURGICAL ONCOLOGY

4

■ Management of the primary tumour   36
■ Combined surgery and radiotherapy   37
■ Management of regional lymph nodes   37
■ Palliative surgery   38
■ Further reading   40
■ Self-assessment questions   41

The local treatment of malignant disease involves the use of surgery, radiotherapy or a combination of the two. Surgery is essentially a local treatment while radiotherapy offers locoregional treatment covering a wider area less constrained by anatomical boundaries and surgical technique. Optimum initial management of the primary tumour and regional metastases is vital if later relapse is to be avoided, and close liaison between surgeon and oncologist is required to enable the best use of each modality.

MANAGEMENT OF THE PRIMARY TUMOUR

Surgery for a malignant tumour may have several components:

- tissue biopsy to establish the diagnosis
- removal of malignant disease with a clear margin of normal tissue
- repair, reconstruction and restoration of function. This may vary according to the extent of resection and anatomical site, from simple primary wound closure to major reconstruction of bone and soft tissue with vascularized grafts and prostheses.

The type of surgery required will be determined by the type of tumour and the anatomical site, and may include:

- wide local excision of the tumour mass, e.g. local excision of a breast lump
- removal of part of an organ and surrounding tissue, e.g. partial glossectomy and neck dissection for a carcinoma of the tongue
- removal of an entire organ, e.g. laryngectomy, cystectomy or hysterectomy.

En bloc removal of the immediate lymphatic drainage areas is usually an integral part of any cancer surgery, e.g. hysterectomy for cervical cancer includes pelvic lymphadenectomy.

Radiotherapy will give equivalent local control rates to surgery for small tumours (<5 cm) in many anatomical sites and has the potential advantage in certain sites of being able to preserve anatomical structure and function, e.g. in the treatment of cancer of the larynx where radical radiotherapy can result in tumour eradication with voice preservation in contrast to the surgical alternative, which is total laryngectomy. However, against this must be balanced the need for close postradiotherapy surveillance, which can be difficult if there are florid late radiation tissue changes, and that a significant

TABLE 4.1 Relative merits of pre- and postoperative radiotherapy

Preoperative RT	Postoperative RT
Early radiotherapy	No delay to surgery
Enables preoperative preparation for planned surgery	True pathological staging may be masked by preoperative RT
Surgery may be easier if tumour shrinks preoperatively	Pathology of surgical specimen may guide later RT
	Lower dose of RT needed for microscopic disease

proportion (around 20 per cent) of patients will still come to surgery. Furthermore, surgery following radiotherapy can be technically more difficult and have a higher complication rate.

As with surgical management, irradiation of a local tumour must include areas of potential spread. A common approach to enable high radiation doses to be concentrated at the site of the tumour mass is to use a shrinking field technique. This involves:

■ initial treatment of a wide area to cover all potential routes of microscopic spread together with the primary tumour and regional lymphatics
■ a boost to the primary tumour site alone with a margin of 1–2 cm.

COMBINED SURGERY AND RADIOTHERAPY

The combination of surgery with radiotherapy has two potential advantages and applications:

■ It enables the extent of surgery to be limited by treating sites of microscopic disease immediately adjacent to the primary site with radiotherapy, e.g. the use of local excision and radiotherapy in place of mastectomy for breast cancer.
■ For large tumours (>5 cm) local control rates are in general better for combined therapy than either modality alone.

Combined treatment may involve the use of preoperative or postoperative radiotherapy. The relative merits of each approach are shown in Table 4.1. There is no evidence that pre- or postoperative radiotherapy is more effective in ultimate tumour control.

MANAGEMENT OF REGIONAL LYMPH NODES

The common epithelial tumours, such as those of the lung, breast, head and neck region and pelvis, metastasize through two routes, the lymphatic system and the blood circulation. Clinically involved lymph nodes and those at high risk of microscopic involvement require active treatment.

Surgery

Surgery is indicated for the immediate draining nodes around a primary tumour. Radical dissection of the involved node chain should be considered, and may involve:

■ axillary dissection for breast cancer
■ radical neck dissection for head and neck sites
■ inguinal node dissection for vulval, anal or penile cancers treated with primary surgery.

A more conservative approach, sentinel lymph node mapping, is now the standard of care for breast cancer and melanoma. This entails identification of the 'sentinel' lymph node. This is the node that is first to receive lymph from the tumour-bearing tissue. A vital blue dye and radiolabelled colloid microspheres are injected preoperatively to allow perioperative identification of the lymph node(s) to be removed. If they are found to be involved by frozen section analysis or on definitive histological examination, a full lymph node dissection is mandatory. If this is negative, it is highly unlikely that other lymph nodes in that group will harbour cancer cells, and the

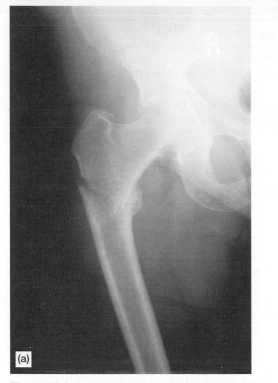 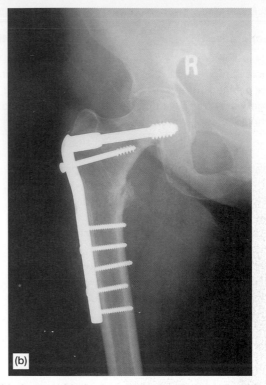

Figure 4.1 Pathological fracture of the right neck of femur (a) before and (b) after internal fixation.

patient may be spared the additional morbidity of the larger operation. The technique can allow identification of unusual patterns of lymphatic spread, e.g. to the internal mammary lymph nodes in breast cancer, or the axilla in truncal melanoma.

Radical excision of nodes is *not* indicated for:

■ lymphomas (Hodgkin's disease or non-Hodgkin's lymphoma) or leukaemias
■ those with metastatic involvement at visceral sites where there may be little or no quality of life gain by removing enlarged lymph nodes.

Radiotherapy

Radiotherapy is indicated for surgically inoperable nodes and might succeed in rendering inoperable lymph nodes operable. Postoperative radiotherapy following surgical dissection is recommended for those patients with multiple node involvement and extension of tumour beyond the capsule of the gland. Prophylactic radiotherapy to sites of potential microscopic disease is often given when a primary site is being treated, e.g. pelvic nodes for gynaecological malignancy, neck nodes for head and neck tumours.

Chemotherapy

Chemotherapy might be indicated for enlarged lymph nodes owing to germ cell tumour, lymphoma, metastatic breast cancer or small cell lung cancer.

PALLIATIVE SURGERY

Even when cure is no longer a realistic aim, surgery can have an important role in the palliation of local symptoms. Specific examples where surgery should be considered include:

■ palliation of obstructive symptoms
■ control of haemorrhage

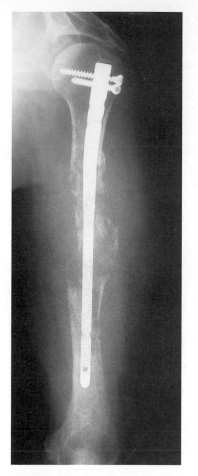

Figure 4.2 Uncontrolled bone metastases. This woman had internal fixation for a pathological fracture of the mid-shaft of the humerus. This was not followed by radiotherapy. She has now developed significant bone lysis compromising the mechanical integrity of the bone.

■ palliation of tumour fungation
■ fracture reduction and fixation.

Palliation of obstructive symptoms

■ Palliative resection of a bowel tumour or a simple bypass procedure such as a gastrojejunostomy will avoid symptoms of intestinal obstruction.
■ Laser or cryotherapy resection of an obstructing tumour mass will restore the lumen of an obstructed bronchus or oesophagus.

■ Intubation of the oesophagus with a rigid tube or flexible stent provides rapid and effective relief of dysphagia.
■ Nephrostomy or passage of ureteric catheters will relieve obstructive hydronephrosis.
■ Biliary stents or choledochojejunostomy will relieve obstructive jaundice owing to extrahepatic bile duct obstruction as in carcinoma of the pancreas.
■ Gastroenterostomy will relieve gastric outflow obstruction.
■ Rectal stents can be used for rectal obstruction.
■ Ventriculoperitoneal shunting of hydrocephalus may result in dramatic improvement of headache and neurological deficits even though the underlying tumour may be incurable.

Control of haemorrhage

■ Diathermy at bronchoscopy or cystoscopy will control haemoptysis or haematuria respectively.
■ Bleeding tumours in the oesophagus, stomach or in the large bowel can be controlled by using diathermy or laser coagulation at endoscopy.

Palliation of tumour fungation

Local resection, even if not complete, may be of value for a locally advanced tumour mass that is necrotic and breaking down. Toilet mastectomy for a progressive breast cancer is perhaps the most common example of this.

Fracture reduction and fixation

Pathological fracture of a weight-bearing bone is best dealt with by internal fixation, as shown in Figure 4.1, followed by postoperative radiotherapy. Radiotherapy consolidates the surgical fixation, maximizing the probability of its security in the longer term (Fig. 4.2). In certain circumstances prophylactic fixation may also be indicated; specific indications for this include diffuse lytic bone disease in a weight-bearing area and destruction of more than 50 per cent of the cortex by a lytic deposit.

FURTHER READING

Pollock RE, Curley S, Ross M, Perrier N. Advanced Therapy. In: *Surgical Oncology*. BC Decker, Hamilton, Ontario, 2008.

Sabel MS, Sondak VK, Sussman JJ. *Essentials of Surgical Oncology*. Mosby, London, 2007.

Schauer A, Becker W, Reiser M, Possinger K. *The Sentinel Lymph Node Concept*. Springer, Berlin, 2005.

SELF-ASSESSMENT QUESTIONS

1. Which three of the following are indications for the surgical treatment of cancer?
   a. Long waiting time for radiotherapy
   b. Fracture of a weight-bearing bone
   c. Acute intestinal obstruction
   d. Hypercalcaemia
   e. Anaemia
   f. Hypoproteinaemia
   g. Intestinal perforation

2. Which one of the following is the most important feature of preoperative radiotherapy?
   a. Allows treatment of regional lymph nodes
   b. Downstages disease to facilitate surgical resection
   c. Removes need for radiotherapy after surgery
   d. Lessens morbidity from radiotherapy
   e. Cost-effective

5

PRINCIPLES OF RADIOTHERAPY

- Types of radiotherapy 42
- Other forms of radiation 44
- Biological actions of ionizing radiation 44
- Clinical use of radiotherapy 45
- Side-effects of radiotherapy 48
- Radiation protection 49
- Further reading 50
- Self-assessment questions 51

Radiotherapy is the use of ionizing radiation to treat disease. Ionizing radiation can be delivered by X-ray beams, beams of ionizing particles, e.g. electrons, or by beta or gamma irradiation produced in the decay of radioactive isotopes.

TYPES OF RADIOTHERAPY

External beam radiotherapy

External beam radiotherapy is the most common form of treatment in clinical use. A range of X-ray beams is available, varying according to their energy.

Superficial voltage

These X-ray beams are of energy 50–150 kV and are, as their name implies, suitable for the treatment of superficial lesions in the skin; their useful treatment energy penetrates no more than 1 cm beneath the surface.

Orthovoltage machines

These produce X-rays of energy 200–300 kV and penetrate to a depth of approximately 3 cm. These are therefore useful for treating structures such as ribs, scapula or sacrum but are not sufficiently powerful to reach deeper internal organs.

Megavoltage machines

These are either linear accelerators producing high energy X-ray beams of 4–20 MV or cobalt machines containing a source of cobalt-60, which decays spontaneously to nickel-60 releasing gamma rays of 1.2 and 1.3 MV. Linear accelerators form the mainstay of modern clinical radiotherapy and have largely replaced older cobalt machines in modern radiotherapy departments. A modern linear accelerator is shown in Figure 5.1.

Electron beams are also produced by linear accelerators and have the advantage that, as particulate radiation beams, they have a defined range in tissue with a sharp cut-off at the point where they deliver their energy. This is of value where a tumour is superficial and particularly when it is overlying a radiosensitive structure such as the spinal cord. In many centres electron beam treatment has replaced older superficial and orthovoltage X-ray machines, providing a wide range of beams with varying effective treatment depths from the linear accelerator.

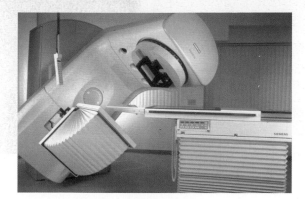

Figure 5.1 A modern linear accelerator.

Brachytherapy

This is the use of radioactive sources placed either on or within a site involved with tumour. The great advantage of this form of treatment is the rapid fall-off in dose at only a short distance from the source (obeying the inverse square law). There are three types of brachytherapy in use:

- *Mould treatment* This uses sources placed directly over a superficial tumour of the skin fixed in a plastic mounting (the mould).
- *Intracavitary treatment* This uses radioactive sources placed within a body cavity. Intrauterine tubes and vaginal sources in the treatment of gynaecological tumours are a common application of this technique.
- *Interstitial treatment* This uses radioactive sources, which may be in the form of needles or wire inserted directly within the area of interest. This technique is used for cancer of the tongue, floor of mouth and breast.

The first isotope to be employed was radium. This is no longer used because it constitutes a major radiation hazard as it has a long half-life (1620 years) and decays to a radioactive gas (radon). It has been superseded initially by cobalt sources and currently by caesium and iridium as the principal isotopes used for brachytherapy.

Live source implants

Direct handling of live sources is most commonly used today when iodine or palladium seeds are used for prostate implants. While the radiation from iodine-125 is short range and poses no major radiation hazard, that from iridium is more penetrating and its use has major disadvantages in exposure of staff and patients within the hospital to radiation from the time of insertion to the time of removal, which may be several days. This means that careful monitoring is required and that there are limits to the time that individuals can spend in caring for the patient. It also means that friends and family are not permitted to be with the patient.

Manual afterloading

In this method, inactive source carriers are used initially to enable accurate siting of the treatment so that the patient can be moved within the hospital from theatre or the X-ray department without radioactive sources in place. The active isotope is introduced manually once the inactive carrier is correctly placed. This enables more accurate placement not constrained by the need for rapid placement and long handled instruments required when a live source is used. Loading can be done in the operating theatre or once the patient has returned to a protected room and postoperative recovery is complete. An example is the use of iridium wire hairpins for tongue and floor of mouth implants.

Remote afterloading

Following placement of the source carriers, the radiation sources are introduced by remote control via pneumatic pipes or a cable connected to the source carriers within the patient. This system minimizes exposure to staff and in practice means that only the patient is exposed to radiation. It is also possible to interrupt the treatment so that the patient can receive attention without further exposing hospital personnel and there are no time limits on their stay. A modern afterloading machine is shown in Figure 5.2.

All such treatments require the patient to be isolated in a protected room with thickened or

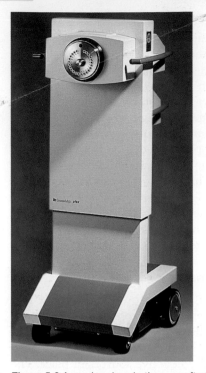

Figure 5.2 A modern brachytherapy afterloading machine, which uses a small iridium source located in the head of the machine that passes out by remote control through a series of channels to deliver radiation into applicators within a tumour area connected to these outlets. (Courtesy of Varian Medical Systems)

shielded walls, floors and ceilings while the source is in position in the patient.

Remote afterloading can deliver radiation at different dose rates but increasingly older 'medium dose rate' systems are being replaced by high dose rate machines, which deliver the dose in only a few minutes. This has substantial advantages in radiation protection and means that the patient no longer needs prolonged periods of isolation to receive brachytherapy.

Internal isotope therapy

Internal isotope treatment involves the administration of a radioactive isotope systemically, which is then concentrated within the body at certain sites. Specific examples of this form of treatment are the use of radioiodine (^{131}I) for thyroid cancer and also neuroblastoma when conjugated in meta-iodobenzyl guanidine (mIBG),

phosphorus (^{32}P) for polycythaemia rubra vera and strontium (^{89}Sr) for bone metastases.

OTHER FORMS OF RADIATION

There are types of radiation other than X-rays or gamma rays that can be used therapeutically. These are either radiation, which causes greater biological damage along each path track it traverses – high linear energy transfer (LET) radiation – or beams that have a highly focused deposition of radiation (*Bragg peak*).

Neutrons

Neutrons have been evaluated extensively in a number of centres across Europe and the US. Their advantages are that they have less dependence on oxygen for cell killing, a recognized limitation for X-rays, and they cause more direct damage to the cellular DNA. While there is little doubt that they are more effective at achieving cell kill, they are not selective for cancer cells and their use has been accompanied by unacceptably high levels of normal tissue damage and severe late side-effects. They are therefore not in routine clinical use.

Protons

Protons are available in an increasing number of centres around the world. Their advantage is the production of a highly localized, high-energy peak of energy deposition, which, by manipulation of the beam energy and the use of absorbing materials, can be focused to a defined position in a patient. Biologically they are similar in action to X-rays. They have been used particularly for tumours in inaccessible sites such as the back of the eye, pituitary and base of skull, and are being applied to many other sites as experience and accessibility increases.

BIOLOGICAL ACTIONS OF IONIZING RADIATION

Ionizing radiation causes damage to cellular DNA by two mechanisms:

- direct damage caused by the passage of the photon through the nucleic acid structure
- indirect damage owing to the production of toxic free hydroxyl radicals from the interaction of radiation with water within the cell. This results in single and double strand breaks in the DNA, which, unless repair occurs, will accumulate, resulting in reproductive death of the cell.

Other factors important in the response to radiation include:

- *Oxygenation* Hypoxic tissues are considered relatively radioresistant. Delivery of radiotherapy in multiple fractions allows reoxygenation to occur between each treatment as the tumour shrinks and blood flow improves.
- *Repopulation* Both tumour tissue and normal tissues continue to divide during a course of radiotherapy and there is even some evidence to suggest that repopulation may increase during this time as cells are lost. Gaps within a radiotherapy schedule should therefore be avoided wherever possible to avoid significant repopulation undoing any effects from irradiation in the previous days.
- *Repair* Much of the damage produced by X-rays and gamma rays is not sufficient to kill the cell immediately (sublethal damage). Repair of such damage will mean that the cell retains its viability. This capacity is better developed in normal tissues than in many malignant tumours, which accounts for much of the differential cell kill between tumour and normal cells.
- *Redistribution* Radiosensitivity varies as cells progress through the cell cycle, being maximum during the periods of active DNA synthesis in late G1 and S phases and least during G2 and early M phases.

There is a spectrum of radiosensitivity for both tumour and normal cell types. Few, if any, tumours are truly radioresistant, although some may require a larger dose of radiation than others to achieve the same effect. There is also a wide spectrum of sensitivity in normal tissues.

Particular care is required with certain normal tissues when irradiation is delivered:

- CNS tissue has a relatively low threshold for damage and has little or no capacity for repair. Radiation damage to the CNS is therefore often irreversible and can result in catastrophic morbidity if, for example, necrosis of the spinal cord or brainstem results.
- The small bowel is also relatively sensitive and doses well below those required to sterilize an epithelial tumour will cause serious damage.
- The lens of the eye will develop cataract after exposure to only small doses and must therefore be carefully shielded whenever possible.
- Bladder and rectum are often dose-limiting tissues when pelvic tumours are treated.
- Lung damage occurs at around half the dose required to treat a lung cancer; damage to a large volume of lung will result in respiratory distress and even death from respiratory failure.

The balance between causing serious normal tissue damage and curing a malignant tumour is termed the 'therapeutic ratio'. Compromise of radiation dose to avoid excessive toxicity is the major limitation in successfully achieving local cure of malignant tumours with radiotherapy.

CLINICAL USE OF RADIOTHERAPY

The patient attending for radiotherapy treatment will pass through a series of steps to ensure that treatment is given as accurately and safely as possible. These include:

- patient positioning and immobilization
- tumour localization
- treatment planning
- verification
- treatment.

Positioning of a patient

This is very important in order to enable an X-ray beam to reach a certain site. It is particularly

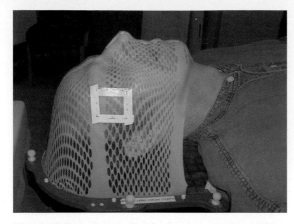

Figure 5.3 Patient in position for treatment to the orbit demonstrating immobilization mask.

the case in the head and neck region where small changes in the position of the neck or chin can greatly affect the tissues included in an X-ray beam.

In order to reproduce a particular position accurately, some form of immobilization may be designed, such as a plastic head shell to hold the head in a fixed position as shown in Figure 5.3.

Tumour localization

Localization can be achieved by simple clinical examination as in the case of a skin tumour; plain X-rays as in bone metastases; or a CT scan

for tumours in the thorax, abdomen or pelvis. Alongside this, it is important to identify vital structures to be avoided such as the spinal cord or kidney.

Treatment planning

This defines the optimal arrangement of X-ray beams to cover the treatment area as evenly as possible while avoiding structures around it. At its simplest level this may be a single direct electron beam for a skin tumour; for internal tumours a more complex arrangement of two, three or four X-ray beams approaching from different directions may be required. Treatment plans of multiple beams are drawn up using computerized data describing the characteristics of the beam and enabling rapid addition of their effects at a point.

Conformal radiotherapy using external X-ray beams shapes the high-dose treatment area as closely as possible to that of the tumour volume, even where this may be a highly irregular shape, while avoiding adjacent sensitive normal structures. This requires accurate three-dimensional reconstruction of the volume to be treated and irregular beam shaping using lead blocks, or more commonly a multileaf collimator shaping the beam typically by 80 or 120 interleaved projections into the beam, which can be adjusted as required. An example is shown in Figure 5.4.

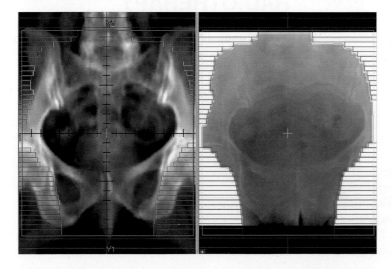

Figure 5.4 On left, beam's eye view (BEV) of planning scan pictures from a radiotherapy plan to treat the pelvis, demonstrating position of the beam and shaping using the multileaf collimator. On the right, an electronic portal image (EPI) has been taken using the high energy linear accelerator beam prior to a treatment exposure to verify the beam size, shape and position. Note the loss of definition between bone and soft tissue characteristic of high energy (megavoltage) X-rays.

Intensity-modulated radiotherapy (IMRT) is a further development, which varies the dose delivered within a tumour volume. This means that a central high-dose region can be defined surrounded by a lower dose region, minimizing inclusion of normal tissues, all within the same treatment volume.

Stereotactic radiotherapy is a means of treating a small spherical volume to a high dose and is typically used for localized lesions in the brain. This can be achieved using a standard linear accelerator with a modified beam producing a small focused field, which builds up the high-dose volume using a series of rotating arc movements. Modern developments of this include tomotherapy and the 'cyberknife', which incorporate a megavoltage X-ray beam in a gantry capable of multiple arcs controlled by software that enables variable beam profiles during the arc to build up a complex localized dose distribution. The alternative approach is to use the Gammaknife®. This is a machine containing multiple cobalt sources each with its independent shield which can be opened to focus on the treatment volume in a spherical pattern. Such machines are only available in a few specialized units.

Verification

Verification entails ensuring that the treatment plan can be translated back to the patient in the defined treatment position. This is usually done on a machine called a treatment simulator, which reproduces precisely the movements of the treatment machine but produces only a diagnostic X-ray beam so that an X-ray picture of the proposed treatment beam can be taken.

Further verification when the actual treatment starts is essential, particularly if complex beam shapes or lead shielding are to be employed. Megavoltage images can be taken using the linear accelerator beam. Their disadvantage is that, because they interact in a different manner to low-energy X-rays, there is no differential absorption between bone and soft tissue, resulting in poor anatomical definition; this is shown in Figure 5.4. Modern linear accelerators also incorporate a kilovoltage X-ray

tube on the gantry, which enables cross-sectional imaging to be acquired at the time of treatment. This has the advantage of providing information on the soft tissues within the beam to be exposed, which cannot be identified from conventional beam verification images.

Treatment only proceeds once it is certain that the defined area to be treated will be encompassed using the planned X-ray beams. During treatment the patient will be continually monitored by the radiographers and seen regularly by the medical staff. In a radical treatment, verification images will typically be repeated daily for the first 3 days and then once a week to ensure the beam positioning is consistent throughout. Specific additional measurements of radiation exposure can be taken using dosimeters placed on vital areas, such as the eye or testes, and further verification X-rays taken during the course of treatment.

Image-guided radiotherapy is the latest development to ensure that the radiation beam follows as closely as possible the planned volume and avoids normal structures. This has evolved with the increasing recognition that, during a few minutes of radiation exposure and between daily exposures, there may be critical changes, for example bladder filling, rectal and bowel distension, respiratory and cardiac movements, which will alter the anatomical relations of the treated radiation volume. The use of imaging immediately prior to exposure with markers, such as small metallic clips or gold grains fixed in the tissue, will allow adjustments to the beam to be made immediately prior to radiotherapy being delivered. Complex techniques for exposure to be matched to phases of the respiratory cycle, termed gating, are also available to optimize delivery to tumours in the lung.

Treatment duration

There is considerable variation in the dose and duration of radiotherapy treatment given to patients, which can appear confusing. Neither the total number of treatments nor the total dose given are necessarily a guide to the biological dose of radiation delivered. There are three components to biological radiation dose:

- total dose
- number of treatments (fractions) of a given dose
- overall time of treatment.

The following general principles can be applied:

- The same total dose given in a short time or fewer fractions has greater effect than the same dose given over a longer time in many fractions.
- Fraction size is an important determinant of normal tissue damage: small fractions minimize normal tissue effects. However, it follows from the previous point that, if used, small fractions demand a longer course of treatment with a higher total dose to have the same effect.
- Overall treatment time is important in achieving tumour control. Delays and interruptions in a course of treatment should be avoided as should overall treatment times of greater than 6–7 weeks.

The unit of radiation dose used is the Gray which is a measure of absorbed energy (1 Gy = 1 joule per kilogram). This has replaced the rad but the conversion is simple: 1 Gy = 100 rads. In some centres in order to keep the actual numbers the same, doses are described in centigray since 1 cGy = 1 rad.

Precise radiation schedules vary from centre to centre and between individual clinicians, however, some generalizations can be made. A fundamental difference lies between palliative and radical doses.

Radical treatments require high doses of radiation to eliminate tumour but are divided into smaller fractions to minimize side-effects and remain within the tolerance of normal tissues. Examples of radical schedules include:

- 60–70 Gy in 30–35 fractions in 6–7 weeks
- 55 Gy in 20 fractions in 4 weeks or 50 Gy in 15 fractions in 3 weeks.

Palliative treatments require short schedules with few acute side-effects. The ideal palliative treatment is a single dose and many centres use

this routinely, while others treat over 1–2 weeks. Examples include:

- 8–10 Gy in a single dose
- 20 Gy in 5 daily fractions over 1 week or 30 Gy in 10 daily fractions over 2 weeks.

SIDE-EFFECTS OF RADIOTHERAPY

The toxicity of radiotherapy is divided into two distinct groups: the early effects, which occur during treatment, and the late effects, which come on months or years following treatment.

Early effects

These develop during treatment usually in the second to third week of a course of radical irradiation. They may be divided as follows:

- *Non-specific effects* Many patients feel tired and lack energy during treatment. There may be many factors in addition to radiation exposure to account for this, including depression, anxiety, travelling daily to treatment and concomitant medication.
- *Specific local effects related to the area being treated* It is important to note that areas outside the irradiation field do not exhibit acute toxicity. Examples are shown in Table 5.1 together with suggested treatment. As a general principle, these are all self-limiting effects, which resolve spontaneously after treatment, their pathogenesis being related to temporary loss of cell division at an epithelial surface.

Late effects

These are potentially the most serious effects of treatment since, unlike the acute effects, they are not self-limiting and indeed tend to be progressive and irreversible. They arise owing to loss of stem cell recovery potential and progressive damage to small blood vessels resulting in their occlusion (endarteritis obliterans).

Fortunately in practice they are rare but any radical treatment dose will carry a risk of late

TABLE 5.1 Acute effects after radical radiotherapy

Site	Effect	Treatment
Skin	Erythema leading, if severe, to desquamation	Minimal; avoid irritants, trauma Aqueous or weak hydrocortisone cream
Bowel	Diarrhoea/colic	Low residue diet Codeine or loperamide
Bladder	Frequency/dysuria	Exclude infection
Scalp	Hair loss	Order wig in advance; hair will regrow after palliative but not radical doses
Mouth/pharynx	Mucositis	Avoid irritants and alcohol; treat candidiasis; topical chlorhexidine or benzydamine

TABLE 5.2 Late effects after radical radiotherapy

Site	Effect	Treatment
Skin	Fibrosis; telangiectasia; rarely necrosis	Usually none
Bowel	Stricture; perforation; bleeding fistulae	If severe, resection of affected segment
Bladder	Fibrosis causing frequency; haematuria; fistulae	If severe, surgical resection
CNS	Myelitis causing paraplegia; cerebral necrosis	None
Lung	Fibrosis	None

damage becoming manifest in the months and years ahead. They are not usually seen before 6 months after treatment but there is an ongoing risk, which is never entirely lost. Examples of late effects are given in Table 5.2.

Finally, the risk of inducing second malignancy should be considered. In practice this is exceedingly rare and invariably outweighed by the risk from the established malignancy for which radiation is given. A clear pattern is recognized with leukaemia or lymphoma seen in the first few years after exposure, reaching a peak incidence around 3 years and not seen after 10 years. In contrast solid tumours have an increasing risk with time, are rarely seen before 10 years and may occur 30 years or more after exposure.

The greatest risk may be associated with low-dose exposure and there are many historical examples after treatment of benign disease such as tinea capitis, goitre and ankylosing spondylitis. After therapeutic radiation the risk is small but there is some evidence that this may be increased in patients who receive combined modality treatment with the addition of chemotherapy. This has recently become apparent in long-term survivors of lymphoma treat-ments in whom the risk of a second tumour after 20 years is around 15 per cent.

RADIATION PROTECTION

Indiscriminate use of radiation is dangerous. There are strict regulations surrounding its use for medical purposes to ensure that exposure to staff, visitors and patients is kept to an absolute minimum. This is achieved by physical separation and protection from the sources of radiation and subsequent monitoring of exposure in those at particular risk.

Separation and protection

Radiotherapy machines are localized in one area or even in a separate hospital. Their design incorporates shielding of scattered radiation to produce a defined beam, the penetration and qualities of which are carefully measured and maintained. They are housed within a room designed to contain the radiation, using lead barriers within the walls for low-energy beams and thick high-density concrete walls for high-energy beams.

Similarly, radioisotopes are stored under carefully controlled conditions in a radiation safe and administered to the patient in a designated area, again designed to contain any radiation exposure. Patients having implants or high doses of radioiodine will be isolated in single rooms that have additional shielding to prevent radiation reaching other areas of the ward. Staff are given strict time limits to be spent with the patient. Visitors are usually not permitted while there are high levels of radioactivity present.

Radiation monitoring

All staff involved in the direct care of patients receiving radiation treatment will be designated as workers who require regular monitoring for radiation exposure. The mainstay of monitoring is the film badge worn by these staff, which, when processed, will detect those who may have been inadvertently exposed to radiation. There are clearly defined exposure limits for adults within which all personnel must remain. All departments must have local rules regarding the handling and use of radiation sources and staff must be fully acquainted with these.

It is important to keep the dangers of radiation as used under controlled medical conditions in context, while not relaxing the rules governing its use. There is no evidence that hospital workers are at greater risk than the general population from malignant disease. The entire population is exposed to levels of background radiation and many other common daily activities carry a greater risk than low-level exposure. For example, it has been estimated that all of the following activities carry a one in a million risk of death:

- driving for 65 miles
- flying in civil aircraft for 400 miles
- smoking less than one cigarette
- drinking half a bottle of wine.

FURTHER READING

Bomford CK, Kunkler IH. *Walter and Miller's Textbook of Radiotherapy*, 6th edn. Churchill Livingstone/Elsevier, London, 2002

Hoskin P (ed.). *Radiotherapy in Practice: external beam therapy*. Oxford University Press, Oxford, 2007

Hoskin P, Coyle C (eds). *Radiotherapy in Practice: brachytherapy*. Oxford University Press, Oxford, 2005

Joiner M, van der Kogel A. *Basic Clinical Radiobiology*. 4th edn. Arnold, London, 2009

SELF-ASSESSMENT QUESTIONS

1. Which of the following best describes radiotherapy?
   a. It uses non-ionizing radiation
   b. It is a useful systemic treatment for cancer
   c. It can use beams of ionizing particles
   d. Toxicity is usually limited to acute effects during treatment
   e. It is suitable for tumours at any site

2. Which of the following applies to megavoltage X-ray machines?
   a. They are useful for diagnostic X-ray production
   b. They are usually portable
   c. They can be used to produce neutrons for superficial radiotherapy
   d. They can have a radioisotope for their radiation source
   e. They are commonly used for brachytherapy

3. Which three of the following are important in modifying the response of radiotherapy in the cell?
   a. White cell count during irradiation
   b. Oxygen levels during irradiation
   c. RNA repair after irradiation
   d. Cell repopulation after irradiation
   e. Phase of cell cycle during irradiation
   f. Water content of the cell during irradiation
   g. Interstitial pressure during irradiation

4. Which of the following statements is correct regarding radiation dose?
   a. Total dose alone will indicate the biological effect
   b. The same dose given over a longer time is more effective
   c. A dose is most effective given in multiple small doses (fractions)
   d. Large doses per fraction are more effective than smaller fractions
   e. The overall time is more important than the dose per fraction

5. When the clinical use of radiotherapy is considered, which of the following is correct?
   a. Palliative treatments will require high total doses
   b. Radical treatments are best given in large daily fractions
   c. A typical radical dose would be 30 Gy in 10 daily fractions
   d. Single doses are the best palliative treatment if effective
   e. Radical doses work best when delivered slowly over a long time

6. Which three of the following are recognized acute effects of radiotherapy?
   a. Constipation
   b. Peripheral neuropathy
   c. Skin erythema
   d. Cataract
   e. Dysphagia
   f. Dysuria
   g. Lymphoedema

7. Which three of the following are recognized late effects of radiotherapy?
   a. Peripheral neuropathy
   b. Skin fibrosis
   c. Cataract
   d. Constipation
   e. Dysuria
   f. Lymphoedema
   g. Fatigue

8. With regard to radiation protection, which of the following is correct?
   a. There is no significant risk from doses used in clinical practice
   b. High energy beams are shielded behind lead screens
   c. Patients receiving radioisotope therapy can be visited regularly
   d. Hospital workers have higher rates of exposure than the public
   e. The entire population is exposed to radiation

6 PRINCIPLES OF SYSTEMIC TREATMENT

■ Chemotherapy agents   52
■ Efficacy and toxicity of
  chemotherapy   54
■ Clinical use of chemotherapy   56
■ Drug resistance   56
■ Administration of chemotherapy   57

■ Hormone therapy   61
■ Biological therapy   63
■ Growth factors   64
■ Experimental chemotherapy   65
■ Further reading   65
■ Self-assessment questions   66

Cancer chemotherapy is the treatment of malignant disease with drugs rather than radiation or surgical removal. The drugs used are often highly toxic since they are rarely totally selective for cancer cells. They should therefore be given within an oncology unit by those experienced in their use.

Systemic therapy can be used alone or, more commonly, in combination with surgery or radiotherapy as an adjuvant to enhance local control and to attack potential sites of metastases.

CHEMOTHERAPY AGENTS

Cancer chemotherapy agents act upon cell division, interfering with normal cell replication. They can be broadly classified as follows:

■ Drugs acting on the structure of DNA
  – antimetabolites
  – alkylating agents
  – intercalating agents
  – topoisomerase inhibitors
■ Drugs acting on mitosis

■ Signal transduction inhibitors
■ Drugs inducing apoptosis
■ Drugs targeting the tumour vasculature
  – antiangiogenesis
  – vascular disrupting agents.

Drugs acting on the structure of DNA

Antimetabolites

These function at the level of DNA synthesis, interfering with the incorporation of nucleic acid bases (cytosine, thymine, adenine and guanine). These can be classified into two groups:

■ Drugs based on chemical modification of a nucleic acid so that the drug rather than the true nucleic acid is incorporated into the DNA, thereby preventing accurate replication of the complementary base sequence. 5-Fluorouracil (5FU) is the classical example now available as an oral prodrug capecitabine. Others include gemcitabine, cytosine arabinoside and fludarabine. These drugs may also have additional modes of inhibiting DNA synthesis, e.g. the inhibition of thymidine synthetase by 5FU and of ribonucleotide reductase by gemcitabine.

- Drugs which inhibit reduction of folic acid (essential for the transfer of methyl groups in DNA synthesis) from its inactive dihydrofolate form to the active tetrahydrofolate, e.g. methotrexate.

Alkylating agents

These directly interfere with the DNA double strand of base pairs by chemically reacting with the structure, forming methyl cross-bridges. These then prevent the two DNA strands coming apart in mitosis to form daughter DNA fragments, and division therefore fails. Drugs in this group include cyclophosphamide, chlorambucil, melphalan, mitomycin C and the nitrosoureas BCNU and CCNU.

Intercalating agents

These act in a similar way to the alkylating agents but, rather than directly forming cross-strands in the DNA molecule, they bind between the base pair molecules, i.e. binding adenine to thymine and cytosine to guanine. This again prevents the DNA double strand from dividing in order to replicate, preventing cell division. Platinum compounds (cisplatin, oxaliplatin and carboplatin) act by binding specifically to guanosine, forming DNA adducts that cross-link either within one DNA strand or across strands. Other compounds, active through DNA intercalation, are the anthracycline group of drugs (Adriamycin, epirubicin and idarubicin).

Bleomycin is not a true intercalating agent but does partially intercalate with DNA and produces direct DNA damage through forming a complex with iron, resulting in the production of reactive toxic products.

Topoisomerases inhibitors

Topoisomerases are enzymes that control the tertiary coiling of DNA molecules. Two main classes are recognized: topoisomerase I and II. The camptothecin group of drugs including topotecan and irinotecan are topoisomerase I inhibitors, and the podophyllotoxins, etoposide and teniposide, are topoisomerase II inhibitors.

Drugs acting on mitosis

Mitosis requires spindle formation essential in the sorting and moving of chromosomes following replication at the end of mitosis. Spindle formation is affected through two mechanisms:

- spindle poisons: the vinca alkaloids (vincristine, vinblastine and vindesine)
- tubulin polymerization resulting in abnormal spindle formation and thereby cell death. The taxane group of drugs (paclitaxel and docetaxel) are cytotoxic through this mechanism.

Microtubule formation is also affected by podophyllin and so etoposide and teniposide both inhibit spindle formation in addition to their effects through topoisomerase.

Signal transduction inhibitors

Communication within and between cells is mediated by extensive biochemical interactions triggered by cell surface receptors. Tyrosine kinases are a frequent component of these cascades, particularly those related to the epidermal growth control receptor (EGFR) and angiogenesis (VEGF and PDGF). They are therefore a potential target for new drug development. Drugs which act primarily through inhibition of tyrosine kinases include imatinib, gefitinib, sorafenib and sunitinib.

Drugs inducing apoptosis

A new class of drugs, proteosome inhibitors, has emerged, which enhance apoptosis in a population of tumour cells. Proteosomes are large protein complexes within the cell, which regulate the degradation and removal of proteins. Inhibitors of proteosomes have been shown to enhance apoptosis by disrupting the ordered degradation of proteins controlling the cell cycle. The most successful agent in this group is bortezomib which is now the recognized treatment for recurrent multiple myeloma.

Drugs targeting the tumour vasculature

New blood vessel formation is an essential prerequisite for a tumour to become established and remain viable. VEGF is an important component in this process. Tumour blood vessels differ from normal vasculature forming a random chaotic network with little structure and variable flow controlled primarily by fluctuations in interstitial pressure. Both the formation of blood vessels (angiogenesis) through VEGF and the new blood vessels themselves are therefore potential targets to inhibit tumour growth.

Antiangiogenic drugs include bevacizumab, which is a monoclonal antibody to the VEGF receptor, and sorafenib which inhibits signalling from the VEGF receptor through tyrosine kinase inhibition. Thalidomide and lenalidomide, both used in multiple myeloma, also have antiangiogenic activity, although their main mode of action may relate to inhibition of IL-6 and immunomodulatory effects.

Vascular disrupting agents (VDAs) target the stucture of the blood vessels and prevent their proliferation. Examples include combretastatin-4 phosphate and its analogues.

Because of their mode of action, certain drugs require cells to be in specific phases of the cell cycle to have any effect. For example, those acting on synthesis of DNA will act only on cells actively synthesizing at the time they are exposed to the drug. Cytotoxic drugs are therefore further classified into:

- *phase-specific drugs*, which act only in a specific phase of the cell cycle, e.g. antimetabolites during S phase and vinca alkaloids in M phase
- *cycle-specific drugs*, which require that cells are only dividing and passing through the cell cycle rather than being in the resting G0 phase. These include the alkylating agents and intercalating agents.

EFFICACY AND TOXICITY OF CHEMOTHERAPY

Although in principle all cycling cells should be sensitive to drugs that act on the cell cycle, in practice chemotherapy for most cancers is only modestly effective. This is due to a variety of reasons related to drug delivery to the cell and activation or deactivation within the target cells. Precise indications for the use of chemotherapy are detailed in the following chapters but in general the common malignant diseases can be broadly classified into three groups:

- those extremely sensitive to chemotherapy where this is the treatment of choice
- those with modest sensitivity where chemotherapy may play a part in their management but usually in combination with other treatment as an adjuvant or for recurrent disease
- those where chemotherapy is only of limited value in the palliation of advanced disease.

Examples of this classification are given in Table 6.1.

TABLE 6.1 Classification of common malignant diseases according to their sensitivity to chemotherapy

Group 1: High sensitivity	Group 2: Modest sensitivity	Group 3: Low sensitivity
Leukaemias	Breast	Prostate
Lymphomas	Colorectal	Kidney
Germ cell tumours	Bladder	Primary brain tumours
Small cell lung cancer	Ovary	Adult sarcomas
Myeloma	Cervix	Melanoma
Neuroblastoma		
Wilms' tumour		
Embryonal rhabdomyosarcoma		

Response and survival

In describing the efficacy of chemotherapeutic agents, there are internationally accepted response criteria, the RECIST (Response Evaluation Criteria in Solid Tumours) criteria (see also page 30), defined as follows:

- Complete response (CR) – complete resolution of all clinically detectable disease
- Partial response (PR) – a reduction in the longest diameter of a tumour of at least 30 per cent
- Stable disease (SD) – small changes with a response less than a partial response or progression less than a 20 per cent increase in measurable disease during the period of observation
- Progressive disease (PD) – an increase in measurable disease of at least 20 per cent during the period of observation, or the development of any new lesions.

It is important to interpret with care response data derived from clinical trials. Unless an agent or drug combination achieves a complete response in a significant proportion of patients, it is unlikely to have any impact on overall survival when used to treat that disease in the general population. Partial responses may be of value in delaying progression of a disease but, since they represent only a very small decrement in total cancer cell burden, significant effects on overall survival are unlikely.

With this in mind, performance status and quality of life measures are becoming an increasingly important measure of the efficacy of cancer treatment. Numerous scales of performance status have been devised, usually based on a 4 or 5 point scale ranging from normal to moribund. A common example is the WHO performance scale shown in Table 6.2.

Quality of life measures are more complex; they should be completed by the patient and will involve a structured questionnaire often divided into domains evaluating different aspects of the patient's activity, e.g. physical activity, pain and specific symptoms, emotional response, social interaction and financial impact. The most widely used quality of life questionnaires are the EORTC QLQ-C30 and

TABLE 6.2 Scales for performance status

Score	Status
Karnofsky	
100	Normal; no complaints; no evidence of disease
90	Able to carry on normal activities; minor signs or symptoms
80	Normal activity with effort, some signs or symptoms of disease
70	Cares for self; unable to carry on normal activity or do active work
60	Requires occasional assistance but able to care for most needs
50	Requires considerable assistance and frequent medical care
40	Disabled; requires special care and assistance
30	Severely disabled; hospitalization indicated although death not imminent
20	Very sick; hospitalization necessary; active supportive treatment necessary
10	Moribund; fatal processes progressing rapidly
0	Dead
WHO	
0	All normal activity without restriction
1	Restricted in physically strenuous activity but ambulatory and able to do light work
2	Ambulatory and capable of all self-care but unable to carry out any work. Up and about >50% of waking hours
3	Capable of only limited self-care, confined to bed or chair >50% of waking hours
4	Completely disabled. Cannot carry on any self-care. Totally confined to bed or chair

the FACT (Functional Assessment of Cancer Therapy).

CLINICAL USE OF CHEMOTHERAPY

Cytotoxic drugs can be given as single agents but are more usually given as multiple drug combinations. The major limitation in using these agents is toxicity to normal tissues. Because the majority are non-specific in their action, both malignant and normal cells are damaged when exposed to a cytotoxic drug. When the drugs are used within their defined dose limits, the normal cells will recover and it is the need for this window of recovery that results in the typical intermittent scheduling of these agents, most being given at 3–4 weekly intervals.

Common limiting toxicities are bone marrow suppression, bowel toxicity, and renal and neurological damage. The major limiting factors for specific drugs are shown in Table 6.3.

Combination chemotherapy

For most malignancies, combinations of drugs are more effective than single agents. These are designed by adding together modestly active agents to give greater overall activity and choosing agents with different dose-limiting toxicities so that the antitumour effect but not the toxic effect is additive or synergistic. Combinations also aim to incorporate drugs from different classes thereby attacking cells with both phase- and cycle-specific agents with the intent of targeting as many cells in the population as possible. An example of spreading limiting toxicities is shown in Table 6.4 with R-CHOP used for non-Hodgkin's lymphoma.

Combination therapy can also involve the use of a non-chemotherapy agent with a cytotoxic drug to enhance its activity. The most common example of this in clinical use is the addition of folinic acid to 5-fluorouracil (5FU), which approximately doubles its response rates in the treatment of colorectal cancer. This works because administered folinic acid increases intracellular concentrations of folate, which is an essential cofactor in the incorporation of 5FU into RNA and also its action in inhibiting thymidylate synthetase, an important enzyme in DNA synthesis.

DRUG RESISTANCE

Resistance to chemotherapy drugs can be an intrinsic property of a malignant cell but can also be acquired after exposure to individual drugs. Mechanisms of resistance include:

- altered biochemical pathways to avoid specific pathway blocks, e.g. modified folate use to avoid dihydrofolate reductase block with methotrexate
- altered cell transport mechanisms to prevent drug concentration in cancer cell by either reduced uptake or enhanced efflux
- altered drug metabolism increasing clearance or reducing drug activation; and
- impaired mechanisms of apoptosis (programmed cell death).

TABLE 6.3 Major toxicities for chemotherapeutic agents

Tissue affected	Toxic agents
Bone marrow*	All drugs, in particular vinblastine, etoposide, carboplatin, cyclophosphamide, melphalan, ifosfamide, paclitaxel
Bowel	Melphalan, cisplatin, 5FU, irinotecan, methotrexate
Renal	Methotrexate, cisplatin, ifosfamide
Neurological	Cisplatin, vincristine, ifosfamide, paclitaxel
Cardiac	Adriamycin, 5FU
Bladder	Cyclophosphamide

* In practice, bone marrow toxicity is becoming less important as a limiting toxicity as techniques for bone marrow support, such as autologous marrow or peripheral stem cell transplantation, become available.

TABLE 6.4 Drugs in R-CHOP

Drug	Action	Main toxicity
Rituximab	Complement activation	Allergy, anaphylaxis
Cyclophosphamide	Alkylating agent	Bone marrow, bladder
Adriamycin	Intercalating	Bone marrow, cardiac
Vincristine	Spindle poison	Neurological (peripheral neuropathy)
Prednisolone	Unknown	Fluid retention and weight gain, gastric irritation, hyperglycaemia

It is often found that resistance to a number of drugs develops together, a phenomenon called 'multidrug resistance' (MDR). This is thought to result from common molecular mechanisms related to specific DNA sequences. Identification of one particular genetic change in drug resistance has led to isolation of the *MDR1* gene and the protein for which it codes, a transmembrane glycoprotein important in cell transport. As mechanisms of resistance are elucidated, strategies to overcome them are emerging. For example, transmembrane transport can be modified by drugs such as verapamil and cyclosporin inhibiting the efflux of drugs away from the cell.

ADMINISTRATION OF CHEMOTHERAPY

Chemotherapy should be administered only in specialized units with the experience and support to do so safely. Most of the agents used can be harmful if there is continuous contact with the skin and even more so if accidentally ingested through contamination of hands and work surfaces. Agents should therefore be prepared by a specialized chemotherapy pharmacist under strictly controlled conditions, and gloves should be worn by the clinical staff when they are administering the drugs.

Prior to administration of drugs, all patients should have a full blood count measured. In varying circumstances and with different drugs the criteria for safe administration will vary but a general guide is that chemotherapy should only be given if the following parameters are met:

- haemoglobin >10 g/dL – although this is rarely a limiting factor and it is acceptable to proceed at lower levels and transfuse if necessary
- total white count $>3.0 \times 10^9$/L and total neutrophil count >1.0–1.5
- platelets >50–80×10^9/L.

For certain drugs renal function must also be carefully checked prior to administration of drugs. It is not usually sufficient to rely on serum urea or creatinine, and a measure of creatinine clearance should be performed. This applies in particular to the following:

- cisplatin
- carboplatin
- ifosfamide
- methotrexate (high dose).

Because of the close relation between serum levels and creatinine clearance, the dose of carboplatin is usually defined by a formula (the *Calvert formula*), which relates the predicted area under the serum concentration versus time curve (AUC) to the clearance. This enables the drug to be given relatively safely, even where renal function is impaired, with a predictable AUC after administration.

Chemotherapy drugs can be given orally, by intravenous or intramuscular bolus injection or by intravenous infusion. Examples of these are shown in Table 6.5.

Many chemotherapy drugs are severe irritants when injected outside a vein and extreme care must be taken during intravenous injections. These should be performed ideally by experienced staff working in a dedicated chemotherapy administration unit. Large

TABLE 6.5 Routes of administration

Oral	IV injection	Infusion	Intrathecal
Chlorambucil	Cyclophosphamide	Cisplatin	Methotrexate
Busulphan	Methotrexate	Carboplatin	Cytosine arabinoside
Melphalan (ld)	5FU	Mitozantrone	
Procarbazine	Adriamycin	Ifosfamide	
Etoposide	Vincristine	Methotrexate (hd)	
Capecitabine	Vinblastine	Melphalan (hd)	
Temozolamide	Vinorelbine	Paclitaxel	
		Gemcitabine	
		Oxaliplatin	
		5FU	

Key: ld, low dose; hd, high dose

visible veins should be chosen as far as possible and it is safest to administer the drugs into a running intravenous drip.

Where venous access is difficult:

■ for schedules requiring lengthy infusions
■ when continuous infusion pumps are to be used
■ in procedures likely to require the administration of many intravenous drugs, and
■ in transfusions such as bone marrow transplantation or high-dose chemotherapy

an indwelling central venous catheter has many advantages. A common type is the Hickman catheter as shown in Figure 6.1. These can be inserted under radiological control with local anaesthetic and remain in situ for many months. Regular flushing with heparinized saline at least weekly is required, and some doctors also recommend continous low-dose warfarin 1 mg daily while the line remains to prevent thrombotic complications. More sophisticated devices place a reservoir under the skin of the chest wall rather than an external line; this enables multiple access with less potential risk of infection, and it is more convenient for the active patient.

An alternative type of central line, which may be less robust but is simpler to insert, is a line such as a PICC line, which enters through the antecubital vein and is then directed through the brachial and subclavian veins into the vena cava; an example is shown in Figure 6.2.

The major complication from central lines in chemotherapy patients is that of infection, and

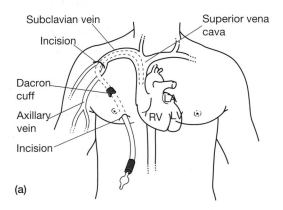

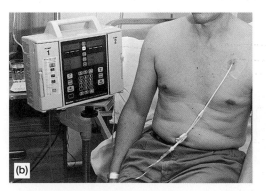

Figure 6.1 Central Hickman line shown (a) diagrammatically and (b) in situ in a patient.

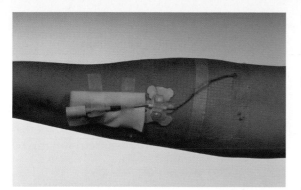

Figure 6.2 A PICC line in situ entering an antecubital vein.

infected lines or subcutaneous tracts require immediate removal of the catheter together with high-dose antibiotic cover. Subclavian vein thrombosis may also occur, particularly around an infected line.

If extravasation of chemotherapy does occur then there should be clear guidelines for its management. Table 6.6 details the drugs for which this is an important issue.

The following principles apply:

- The chemotherapy injection or infusion must be stopped immediately.
- The cannula is left in situ, residual drug is aspirated and the area flushed with saline.
- Ice packs may be applied and some recommend administration of local steroids or hyaluronidase, except for vincristine and oxaliplatin when gentle warming of the area is recommended.

In severe cases with irritant drugs such as Adriamycin or epirubicin, there may be extensive soft tissue damage as shown in Figure 6.3, particularly if the problem is not identified immediately and action taken. Liaison with a plastic surgery unit for such eventualities is of great value. Occasionally damage may be such as to require surgical repair.

Avoiding side-effects

As a general rule side-effects are best anticipated and prevented. Chemotherapy agents vary in their emetic potential but all may cause nausea and some severe vomiting. Anti-emetics

TABLE 6.6 Vesicant properties of common cytotoxic drugs

Vesicants	Exfoliants	Irritants	Inflammatory agents	Neutral
Causing pain, inflammation and blistering, leading to tissue death and necrosis	*Causing inflammation and shedding of skin*	*Causing inflammation and irritation*	*Causing mild to moderate inflammation and flare in local tissues*	*Causing no inflammation or damage*
Carmustine	Cisplatin	Carboplatin	Fluorouracil	Aspariginase
Dacarbazine	Docetaxel	Etoposide	Methotrexate	Bleomycin
Dactinomycin	Mitozantrone	Irinotecan		Cyclophosphamide
Daunorubicin	Oxaliplatin			Cytarabine
Doxorubicin	Topotecan			Fludarabine
Epirubicin				Gemcitabine
Idarubicin				Ifosfamide
Mitomycin				Melphalan
Mustine				
Paclitaxel				
Vinblastine				
Vincristine				
Vindesine				
Vinorelbine				

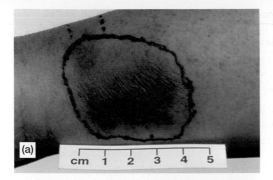

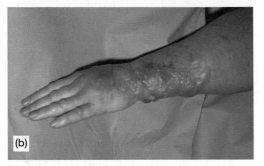

Figure 6.3 (a) Erythema following minor extravasation of epirubicin and (b) more severe soft tissue damage following extravasation of chemotherapy given intravenously into the back of the hand.

should therefore be considered for all but the most gentle of agents. A three-stage anti-emetic policy based on emetic potential will work for most patients.

Emetic potential of common chemotherapy agents

Chlorambucil and vincristine/vinblastine, used as single agents, rarely cause significant nausea and either anti-emetics are not required or simple oral agents are sufficient. Other drugs or combinations fall into the groups shown in Table 6.7

The use of specific anti-emetic drugs will vary but a simple anti-emetic protocol is as follows.

- Low potential schedules
  - metoclopramide 10 mg orally or prochlorperazine 25 mg rectally preceding chemotherapy
- Moderately emetogenic schedules
  - dexamethasone 8 mg and metoclo-

pramide 10 mg intravenously preceding chemotherapy followed by dexamethasone 2 mg tds orally for 2–3 days with metoclopramide 10 mg tds orally
- Highly emetogenic schedules
  - dexamethasone 8 mg and ondansetron 8 mg orally or intravenously preceding chemotherapy followed by dexamethasone 4 mg bd and ondansetron 8 mg bd orally daily for 2–3 days.

Anticipatory nausea and vomiting may be a particular problem for some patients. This occurs when they experience symptoms with any visit to the hospital, often on arrival, without exposure to the drugs. Lorazepam may be helpful in these instances. It is also often easier for inpatients to receive chemotherapy in the evening when they can receive added sedation and sleep through the administration.

Other side-effects must also be anticipated and steps taken to prevent them. For example:

- diarrhoea (e.g. from cisplatin, 5FU or irinotecan) – prescribe loperamide or codeine phosphate
- mucositis (e.g. from 5FU, methotrexate) – use regular chlorhexidine and benzydamine mouthwashes
- alopecia (e.g. from Adriamycin) – use of scalp cooling and provision of wig.

Scheduling

Chemotherapy schedules vary from simple single oral drugs to complex multiple drug regimens. The design of drug schedules is based on a consideration of the effects on both normal tissues and the tumour cells as discussed above.

Normal tissues are inevitably damaged by chemotherapy agents. Particularly sensitive are the dividing cells of the bone marrow and mucosal epithelial cells lining the oropharynx, gut and bladder. The general principle of scheduling chemotherapy is that each successive course should be given only when damage from the previous drug exposure has been repaired. Fortunately both bone marrow and epithelial lining cells have a large capacity for tolerating and recovering from damage and usually do so

TABLE 6.7 Classification of chemotherapy drugs according to their potential to provoke emesis

Low (<10%)	Moderate (10–30%)	High (31–90%)	Very high (>90%)
Vincristine	Cyclophosphamide	Adriamycin	Cisplatin
Vinblastine	Methotrexate	Epirubicin	Dacarbazine
Bleomycin	Mitomycin	Ifosfamide	Carmustine
Fludarabine	Mitozantrone	Carboplatin	Mustine
Rituximab	Etoposide	Oxaliplatin	Cyclophosphamide (>1.5 g/m^2)
Bevacizumab	5FU	Irinotecan	
	Paclitaxel		
	Gemcitabine		
	Cetuximab		
	Transtuzumab		

within 2–3 weeks. On this basis most chemotherapy is given at 3–4 weekly intervals.

Damage to tumour cells may depend on both the absolute levels of drug that can be achieved within them and the duration of exposure. In order to achieve the maximum levels possible, a fine line may be drawn between serious side-effects and maximizing tumour cell kill. In some circumstances where there is evidence that very high doses of drugs beyond normal tolerance will achieve more, e.g. in acute leukaemia, then bone marrow, or more usually bone marrow stem cells, can be removed prior to chemotherapy and stored to be used as an autograft once high-dose therapy has been given.

In order to achieve maximum levels for a suitable duration a knowledge of the pharmacokinetics of the drug is important. Drugs with short half-lives, such as 5FU, may have a greater effect when given by infusion or in divided doses.

The design of chemotherapy drug schedules is often a combination of elegant hypothesis, serendipity and pragmatism. However, when the results of chemotherapy trials are assessed and translated into general oncological practice, careful attention to the drug dosing and scheduling is important. There is some evidence that patients who fail to receive full doses of drugs at the designated minimum intervals have a reduced benefit from the treatment and this is a strong argument for chemotherapy being managed only in experienced units familiar with the complications and tolerance for each schedule.

HORMONE THERAPY

A small number of tumours are influenced by therapeutic changes in their hormone environment. In practice, hormone therapy is of value for breast and prostate cancer and to a lesser extent endometrial cancer. The response of breast cancer is based primarily upon the influence of oestrogen, and that of prostate cancer upon the influence of androgens.

Occasional responses with other tumour types have been reported, particularly to the drug tamoxifen, but their basis remains uncertain.

Breast cancer

Oestrogen exerts its effect by binding to a receptor within the cell nucleus called the 'oestrogen receptor'. This process is thought to be fundamental to the way in which oestrogen can influence the development of breast cancer. Drugs that alter the balance of activity at the oestrogen receptor are therefore often of value in the treatment of breast cancer. Such drugs may act directly by binding to the receptor and thereby blocking its activity as typified by tamoxifen, or indirectly on the production and peripheral activation of oestriol and oestrone to oestradiol by inhibiting the enzyme aromatase; commonly used aromatase inhibitor drugs include anastrozole and letrozole.

The presence of oestrogen receptors can be demonstrated histologically using immunohistochemistry and the demonstration of oestrogen receptors (ER) in an individual tumour is important in predicting the likelihood of response to hormonal treatment. Overall around 50 per cent of patients with breast cancer will respond to hormone therapy, but this figure reflects a response rate of up to 80 per cent when oestrogen receptors are positive compared with around 10 per cent where they are negative.

The observation that some patients who have no demonstrable receptors will respond may be explained by the presence of receptors in these cancer cells that have a slightly different structure not detected by the routine methods of assay.

Characteristically, hormone responses have a finite duration and it would seem that all breast cancers eventually become resistant to the first hormone treatment to which they are exposed. This may, however, be followed by second, third and even fourth successive responses to further hormone manipulations.

The basis for hormone resistance developing is thought to be changes in the characteristics of the oestrogen receptor, varying from complete loss of receptor to alterations in its binding sites or in its transcriptional properties within the nucleus. In other cases access to the receptor may be denied because of alterations of transport mechanisms and metabolism within the cell. Exposure to an alternative hormone therapy may in many cases achieve a second response, which will be seen in up to 45 per cent of patients after an initial exposure.

Progestogens and androgens can also be effective as second- and third-line treatments in breast cancer. Drugs such as megestrol and medroxyprogesterone do indirectly affect activity at the oestrogen receptor causing downregulation (i.e. making them less sensitive to stimulation by oestrogen), but in addition specific progestogen receptors have been identified in breast cancers and found to correlate with response to treatment.

An overview of hormone therapy in breast cancer is given in Table 6.8.

Prostate cancer

The basis of hormone therapy in prostate cancer is the dependence on androgen for its growth. The drugs used to treat prostate cancer therefore are anti-androgens working either directly by antagonism at the androgen receptor or indirectly on the hypothalamic–pituitary axis regulation of androgen release. Similar effects are also achieved by surgical orchidectomy removing the main site of androgen production. An overview of androgen blockade is shown in Figure 6.4. The relative clinical merits of the available antiandrogen therapies are shown in Table 10.1 (see Chapter 10, page 171).

None of the individual anti-androgen treatments offer complete blockade of both testicular and adrenal androgens. This may be achieved by combining a centrally acting gonadotrophin-

TABLE 6.8 Hormone therapy in breast cancer

Drug	Mode of action	Other actions and common side-effects
Tamoxifen Faslodex	Anti-oestrogen	Hot flushes, fluid retention, vaginal dryness/discharge, uterine bleeding, deep vein thrombosis
Exemestane Anastrozole Letrozole	Aromatase inhibitor	Hot flushes, nausea, rashes, joint stiffness, vaginal dryness, raised cholesterol, osteoporosis
Medroxyprogesterone Megestrol	Progestogen	Nausea, fluid retention, weight gain

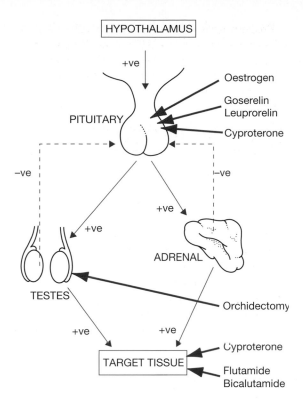

Figure 6.4 Mechanisms of androgen release and blockade.

releasing hormone agonist/antagonist, e.g. goserelin, with a peripherally acting drug such as cyproterone or bicalutamide, and is known as 'maximal androgen blockade – MAB'. This may be slightly more more effective than single drug therapy in advanced disease, particularly in younger patients but will be associated with more severe toxicity from androgen withdrawal, including lethargy, hot flushes, gynaecomastia and loss of sexual interest and function.

An important distinction between the hormone response of prostate cancer and that of breast cancer is seen on relapse to first-line anti-androgen therapy; second responses with prostate cancer are seen only occasionally.

Endometrial cancer

Endometrial cancer is recognized as a tumour related to high levels of circulating oestrogen. Both oestrogen and progesterone receptors can be demonstrated in cells of endometrial cancer and treatment with progestogens or gonadotrophin-releasing hormone agonist/antagonists such as goserelin or leuprorelin can be effective in metastatic disease. Response is predicted by the presence of oestrogen or progestogen receptors with around 65 per cent of patients having positive receptors responding to treatment. A reduction in oestrogen receptor concentration has been seen after progestogen treatment, suggesting that the efficacy of hormone treatment in endometrial cancer reflects inhibition of oestrogenic stimulus at the tumour cell.

BIOLOGICAL THERAPY

A number of the chemicals produced by the body in response to injury or infection have been explored as potential new treatments to eradicate cancer cells. Unfortunately only limited success has so far been achieved. Invariably such preparations are immunogenic and are therefore associated with side-effects such as malaise and low-grade fever. These are often debilitating but major toxicities are rare with commercially available compounds. In clinical practice only α-interferon is in occasional use.

α-Interferon

This has been the treatment of choice in the rare haematological malignancy hairy cell leukaemia (see Chapter 17). In renal cancer a modest impact in high-risk and advanced disease is seen and some responses are also seen in melanoma. In each of these instances interferon is believed to function by enhancing the natural defences available within the body, facilitating removal of malignant cells.

Alpha-interferon is given by subcutaneous injection three times per week. In doses above 3 megaunits side-effects of fever and malaise can be dose limiting. Treatment can be continuous for many months or even years.

Monoclonal antibody treatments

Monoclonal antibodies (MABs) are the equivalent of the magic bullet, their principle being to carry a toxic agent to a cell defined by specific surface antigens against which the antibody is targeted. In recent years this approach has resulted in a number of new clinical agents becoming available.

Rituximab is targeted against the CD20 antigen on B-cell lymphomas; in addition to standard chemotherapy it improves survival. Ibritumomab is an anti-CD20 antibody tagged with a radioisotope yttrium-90, which is highly effective in follicular lymphoma.

Herceptin is targeted against the HER2 antibody on breast cancer cells. and is now a valuable additional treatment option for patients with breast cancer which is HER2 positive; this can be demonstrated immunohistochemically and the extent of staining can be graded to predict the likelihood of response, as shown in Figure 6.5.

Alentuzumab is an anti-CD52 antibody, which is highly active in chronic lymphocytic leukaemia.

Bevacizumab, discussed earlier, is a monoclonal antibody, targeting tumour vasculature through VEGF.

Clinical trials are underway to define the precise role of these new agents in the management of these diseases; they will probably be incorporated into existing chemotherapy regimens both in the adjuvant setting and in primary treatment.

GROWTH FACTORS

One of the major dose-limiting toxicities encountered in the use of chemotherapy is that of bone marrow toxicity. In recent years the availability of colony-stimulating factors (CSF), in particular granulocyte colony-stimulating factor (G-CSF) has enabled chemotherapy dose to be intensified within the limits of tolerance of bone marrow. G-CSF is an analogue of naturally occurring growth factors given by subcutaneous injection following exposure to chemotherapy. It stimulates the granulocyte production lines in the bone marrow, reducing the period of neutropenia after intensive chemotherapy. The growth factors currently available have no significant effect upon platelet and red cell lines. Their use has also facil-

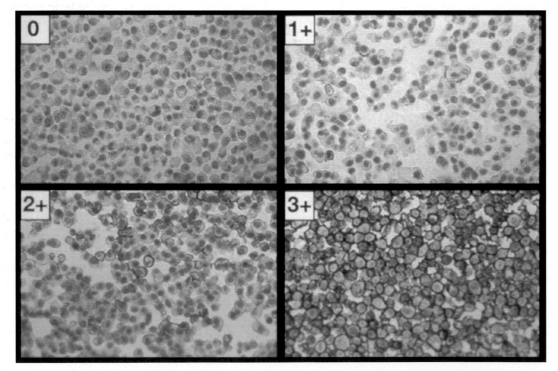

Figure 6.5 Histological section showing breast cancer cells with a range of positive staining for the HER-2 receptor, which may be seen to predict varying degrees of response to the monoclonal antibody transtuzumab (Herceptin®).

itated the process of peripheral blood progenitor cell (PBPC) harvesting, thereby simplifying the use of ultra-high-dose chemotherapy which is being increasingly applied to the treatment of solid as well as haemopoietic tumours.

EXPERIMENTAL CHEMOTHERAPY

The chemotherapy drugs and combination regimens widely used in routine oncological practice today have arisen out of carefully designed and regulated drug development programmes. From discovery of a promising new drug in the laboratory a lengthy and expensive period of evaluation starting with animal pharmacology and toxicology studies and ending in successful drug marketing has to be embarked on. The clinical studies within which new drugs may be given are outlined below and discussed in greater detail in Chapter 3.

- *Phase 1 studies* These are studies in which the new agent is first tried in patients. Such agents are offered only to patients for whom there is no other recognized effective treatment and who may wish to try other drugs in the slim hope of benefit. In phase 1 studies activity against the tumour is not an endpoint but these studies are designed to assess the maximum tolerated doses and define the toxicity profile in humans.
- *Phase 2 studies* These are the earliest studies in which antitumour activity is sought, giving the drug in doses and schedules defined from the phase 1 studies to patients who have failed previous conventional therapy or for whom there may be no effective recognized treatment.
- *Phase 3 studies* With activity in phase 2 established, the new agent is compared with the standard best treatment (or, if there is none, with placebo) in a large prospective randomized trial. Large numbers of patients are entered into such trials in order to achieve statistically robust

results and most of these studies are therefore multicentre studies.

Only following satisfactory passage through the above steps is a drug incorporated in the routine treatment of cancer; this may be many years after the first identification of the compound and will be followed by further evaluation of the drug to establish its full potential and application in adjuvant and primary treatment and its role in palliation both alone and in combination. Its toxicity in wider use must also be continuously monitored and notified (*post-marketing surveillance*).

Current areas of research in drug development alongside the more conventional classes of chemotherapy drugs include the following:

- drugs targeted against specific biochemical pathways involved in cellular growth control, for example the epithelial growth factor receptor (EGFR), tyrosine kinases and proteosomes
- anti-angiogenic agents and vascular targeting agents exploiting the different characteristics of tumour vasculature from normal blood vessels to selectively damage tumour blood supply
- immunotherapy through the development of vaccines against tumour antigens.

FURTHER READING

Brighton D, Wood M. *Royal Marsden Hospital Handbook of Chemotherapy*. Churchill Livingston, London, 2005

Buzdar AU (ed.). *Endocrine Therapies in Breast Cancer*. Oxford University Press, Oxford, 2007

Hesketh PJ. Chemotherapy-induced nausea and vomiting. *New England Journal of Medicine* 2008; **358**:2482–92

Summerhayes M and Daniels S. *Practical Chemotherapy: a multidisciplinary guide*. Arnold, London, 2003

Young A, Rowett L, Kerr D (eds). *Cancer Biotherapy: an introductory guide*. Oxford University Press, Oxford, 2006

SELF-ASSESSMENT QUESTIONS

1. Which three of the following drugs are antimetabolite chemotherapy agents?
   a. Gemcitabine
   b. Topotecan
   c. Cisplatin
   d. Fludarabine
   e. Adriamycin
   f. Cyclophosphamide
   g. Cytosine arabinoside

2. Which of the following applies to intercalating agent chemotherapy drugs?
   a. They act by alkylation of DNA
   b. They inhibit RNA synthesis
   c. They prevent separation of the DNA strands
   d. They are topoisomerase inhibitors
   e. They include irinotecan

3. Which of the following statements is true regarding those chemotherapy agents acting on mitosis?
   a. They interfere with synthesis of DNA
   b. They affect spindle formation
   c. They are independent of topoisomerase
   d. They include cisplatin
   e. They are independent of the cell cycle

4. The following is true of signal transduction inhibitors:
   a. They act through tyrosine synthase
   b. They can inhibit angiogenesis
   c. They include bortezomib
   d. They are cell cycle dependent
   e. They act on cell division

5. Which three of the following are true of drugs targeting the tumour vasculature?
   a. They will reduce blood flow to normal tissues
   b. They can act through VEGF
   c. They include thalidomide
   d. They cause extensive thrombosis
   e. Their effect is reversed by heparin
   f. They can alter blood vessel structure

6. Which three of the following are highly sensitive to chemotherapy?
   a. Breast cancer
   b. Non-Hodgkin's lymphoma
   c. Small cell lung cancer
   d. Neuroblastoma
   e. Renal cell carcinoma
   f. Phaeochromocytoma
   g. Glioblastoma

7. For which three of the following drugs is neurological toxicity a major concern?
   a. Cyclophosphamide
   b. Carboplatin
   c. Paclitaxel
   d. Irinotecan
   e. Cisplatin
   f. Ifosphamide

8. For which of the following drugs must renal function be measured before administration?
   a. Vincristine
   b. Adriamycin
   c. Carboplatin
   d. Etoposide
   e. Epirubicin

9. Which of the following drugs are used for anti-androgen activity?
   a. Fluoxetine
   b. Tamoxifen
   c. Exemestane
   d. Bicalutamide
   e. Cyclophosphamide

10. Which three of the following are monoclonal antibodies used in cancer treatment?
    a. Rituximab
    b. Bortezomib
    c. Herceptin
    d. Lapatinib
    e. Erythropoietin
    f. Combretastatin
    g. Bevacizumab

7   LUNG CANCER AND MESOTHELIOMA

■ Lung cancer   67   ■ Further reading   87
■ Mesothelioma   84   ■ Self-assessment questions   88

LUNG CANCER

Epidemiology

Each year in the UK there are 38 000 cases of lung cancer, 22 000 cases in men and 16 000 cases in women, making it the second commonest form of cancer, accounting for 14 per cent of all cancer cases and leading to a total of 34 000 deaths per annum. It is the prime cause of cancer mortality in Europe with a peak incidence at 60–70 years. It is three times more common in men, in whom it is the most common cancer. The mortality is declining in men, but increasing in women owing to changes in smoking habits in recent decades.

Aetiology

The majority of cases of lung cancer can be attributed to exposure of the bronchial epithelium to inhaled carcinogens. There is a strong causal relationship between smoking and lung cancer, with 90 per cent of cases attributable to the use of tobacco in males and 80 per cent in females. The bronchial tree and alveoli are directly exposed to the inhaled smoke and it is the hydrocarbon carcinogens such as benzpyrene liberated by the combustion of tar that are responsible, rather than nicotine. These lead to metaplasia of the bronchial epithelium from a columnar pattern to a squamous one, eventually leading to dysplasia and carcinoma. The risk of developing lung cancer is related to the duration and intensity of smoking, increasing with the rise in number of cigarettes or weight of tobacco smoked per day, increasing tar content, shorter cigarette stubs and use of non-filter brands. The tumours tend to be found adjacent to the larger airways of the lung comprising mainly squamous cell carcinoma and small cell lung cancer. Evidence suggests that passive smoking leads to an increased risk if a partner smokes 20 cigarettes per day or more. The lung cancer risk declines towards that of non-smokers after 10–20 years of abstinence, although there is a persistent risk in those who have smoked more than 20 per day. Particulate air pollution in cities is weakly associated with lung cancer.

It is important to elicit a history of occupational asbestos exposure in patients with lung cancer as they may be eligible for industrial injuries compensation. The carcinogenic potential of asbestos is synergistic with that of tobacco smoking and, of the many types of asbestos, the blue variant is the most powerful carcinogen. Asbestos-induced cancers are more common in the lower lobes, usually squamous carcinomas, and may be multicentric.

During the nineteenth century, cobalt miners in Eastern Europe were noted to have a very high mortality from lung cancer owing to high levels of radon gas released from the granite-bearing rocks by the radioactive decay of naturally occurring uranium, which in turn led to high doses of radiation to the bronchial tree and eventual malignant transformation. There is evidence that the level of radon in dwellings may account for a small proportion of deaths from lung cancer each year, particularly for non-smokers, and an increased incidence of lung cancer has also been noted in patients who have had previous spinal irradiation for ankylosing spondylitis.

Nickel, arsenic and chromates have all been implicated as causes of lung cancer. Tuberculous scars, subpleural blebs/bullae or the site of a previous pulmonary embolus may occasionally account for peripheral carcinomas, particularly adenocarcinoma. Cytogenetic studies have shown loss of a tumour-suppressor gene on part of the short arm of chromosome 3 in some cases of small cell lung cancer.

Pathology

Macroscopically, lung cancers arise within the bronchial epithelium and therefore usually have an endobronchial component. They may be multifocal and may arise anywhere in the bronchial tree, although squamous and small cell carcinomas often arise centrally in the larger airways, while adenocarcinomas usually arise peripherally, particularly at the apices. Central necrosis leads to cavitation in the larger tumours. Microscopically, lung cancers may be divided into two groups:

- small cell carcinoma (SCLC) – 25 per cent
- non small cell lung cancer (NSCLC):
    - squamous cell carcinoma – 50 per cent
    - adenocarcinoma – 15 per cent
    - large cell anaplastic carcinoma – 10 per cent

Squamous cell carcinoma may be preceded by the stepwise progression from squamous metaplasia to dysplasia followed by carcinoma in situ and frankly invasive cancer. The tumour cells have the morphology of squamous epithelial cells, stain for keratin, and intercellular bridges are visible under the electron microscope, these features being more evident in well-differentiated tumours.

Small cell carcinoma arises from the Kulchitsky cells of the basal layer of the bronchial epithelium and is characterized histologically by small, uniform cells containing neurosecretory granules, and staining for neurone-specific enolase (NSE), reflecting their origin from cells derived from the neural crest of the fetus. The ectopic production of peptides and hormones will be reflected in their immunocytochemical staining. There are several subtypes, the best known of which is the oat cell carcinoma, which is composed of sheets of fusiform cells.

Adenocarcinoma cells stain for mucin, reflecting their glandular origin, and may be arranged in an acinar pattern. Large cell anaplastic carcinoma is poorly differentiated and cannot be recognized under the light microscope as belonging to any of the other subgroups. Clear cell and giant cell tumours are included in this group.

Natural history

The pattern of growth of a lung cancer is related to the histological subtype. The anaplastic carcinomas are the most rapid growing, while adenocarcinomas grow slowly and may be seen to have been present over several years prior to diagnosis. SCLC has a propensity to early and widespread metastatic dissemination with 80–90 per cent having spread beyond the thorax by the time of diagnosis.

Lung cancer spreads circumferentially and longitudinally along the bronchus of origin, eventually leading to bronchial occlusion, which causes lobar or segmental pulmonary collapse owing to resorption of air distal to the tumour. Stasis of pulmonary secretions in turn leads to secondary infection manifesting as pneumonia and occasionally lung abscess and empyema. Proximally the tumour may extend to the carina and trachea while distally it may reach the

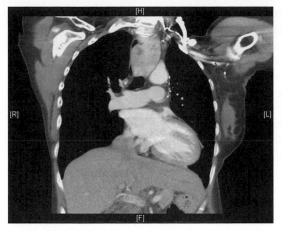

Figure 7.1 Mediastinal lymphadenopathy. Coronal CT image of the thorax. There is a large central mass of lymph nodes.

visceral pleura from where it may invade the chest wall, interlobar fissures or pleural space, resulting in a blood-stained exudative pleural effusion. A pneumothorax may result from a tumour that breaches the visceral pleura and allows a direct connection between the pleural space and the bronchial tree, i.e. a bronchopleural fistula. Mediastinal structures such as the oesophagus, pericardium, heart and great vessels, and occasionally the vertebral bodies and diaphragm, may be invaded. The tumour frequently involves the regional lymphatics, spreading to ipsilateral peribronchial and hilar nodes, followed by subcarinal, contralateral hilar, paratracheal and supraclavicular nodes (Fig. 7.1). Lung cancer has a propensity to disseminate widely via the bloodstream and virtually any site can be involved. There is an unusual and unexplained involvement of the adrenal glands in a high proportion of cases. Other common sites include the liver, skeleton, brain (especially SCLC), skin and contralateral lung (Fig. 7.2).

Symptoms

A small proportion of patients will present with no symptoms, having been diagnosed on a chest X-ray either as part of a routine screen or as part of the investigation of another disease. Most, however, present owing to intrathoracic symptoms:

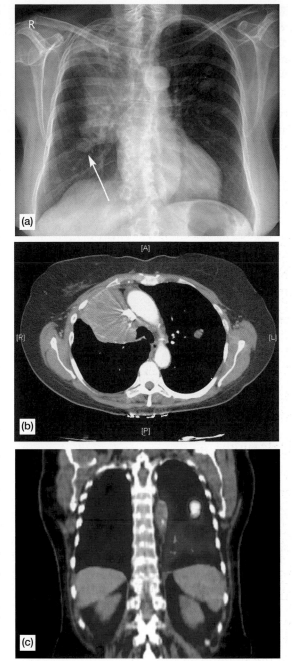

Figure 7.2 Transpulmonary spread of lung cancer. (a) Chest radiograph demonstrating a large carcinoma arising in the right upper lobe. There is a smaller mass in the right lower lobe (arrowed) representing an ipsilateral lung metastasis. (b) Corresponding CT image – note the occult metastasis in the contralateral lung. (c) Coronal PET image of thorax showing the primary tumour in the left mid-zone, and four small adjacent areas of glucose uptake consistent with intrapulmonary spread.

- cough
- haemoptysis
- dyspnoea
- chest pain
- recurrent chest infections.

Cough is due to bronchial irritation by the tumour and is often unproductive unless associated with secondary infection. Bronchoalveolar tumours (see Rare tumours section below) characteristically result in the expectoration of large quantities of mucoid sputum. The cough will have a 'bovine' character if there is also a vocal cord palsy.

Haemoptysis varies in severity from slight streaking of the sputum with blood to frank haemorrhage where there is a large intra-bronchial component to the tumour with mucosal ulceration. It is a common presenting symptom. Massive intrapulmonary haemorrhage may occasionally lead to the death of the patient.

Dyspnoea reflects a deficiency in pulmonary ventilation owing to a restrictive defect (e.g. pleural effusion, diffuse parenchymal infiltration), obstructive defect (e.g. bronchial obstruction by tumour or secondary infection) or a combination of the two. It will first be noticed on mild exertion, progressing to dyspnoea at rest. It usually indicates locally advanced disease.

Chest pain may be pleuritic or aching in nature and localized to the involved hemithorax, reflecting pleural involvement by tumour, secondary infection of the pleura or direct invasion of the chest wall.

Recurrent chest infections are a common presenting feature and carcinoma of the lung should be considered in anyone of the appropriate age who has had recurrent chest infections for no apparent cause or an infection that has failed to resolve following one or more courses of the appropriate antibiotic.

Dysphagia may result from extrinsic compression from the primary tumour, particularly if the tumour is arising from the left main bronchus as the oesophagus is a close anatomical relation posteriorly. A large mass of *involved lymph nodes* (usually subcarinal) should also be considered as a cause. A *hoarse voice* suggests invasion of the recurrent laryngeal nerve, giving rise to a vocal cord paralysis, which in turn results in a hoarse voice and 'bovine' cough owing to failure to adduct the vocal cords. Indirect laryngoscopy in the clinic or visualization of the cords at bronchoscopy will be diagnostic.

Tumours arising at the lung apex may cause nerve root pain as they lead to direct invasion of the T1 nerve root, leading to pain radiating down the ipsilateral arm to the medial aspect of the forearm, and may lead to infiltration of the spinal cord itself. Non-specific extrathoracic symptoms include anorexia, weight loss, malaise and lethargy.

Signs

No physical signs at all may be elicited, particularly in those presenting without symptoms after a routine chest X-ray. Pulmonary collapse and/or consolidation is the most frequent finding. Examination of the hands frequently reveals clubbing, characterized by an increase in nail convexity in the transverse and longitudinal planes, loss of the nail fold angle and sponginess of the nail bed on compression of the nail (Fig. 7.3). There may be nicotine staining of the fingers. The supraclavicular lymph nodes should be checked as these are the only palpable nodes that are in continuity with the regional lymphatics. The syndrome of superior vena cava

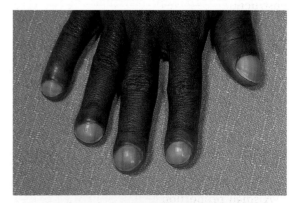

Figure 7.3 Clubbing of the fingers. This is a common non-metastatic manifestation of squamous carcinoma . There are many non-malignant causes, e.g. chronic pulmonary and cardiac disease.

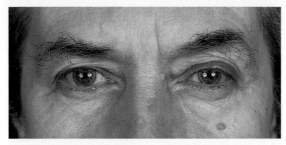

Figure 7.4 Horner's syndrome affecting the left eye. There is a partial ptosis, enophthalmos and miosis of the pupil.

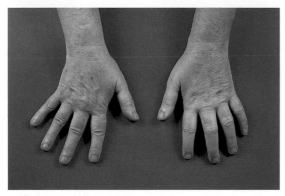

Figure 7.5 The hands of the patient in Figure 7.4. Note the clawing of the left hand owing to a T1 nerve root lesion. This has weakened the extensor muscles of the fingers leading to unopposed action of the muscles, which causes finger flexion.

obstruction deserves special mention (see Chapter 22). Involvement of the cervical sympathetic nerves at the level of T1 leads to Horner's syndrome (Fig. 7.4) characterized by partial ptosis, miosis (pupillary constriction), enophthalmos (indrawing of the globe of the eye relative to the orbit) and anhydrosis (loss of sweating on the ipsilateral side of the face). The ipsilateral hand may be warmer owing to vasodilation, and there will be wasting of the small muscles of the hand as these are partly innervated by the T1 nerve root (Fig. 7.5).

A small proportion will present with one or more of a variety of clinical syndromes which are unassociated with metastases. These are the so called non-metastatic manifestations of malignancy (Table 7.1). Other signs will

TABLE 7.1 Non-metastatic manifestations of lung cancer

Type	Manifestions
Cutaneous	Dermatomyositis
	Acanthosis nigricans
	Erythema gyratum ripens
	Hypertrichosis languinosa
	Clubbing
	Hypertrophic pulmonary osteoarthropathy (HPOA)
	Scleroderma
	Herpes zoster
	Urticaria
Neuromuscular	Myositis
	Proximal myopathy
	Peripheral neuropathy
	Mononeuritis multiplex
	Cortical degeneration
	Progressive multifocal leukoencephalopathy
	Transverse myelitis
	Cerebellar degeneration
	Eaton–Lambert myasthenic syndrome
Ectopic hormone production	Hyponatraemia and water retention (ADH)
	Hyperpigmentation and hypokalaemic alkalosis (ACTH)
	Hypercalcaemia (PTH)
	Carcinoid (5-HT)
	Hypoglycaemia (insulin-like peptides)
	Hyperglycaemia (glucagon, growth hormone)
	Gynaecomastia and testicular atrophy (gonadotrophins, HCG)
	Hypertension (renin)
Haematological	Anaemia (may be sideroblastic)
	Disseminated intravascular coagulation
	Eosinophilia
	Thrombocytosis
	Thrombocytopenia
	Leucocytosis/leukaemoid picture
	Red cell aplasia
	Bone marrow plasmacytosis
Miscellaneous	Murantic endocarditis (may lead to systemic emboli)
	Membranous glomerulonephritis
	Hypouricaemia
	Hyperamylasaemia
	Migratory thrombophlebitis (Trousseau's syndrome)

depend on the tumour burden and sites of spread.

Differential diagnosis

This includes:

- benign tumours – papilloma, hamartoma, carcinoid, fibroma, leiomyoma
- other malignant primary tumours – mesothelioma, bronchial gland carcinomas, soft tissue sarcomas
- metastases
- non-neoplastic diseases, e.g. aspergilloma, chronic lung abscess, Wegener's granulomatosis
- radiographic artefact, e.g. nipple shadow.

Investigations

Chest X-ray

This has the advantage of providing a relatively rapid, non-invasive, widely available means of ascertaining the position, size and number of tumours. For optimal assessment, a postero-anterior and lateral view should always be requested. Common features of lung cancer include a discrete opacity (Fig. 7.6), which may be cavitating, hilar lymphadenopathy, pulmonary collapse, consolidation and pleural effusion. Associated intrathoracic complications owing to local invasion can be assessed, special care being taken to look for rib erosion in peripherally placed tumours. The hemidiaphragms should be inspected, looking for excessive elevation – the right is usually slightly higher than the left owing to the underlying liver. An elevated hemidiaphragm suggests palsy of the ipsilateral phrenic nerve, which in turn suggests mediastinal infiltration and therefore an inoperable tumour.

Sputum cytology

This is a rapid means of obtaining a tissue diagnosis with minimal patient inconvenience and distress, having the advantage of being suitable for outpatients awaiting a definitive investigation such as a bronchoscopy. The sensitivity of the test increases with the number of sputum specimens collected and so at least three speci-

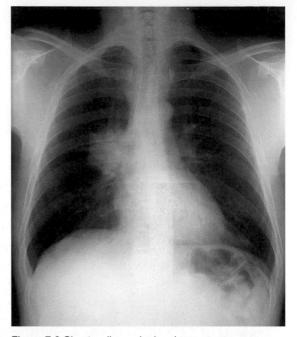

Figure 7.6 Chest radiograph showing a squamous carcinoma arising adjacent to the right hilum. In this example, there is no associated pulmonary collapse, suggesting patency of the bronchi.

mens are desirable. Samples should represent bronchial secretions rather than saliva and the best time for collection is early in the morning. Prior to collection, 5 mL of nebulized saline and physiotherapy might help a patient who has a non-productive cough. Central tumours are most likely to be detected in this way, particularly those associated with a large endo-bronchial component, e.g. squamous carcinoma. It should be noted that sputum containing squamous carcinoma cells could be related to an underlying primary cancer of the upper respiratory tract e.g. larynx.

Bronchoscopy

This should be performed whenever active treatment is indicated. A fibreoptic broncho-scope is passed down the respiratory tract via the nose under topical anaesthesia, although rigid bronchoscopy under general anaesthesia is sometimes performed by the thoracic surgeon. Detailed anatomical information is gained regarding the precise location of the tumour

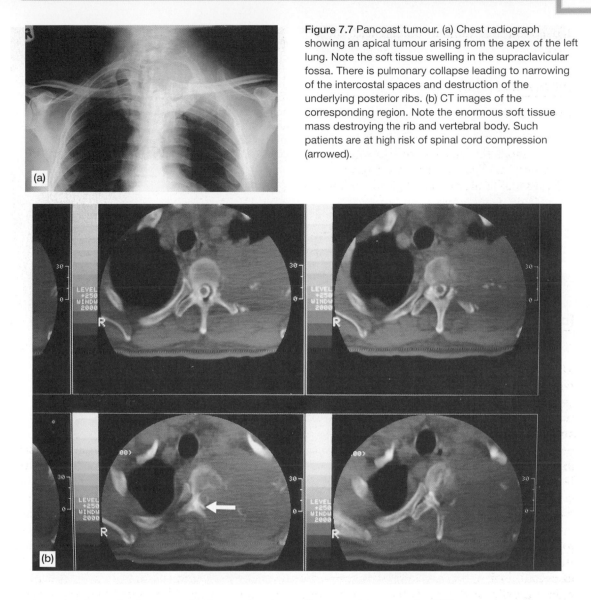

Figure 7.7 Pancoast tumour. (a) Chest radiograph showing an apical tumour arising from the apex of the left lung. Note the soft tissue swelling in the supraclavicular fossa. There is pulmonary collapse leading to narrowing of the intercostal spaces and destruction of the underlying posterior ribs. (b) CT images of the corresponding region. Note the enormous soft tissue mass destroying the rib and vertebral body. Such patients are at high risk of spinal cord compression (arrowed).

within the bronchial tree, which is of value when surgery or radiotherapy is contemplated; vocal cord palsy also may be confirmed on entry into the lower respiratory tract with the scope. Once visualized, the tumour can be biopsied or, if the tumour is located too peripherally for the bronchoscope to reach it, saline can be injected and aspirated, and the 'washings' sent for cytology; a small brush can be used to obtain 'brushings' from the epithelial lining of the bronchi. Bronchoscopy also allows emergency procedures to be performed such as diathermy or laser of a bleeding tumour.

Computed tomography (CT)

CT is indicated in all cases. It is the investigation of choice for detecting chest wall invasion, particularly in the case of apical tumours, which may not be well visualized with plain radiographs (Fig. 7.7), and for detecting mediastinal lymphadenopathy, both of which individually are contraindications to surgical resection. The thorax is scanned to supplement the findings on plain X-rays and bronchoscopy, as the superior soft tissue contrast of CT more precisely defines the local extent of the tumour and distinguishes

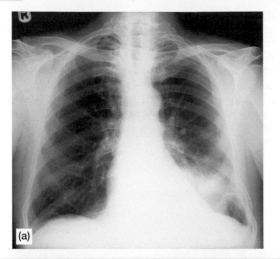

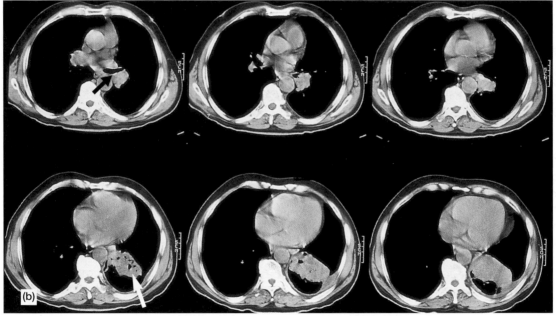

Figure 7.8 Locally advanced lung cancer. (a) Chest radiograph in a patient with a carcinoma causing obstruction of the left lower lobe bronchus leading to collapse and consolidation distally. (b) CT images of the thorax from the same patient demonstrating the primary tumour near the left hilum (top left arrow). The collapse and consolidation can be seen distal to this (bottom left arrow). There is also a left basal pleural effusion. These images demonstrate the greater detail seen with CT compared with plain radiographs.

tumour from collapsed/consolidated lung tissue (Fig. 7.8). The brain, liver and adrenals (Fig. 7.9) are included to exclude distant metastases as they are frequent sites of soft tissue spread. A limited CT scan can also be used to facilitate percutaneous needle biopsy in those patients in whom a tissue diagnosis cannot be obtained by less invasive means.

Magnetic resonance imaging (MRI)

MRI can be used in staging prior to surgery, providing images that are complementary to those obtained by CT. It is of particular value in pro-viding high resolution images of soft tissues, which may clarify the extent of local tumour invasion, e.g. when CT has suggested equivocal large blood vessel infiltration.

Isotope bone scan

This is performed to exclude bone metastases in those who are being considered for curative therapy.

Positron emission tomography (PET)

This is now routinely performed to complete whole body staging prior to curative surgery. It

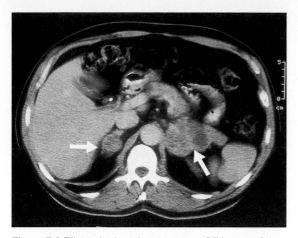

Figure 7.9 Bilateral adrenal metastases. CT image of the upper abdomen.

has the advantage of disclosing the presence of metastatic disease at occult sites in the body (e.g. adrenal glands) and can show foci of active cancer in mediastinal lymph nodes or indeterminate pulmonary nodules, areas where CT can be equivocal or negative.

Biopsy/aspiration of palpable metastases

Biopsy or fine needle aspiration of palpable metastatic deposits, such as a supraclavicular lymph node or a cutaneous nodule, is a relatively atraumatic means of obtaining a tissue diagnosis.

Mediastinotomy and/or mediastinoscopy

These are invasive surgical investigations to determine whether the tumour is operable by allowing the surgeon to visualize and sample the mediastinal lymph nodes. Such procedures have been superseded by the CT scan.

Thoracotomy

This is the most invasive means of obtaining tumour tissue for histopathology, and is reserved for the very small proportion of patients who are not diagnosed after routine investigations. Unless the tumour has been shown to be inoperable during preoperative assessment, the surgeon will aim to proceed to radical resection after frozen section has been performed, particularly for non-small cell lung cancer.

Lung function tests

These are performed to assess the patient's ventilatory capacity with regard to the compliance of the lungs and degree of airway obstruction, and are required only prior to definitive lung resection as a guide to how disabled the patient would be postoperatively. A simpler guide is the patient's exercise tolerance – inability to climb a flight of stairs without stopping would be considered a contraindication to surgery.

Indirect laryngoscopy

This is indicated if the patient has an unexplained vocal abnormality and entails visualization of the position and mobility of the two vocal cords using a laryngeal mirror in the ENT clinic. Partial or complete palsy suggests pressure on the recurrent laryngeal nerve.

Staging

The TNM staging is the most frequently used and can be used as a guide to management and prognosis:

- TX – Primary tumour cannot be assessed, or tumour proven, by the presence of malignant cells in sputum or bronchial washings, but not visualized by imaging or bronchoscopy
- T0 – No evidence of primary tumour
- Tis – Carcinoma in situ
- T1 – A tumour that is 3 cm or less in greatest dimension, surrounded by lung or visceral pleura, and without bronchoscopic evidence of invasion more proximal than the lobar bronchus (i.e. not in the main bronchus)
- T2 – A tumour with any of the following features of size or extent:
  - more than 3 cm in greatest dimension
  - involves the main bronchus, 2 cm or more distal to the carina
  - invades the visceral pleura
  - associated with atelectasis or obstructive pneumonitis that extends to the hilar region but does not involve the entire lung
- T3 – A tumour of any size that directly invades any of the following: chest wall

(including superior sulcus tumours), diaphragm, mediastinal pleura, parietal pericardium; or tumour in the main bronchus less than 2 cm distal to the carina but without involvement of the carina; or associated atelectasis or obstructive pneumonitis of the entire lung

- T4 – A tumour of any size that invades any of the following: mediastinum, heart, great vessels, trachea, oesophagus, vertebral body, carina; or separate tumour nodules in the same lobe; or tumour with a malignant pleural effusion
- NX – Regional lymph nodes cannot be assessed
- N0 – No regional lymph node metastasis
- N1 – Metastasis to ipsilateral peribronchial and/or ipsilateral hilar lymph nodes, and intrapulmonary nodes including involvement by direct extension of the primary tumour
- N2 – Metastasis to ipsilateral mediastinal and/or subcarinal lymph node(s)
- N3 – Metastasis to contralateral mediastinal, contralateral hilar, ipsilateral or contralateral scalene, or supraclavicular lymph node(s)
- MX – Distant metastasis cannot be assessed
- M0 – No distant metastasis
- M1 – Distant metastasis present.

AJCC stage groupings, based on TNM, are frequently used in lung cancer:

- Occult – TX, N0, M0
- Stage 0 – Tis, N0, M0
- Stage IA – T1, N0, M0
- Stage IB – T2, N0, M0
- Stage IIA – T1, N1, M0
- Stage IIB – T2, N1, M0 – T3, N0, M0
- Stage IIIA – T1, N2, M0 – T2, N2, M0 – T3, N1, M0 – T3, N2, M0
- Stage IIIB – Any T, N3, M0 – T4 – Any N, M0
- Stage IV – Any T – Any N – M1

With SCLC, a two-category staging system is still used, which correlates well with prognosis and serves as a guide to determining the most appropriate therapy in clinical trials:

- Limited (30 per cent) – extent of tumour as defined by physical examination and radiological investigations is confined to the ipsilateral hemithorax and ipsilateral supraclavicular nodes; most 2-year survivors will be in this group
- Extensive (70 per cent) – defined as disease other than limited stage.

Management

Radical treatment of non-small cell lung carcinoma (NSCLC)

Surgery

Complete surgical excision is desirable and offers the best chance of cure, although only about 25 per cent of patients will be suitable candidates. Surgery will involve either lobectomy or pneumonectomy depending on the site of the tumour, its size and the patient's respiratory reserve. Both procedures have a significant mortality of approximately 5 and 10 per cent, respectively. A more conservative segmental resection could be considered for those with very small tumours or limited respiratory reserve, although the rate of local recurrence is higher than that following lobectomy, especially for larger cancers. Complete mediastinal lymph node dissection seems superior to node sampling when combined with definitive lung resection. Only 25 per cent of those selected for radical resection will be cured because of either occult persistence of local disease or distant metastases at the time of surgery. The survival rate following surgery varies greatly from series to series but is in the region of 20–30 per cent at 5 years, and reflects the selection criteria used by the surgeon to determine which patients undergo surgery and the skill of the surgeon concerned. Table 7.2 outlines the contraindications to surgery.

Radiotherapy

Comparisons of radiotherapy versus surgery have often been confounded by the majority of poor performance status patients being treated with radiotherapy. This is partly because radiotherapy has the advantage of treating tumours

CASE HISTORY: LUNG CANCER 1

A 65-year-old female smoker with no prior history of pulmonary disease presents to her GP during the winter months with a chest infection manifest as cough productive of purulent sputum and mild shortness of breath on exertion. She receives a course of amoxycillin to good effect but remains slightly short of breath, which she attributes to her age. Four weeks later, the cough and sputum return. Once again she responds to a broad spectrum antibiotic but this time the cough persists. She attributes this to her smoking. She then presents 6 weeks later with increasing cough, sputum with some blood streaking, and more significant shortness of breath. Auscultation of the chest is inconclusive. In view of persistent pulmonary symptoms in a smoker, a chest X-ray is arranged and this reveals collapse and consolidation of the right middle lobe. An urgent referral is made to a chest physician. Bronchoscopy is performed and this indicates a polypoid tumour almost completely obstructing the right middle lobe bronchus with some ulceration and bleeding. Biopsies are taken and laser resection used to restore patency to the bronchus and achieve haemostasis. Histology confirms small cell carcinoma.

She is staged with a CT scan of the brain, thorax and abdomen, which shows bulky right hilar lymphadenopathy but no evidence of distant metastatic disease. Following the scan, she complains of headache and lethargy. Serum biochemistry profile indicates a sodium level of 118 mmol/L. Serum osmolarity is low at 230 mosml/L (normal range 275–295) and urine osmolarity inappropriately low at 300 mosm/L (normal range 400–1000). A diagnosis of inappropriate antidiuretic hormone secretion is made and she is commenced on fluid restriction and demeclocycline to good effect.

Once well, she commences systemic chemotherapy with doxorubicin, cyclophosphamide and etoposide. After three cycles, CT scan of the thorax shows re-expansion of the right middle lobe and a dramatic reduction in the size of the hilar lymphadenopathy. After a further three cycles, there is no further measurable disease. The demeclocycline is withdrawn and the fluid restriction successfully relaxed. Her excellent response to induction chemotherapy is therefore consolidated by a course of radiotherapy to the site of the original bronchial tumour and adjacent hilum, given concurrently with a course of prophylactic cranial irradiation.

She remains well until 8 months later when she experiences further cough and dyspnoea. This is now associated with malaise and lethargy, and her performance status is rapidly deteriorating. Chest X-ray confirms recurrent bronchial obstruction and CT scan indicates liver metastases. She declines further chemotherapy. She requires two bronchoscopic laser treatments within a 2-week period. In order to reduce the need for continual bronchoscopies, she is treated with endobronchial brachytherapy as a day-case procedure. This successfully palliates the local symptoms of her disease. She is referred to the community multidisciplinary team affiliated to her local hospice and dies 6 weeks later.

adjacent to or directly involving vital thoracic structures, which cannot be sacrificed at operation. Five-year survivals of 10–30 per cent have been achieved with radiotherapy alone, even higher for T1N0 tumours. Preoperative and postoperative radiotherapy has not produced any significant prolongation of survival and is not routinely practised. Indeed, meta-analysis of the randomized trials of postoperative radiotherapy suggest a 7 per cent 2-year survival disadvantage for this approach, which should therefore be used only within the context of further clinical trials. The greatest advance in recent years has been the development of

TABLE 7.2 Contraindications to radical surgery for lung cancer

Patient parameter	Preoperative investigation
Poor lung function	Routine lung function testing
Phrenic nerve palsy	Diaphragmatic screening
Recurrent laryngeal nerve palsy	Indirect laryngoscopy
Invasion of trachea, aorta, heart, superior vena cava, oesophagus	CT/MRI scan of thorax
Distant metastases	Relevant imaging studies and/or biopsies

CHART – continuous, hyperfractionated, accelerated radiotherapy. This regimen was developed to exploit the radiobiological advantages conferred by rapid completion of treatment and avoidance of breaks in radiotherapy at weekends. This entails treatment three times daily, 7 days a week for 2.5 weeks (54 Gy in 36 fractions). In the pivotal randomized trial of CHART which enrolled over 500 patients with NSCLC, the 2-year survival was 29 per cent for CHART versus 20 per cent for conventional (2 Gy/day) radiotherapy. The acute side-effects were similar apart from a rapid onset of severe dysphagia in the CHART group.

Chemotherapy

Platinum agents are still considered the cornerstone of chemotherapy for NSCLC. Meta-analysis indicates that cisplatin-based chemotherapy leads to small but consistent improvements in overall survival in all patient groups. In early NSCLC, chemotherapy in combination with surgery yields a 13 per cent reduction in the odds of death and 5 per cent absolute survival advantage at 5 years compared with surgery alone. Comparable benefits are seen for the comparison of radiotherapy and chemotherapy versus radiotherapy alone. The optimal sequencing of modalities and schedule of drug administration remains to be determined and is under study in ongoing clinical trials. Chemotherapy is being used increasingly in a preoperative (neoadjuvant) role to try to downstage disease in order to facilitate surgery or high-dose radiotherapy, again with promising results. As with other solid tumours, synchronous chemoradiotherapy (CRT) protocols are in widespread use to maximize locoregional control and to treat occult metastatic disease at distant sites. Meta-analyses of trials of CRT versus radiotherapy alone for locally advanced disease indicate an improvement in local and distant progression-free survival translating into a 7 per cent reduction in the odds of death at 2 years at the expense of short-term increases in oesophagitis and anaemia. Concurrent chemotherapy appears to be superior to sequential chemoradiotherapy.

Radical treatment of small cell lung cancer (SCLC)

Surgery

There is no proven role for radical surgery in the treatment of SCLC.

Radiotherapy

Thoracic radiotherapy is of value in the combined modality treatment of those with limited stage disease. It has also gained wider acceptance in decreasing the risk of intrathoracic recurrence in those who have had induction chemotherapy, and is associated with a 5 per cent absolute 3-year survival advantage.

Of those with controlled local, regional or visceral disease, 60 per cent will sustain an intracerebral relapse within 2 years. This is often the sole site of disease relapse and frequently proves to be a fatal manifestation of their disease. Prophylactic cranial irradiation (PCI) decreases the incidence of cerebral metastases by approximately 50 per cent. Meta-analysis data suggest a 5 per cent absolute 3-year survival advantage for PCI. There is some evidence suggesting the possibility of neuro-psychiatric sequelae from PCI.

Chemotherapy

The propensity for SCLC to disseminate early and its inherent chemosensitivity means that systemic treatment with chemotherapy is the most appropriate initial management for both limited and extensive stages of disease. Median survival for untreated limited SCLC is only 14 weeks, falling to 7 weeks for those with extensive disease. Combination therapy is more efficacious than single-agent chemotherapy. Objective responses in the order of 70–80 per cent have been reported for a variety of schedules, the active drugs being cisplatin/carboplatin, cyclophosphamide, ifosfamide, etoposide, vincristine, doxorubicin and irinotecan. Complete responses of 30–40 per cent can be expected in limited stage disease, and 20–30 per cent for extensive stage disease. There is no benefit in prolonging chemotherapy beyond 6 months in duration. Chemotherapy improves the median survival significantly to 6–12 months in extensive stage disease and 16–24 months in limited stage disease. In recent years, published data have emerged suggesting a benefit for chemotherapy (e.g. etoposide and cisplatin) given concurrently with thoracic radiotherapy for limited stage disease. Chemotherapy drugs do not cross the blood–brain barrier to a substantial degree, hence the need for PCI in complete responders.

Palliative treatment

The priority of treatment is to relieve symptoms for the patient's remaining lifespan with as little inconvenience and discomfort as possible. There is published evidence confirming that immediate chemotherapy confers a survival advantage for patients with metastatic disease versus best supportive care.

Radiotherapy

Radiotherapy is employed for local symptoms from both NSCLC and SCLC when chemotherapy is deemed inappropriate, and is very effective at relieving cough, chest pain and haemoptysis with palliation lasting for much of the patient's remaining lifespan. Dyspnoea can be helped if it is due to bronchial obstruction. Treatment can be delivered using external beam radiotherapy or high-dose rate brachytherapy using an endobronchial catheter placed adjacent to the tumour under bronchoscopic guidance. Large single doses of thoracic radiation are as effective as a more prolonged course, e.g. 10 fractions in 2 weeks, in terms of onset, quality and duration of response, at least for patients in poor general condition. Median survival in such cases is only 6 months, with a 1-year survival of 20 per cent falling to 5 per cent at 2 years. Palliative thoracic irradiation can be repeated if symptoms recur, providing care is taken not to exceed the radiation tolerance dose of the spinal cord.

Chemotherapy

A rather pessimistic aura has pervaded the management of advanced NSCLC for too long. The emergence of new drugs and the resulting combination therapy has led to increased response rates, disease-free survival and overall survival prolongations. Cisplatin/carboplatin remains the standard treatment for NSCLC. In advanced NSCLC, cisplatin-based chemotherapy reduces the risk of death at 1 year by 27 per cent (10 per cent absolute survival advantage, increase in median survival of 6 weeks) compared with best supportive care. Combination chemotherapy yields an approximate doubling in response rates compared with single agents, but is significantly more toxic. In recent years, a number of other agents used alone or in combination with cisplatin have demonstrated activity in NSCLC:

- vinorelbine
- gemcitabine
- paclitaxel/docetaxel
- premetrexed (Alimta®).

Objective responses are often lower than the rate of symptom relief in lung cancer patients. Combinations are associated with higher response rates than single-agent therapy. A randomized trial comparing five cisplatin-containing regimens showed no significant difference in response, duration of response, or survival. Controversy therefore still exists regarding the optimum combination of these drugs.

For SCLC, the drug regimens are similar to those used for primary treatment. It is sound practice to use drug combinations with constituent drugs to which the patient has not previously been exposed.

Biological therapies

Cetuximab (Erbitux®) is a monoclonal antibody. It inhibits the epidermal growth factor receptor (EGFR) which is often overexpressed in NSCLC. Cetuximab is synergistic with cisplatin/carboplatin, vinorelbine and paclitaxel, which are active agents in NSCLC and radiotherapy. The commonest side-effect is an acne-like rash. Its precise role though is yet to be defined, although it remains a promising addition to standard chemotherapy in advanced disease. *K-ras* is involved in signal transduction 'downstream' from EGFR. Testing for mutations of the *K-ras* oncogene can be undertaken on tissue from diagnostic biopsy and this may predict those patients unlikely to respond to cetuximab. Bevacizumab (Avastin®) is an inhibitor of vascular endothelial growth factor (VEGF), which is involved in tumour angiogenesis. When added to chemotherapy, it leads to modest improvements in response rates, time to progression and overall survival.

Tyrosine kinase inhibitors such as gefitinib (Iressa®) and erlotinib (Tarceva®) are orally delivered treatments that inhibit the intracellular pathways involved in cell signalling and may have a role to play in the management of advanced NSCLC, but this is yet to be defined clearly and is the subject of ongoing research.

Other treatment modalities

Endobronchial laser therapy

This is particularly useful for proximal endobronchial tumours in relieving haemoptysis by permitting direct coagulation of the bleeding tumour and in relieving bronchial obstruction by acting as a cutting diathermy. It is frequently used in patients who have already received a maximal dose of radiation to the thorax.

Endobronchial stent insertion

This can provide instantaneous symptomatic relief when a tumour is occluding one of the main bronchi. By the opening up of an obstruced bronchus, the collapsed lung distally can re-expand.

Vocal cord apposition

Teflon injection into the posterior two-thirds of the vocal cord leads to approximation of the vocal cords. It is indicated for recurrent laryngeal nerve palsy when there is persistent aspiration of food and pharyngeal secretions into the bronchial tree, leading to recurrent chest infections or respiratory distress.

Pleuropericardial aspiration

Drainage of pleural and pericardial effusions will rapidly relieve dyspnoea and sometimes any associated chest pain or dry cough. Talc or bleomycin may be instilled into the pleural cavity to obliterate the pleural space (pleurodesis) and thereby prevent further fluid accumulation.

Other medical measures include:

- antibiotics for chest infections
- codeine or methadone linctus as a cough suppressant
- analgesics for chest pain
- treatment of biochemical abnormalities resulting from non-metastatic manifestations.

Tumour-related complications

Complications can be divided into thoracic and extrathoracic. Thoracic complications include:

- pneumonia
- pleural effusion
- lung abscess
- empyema
- pneumothorax
- massive pulmonary or pleural haemorrhage
- atrial fibrillation
- pericardial effusion
- dysphagia
- broncho-oesophageal fistula
- sudden death from rupture of one of the great vessels

- Horner's syndrome
- spinal cord compression (Fig 7.10)
- superior vena cava obstruction (Fig. 7.11).

Extrathoracic complications can be inferred from Table 7.1. Ectopic hormone production is most common with SCLC although squamous carcinomas may produce a parathyroid hormone-like peptide leading to hypercalcaemia or a syndrome of inappropriate antidiuretic hormone secretion (SIADH).

Treatment-related complications

Radiotherapy

Radiation oesophagitis is characterized by a feeling of retrosternal discomfort on swallowing food or fluids, particularly if hot or spicy, and beginning 2 weeks after commencing radiotherapy. Sucralfate and local anaesthetic lozenges may be of symptomatic benefit. Symptoms are rarely severe enough to interfere significantly with the patient's nutrition and usually subside within 2 weeks of finishing radiotherapy. Radiation pneumonitis has an acute phase beginning 6 weeks to 3 months after radiotherapy and is characterized by dry cough, fever, dyspnoea and chest pain. Radiologically there is a diffuse opacification of the lung corresponding to the applied radiation fields, which is often more severe than the symptoms would suggest. Mild cases resolve spontaneously but more severe cases will require treatment with a broad spectrum antibiotic together with prednisolone 20–40 mg daily. Some will progress to a chronic phase characterized by increasing pulmonary fibrosis leading to a restrictive defect and some degree of permanent respiratory compromise. The probability of pneumonitis can be minimized by using a small radiation dose per fraction and treating as small a lung volume as possible. As a consequence of the large doses per fraction used for palliative radiotherapy, some patients surviving long enough can be at risk of developing radiation myelitis.

Surgery

Potential complications include:

- empyema owing to infection within the pleural space

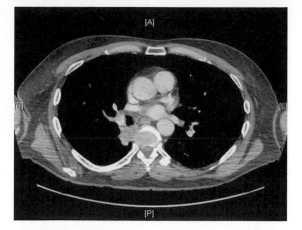

Figure 7.10 Vertebral body erosion from lung cancer. CT image of the thorax. A tumour arising from the right main bronchus has invaded posteriorly causing incipient spinal cord compression.

- decrease in respiratory reserve owing to resection of lung tissue
- persistent bronchopleural fistula
- seeding of the tumour into the thoracotomy scar and subcutaneous tissues; and
- discomfort related to the scar, which may lead to an unremitting neuralgia.

Chemotherapy

Many of the drugs used for SCLC cause alopecia. Radiotherapy can increase the toxicity of drugs such as cyclophosphamide leading to pulmonary fibrosis and Adriamycin leading to heart failure.

Prognosis

The prognosis from lung cancer remains poor and, despite advances in surgery, radiotherapy and chemotherapy, it has not changed for several decades. The three main poor prognostic factors include:

- advanced stage, e.g. large tumour size, extrathoracic disease
- small cell histology
- poor performance status.

Patients with disease not amenable to radical therapy have a median survival of 6 months or

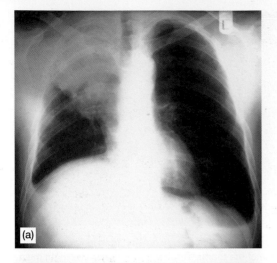

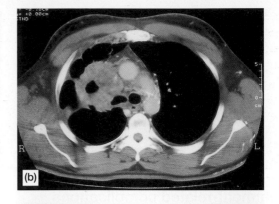

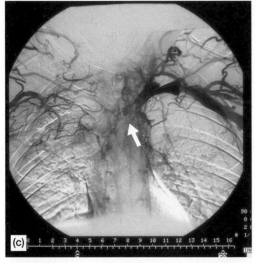

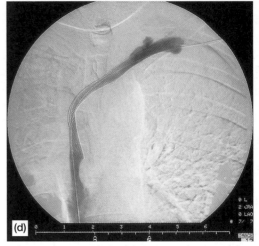

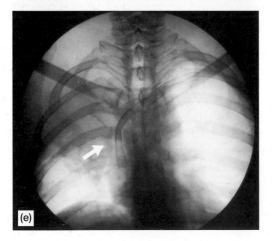

Figure 7.11 Superior vena cava (SVC) obstruction.
(a) Chest radiograph showing collapse of the right upper
lobe. (b) CT image of the same patient showing a soft
tissue mass in the medial segment of the right upper
lobe. It is impinging on the SVC. (c) SVC venogram. The
left brachiocephalic vein is patent. Blood flow is
obstructed at the SVC. (d) Flow in SVC restored. (e) SVC
stent in situ.

less. Only about 5 per cent of SCLC patients survive 5 years. The pretreatment prognostic factors that consistently predict for prolonged survival include good performance status, female gender, and limited stage disease. Patients with involvement of the central nervous system or liver at the time of diagnosis have a significantly worse outcome. Median survival with current treatment of limited stage SCLC is 18–24 months, compared with 6–12 months for those with extensive disease.

Ten to twenty per cent of patients with NSCLC survive 5 years. Stage at presentation is the most important prognostic factor in this disease.

Among surviving smokers, there is a significant risk of second primary cancers of 3–4 per cent per annum, about half of which will be second lung primary cancers.

Screening

Several large prospective screening projects have been completed that have entailed regular chest X-rays or sputum cytology. These have not shown early detection by screening to improve survival in the screened population. Lung cancer survivors can be screened to reflect their risk profile for second malignancies.

Prevention

Lung cancer is predominantly caused by smoking tobacco, implicated in 90 per cent of cases. Better health education, legislation to reduce cigarette advertising and punitive taxes on tobacco may decrease consumption and in turn reduce the incidence significantly. Avoidance of passive smoking in the social and work environment will be of benefit. Ventilation of dwellings in regions where radon gas levels are high and avoidance of industrial carcinogens can also contribute to a reduction in lung cancer incidence, particularly for non-smokers. Reducing particulate air pollution in our cities could also have a small impact. There is currently no evidence to support recommending vitamins such as α-tocopherol, β-carotene or retinol, alone or in combination, to prevent lung cancer.

Rare tumours

Bronchoalveolar carcinoma

This arises more often in women with a peak incidence at 40–50 years. It accounts for 2 or 3 per cent of NSCLC cases. A higher proportion will be non-smokers (one-third) compared with other lung cancer types. It is a pure adenocarcinoma. The cell of origin is the type 2 pneumocyte of the alveoli. It arises peripherally and the expectoration of large quantities of mucus is characteristic. It more frequently remains confined to the lung and may mimic non-malignant conditions such as pneumonia and pneumonitis. Stage for stage it has a better outlook than other forms of NSCLC and may be more responsive to some of the newer biological therapy approaches.

Carcinoid

Bronchial carcinoids are the most common benign tumours, arising in the major bronchi. They are more common in the right lung and usually metabolically inactive but can produce carcinoid syndrome without liver metastases. They occasionally are the site of ectopic ACTH production.

Thymoma

This arises from the adult remnants of the thymus rather than the lung parenchyma; 90 per cent are found in the anterior mediastinum. They are often detected incidentally when the thorax is surveyed by imaging, such as CT, for another purpose. There is a mixture of lymphocytic and epithelial components. Atypical cells or frank malignant change in the latter alters the diagnosis to thymic carcinoma. Thymomas are often slow growing with invasion and expansion at the site of origin. Thymomas are associated with paraneoplastic autoimmune syndromes such as myasthenia gravis (50 per cent), polymyositis, lupus erythematosus, rheumatoid arthritis, thyroiditis, Sjögren's syndrome and autoimmune pure red cell aplasia. Thymic carcinoma is potentially more aggressive with a tendency to metastasize. Both are best treated by surgical thymectomy. Post-thymectomy radiotherapy is reserved for individuals with the more advanced stages of

CASE HISTORY: LUNG CANCER 2

A 44-year-old male smoker presents with two episodes of haemoptysis. A chest X-ray shows a 2 cm rounded density adjacent to the right hilum. Sputum cytology confirms squamous carcinoma. Bronchoscopy indicates a localized mucosal roughening 4 cm distal to the origin of the right main bronchus. CT scan of the brain, thorax and abdomen shows no evidence of distant metastases and a bone scan is clear. A PET scan is also normal apart from a focus of hypermetabolism corresponding to the primary lung tumour. Lung function tests show normal levels of FVC and FEV1. He is referred to a thoracic surgeon. A segmental lobectomy is performed. Pathology indicates a 2.5 cm squamous cell carcinoma. The margins of excision are clear.

Two years later, he presents with a 2-week history of nausea, increasing confusion and polyuria. The corrected serum calcium is measured at 3.85 mmol/L. After a dose of zoledronic acid to correct the calcium, his condition improves. A CT scan confirms metastatic disease in the left adrenal gland and liver. There are no bone metastases on an isotope bone scan suggesting a retrospective diagnosis of inappropriate parathyroid hormone secretion. Rather than electing to be treated with best supportive care, the patient elects to be treated actively. After an EDTA clearance scan to determine the glomerular filtration rate, he receives six cycles of gemcitabine in combination with carboplatin. Prospective imaging confirms disease stabilization. After stopping chemotherapy, he remains on 4-weekly infusions of zoledronic acid; 3 months after stopping chemotherapy, a surveillance CT scan confirms significant hepatic disease progression and bilateral adrenal metastases. He feels very weak to a degree out of context with his disease activity and this precludes further active treatment. A random cortisol analysis suggests a very low value. A diagnosis of adrenal insufficiency is made. He is started on hydrocortisone replacement therapy and regains his strength with a corresponding improvement in performance status. He then starts second-line chemotherapy with single agent vinorelbine. He responds to this by RECIST criteria but develops cerebral metastatic disease. He derives some benefit from whole brain radiotherapy but profound somnolence precludes further active treatment. He is referred to the community palliative care team and dies of progressive disease 3 years after diagnosis.

thymic carcinoma. There is an increased risk of second malignancies.

MESOTHELIOMA

Epidemiology

Each year in the UK there are 2200 cases of mesothelioma, 1800 cases in men and 400 cases in women, accounting for 0.8 per cent of all cancer cases and leading to a total of 2000 deaths per annum. They can arise at any age but are most common in the 50–70-year age group. There is a male predominance (5:1) reflecting occupational exposure to asbestos, e.g. in miners, builders, naval dockyard workers. Only three-quarters of patients actually give a history of asbestos exposure. Case clustering has been described around asbestos mines (e.g. central Turkey, Cyprus, Greece) and in those who used to live near the asbestos processing factories of East London.

Aetiology

Mesothelioma is not caused by smoking. It is now recognized that asbestos exposure is the main risk factor for both pleural and peritoneal mesothelioma. Blue asbestos (crocidolite) is more carcinogenic than white and brown types, and this is due to the size and shape of the asbestos fibres. Not only are asbestos workers at risk, but also their spouses as the fibres are carried on clothing. There is a long latent period (often 30–40 years) between asbestos exposure and development of mesothelioma, and cancer risk is dependent on duration and intensity of fibre exposure. Most patients have no evidence of asbestosis. About half will give a history of occupational exposure to asbestos. Patients with a possible occupational history of asbestos exposure should be identified as they may be eligible for industrial injuries compensation. Such patients should have a post-mortem examination.

Pathology

Mesothelioma arises from mesothelial cells of the pleura, much less commonly the peritoneum, and very occasionally the pericardium or tunica vaginalis around the testicle. Pleural tumours are slightly commoner on the right, probably owing to the greater surface area of pleura at risk. Evidence of pulmonary asbestosis is more common in those with peritoneal mesothelioma, who often have a history of heavy asbestos exposure. Macroscopically, there are multiple, small, pale tumour nodules diffusely involving visceral and parietal layers of the pleura, particularly at the cardiophrenic angle medially. These nodules coalesce to form plaques, which encase the underlying lung and infiltrate into the fissures and intralobular septae. Eventually, the pleural space is obliterated. There may be an associated pleural effusion, usually rich in protein and blood-stained.

Microscopically, the tumours contain varying proportions of epithelial and spindle cell elements (resembling adenocarcinoma and sarcoma, respectively). Approximately two-thirds are epithelial, and one-quarter mixed epithelial/sarcomatous. Asbestos bodies might be found in the underlying lung, and asbestos fibres identified in the tumour by electron microscopy.

Natural history

Mesothelioma relentlessly invades adjacent thoracic structures such as the underlying lung, overlying chest wall, pericardium and contralateral hemithorax. The tumour eventually invades through the diaphragm to involve the peritoneum and abdominal viscera. It also has a propensity to invade the chest wall and skin at the site of a previous thoracocentesis owing to direct implantation of tumour cells. Sarcomatous tumours have a more rapidly progressive natural history compared with epithelial types. Lymphatic spread is uncommon. Symptomatic distant metastases are also uncommon, even during the terminal phase of the disease, but are a greater problem in those with sarcomatous histology and the very few, highly selected patients treated by radical surgery.

Symptoms

Ninety per cent of patients with pleural mesothelioma present with increasing dyspnoea on exertion and/or chest discomfort on the affected side: 70 per cent will have symptoms of less than 6 months in duration at presentation. Dry cough and systemic symptoms, such as anorexia, weight loss and fever, may occur. Haemoptysis is very uncommon, in contrast to lung cancer.

Signs

Finger clubbing and signs of chronic respiratory compromise can occur if there has been prior asbestosis. There is usually reduced expansion, dullness to percussion and reduced breath sounds over the affected region of the chest. This can be difficult to distinguish from a pleural effusion.

Differential diagnosis

Asbestos can also cause a primary lung cancer, which may present with similar symptoms and signs. Other cancers, particularly adenocarcinomas, occasionally demonstrate a pleural pattern of spread and are difficult to distinguish on pleural fluid cytology alone or on analysis of small fragments of pleura.

Investigations

Chest X-ray

This usually shows a lobulated pleural mass with loss of volume of the affected hemithorax and there can be an associated pleural effusion (Fig. 7.12). The changes are commoner in the lower zones and may be bilateral. An underlying asbestosis may be seen. The chest X-ray is best taken after drainage of an effusion, which may obscure the subtle signs of pleural thickening.

Pleural fluid cytology

This can be performed in the outpatient clinic by inserting a hypodermic needle into an inter-costal space under local anaesthetic. The fluid is often heavily blood-stained and high in protein. A high (>50 ng/L) level of hyaluronic acid is common. Cytological examination may reveal malignant mesothelial cells, although the sensi-tivity is not high (approximately 40 per cent).

Pleural biopsy

This is more invasive than obtaining fluid for cytology. It does, however, give a more reliable tissue diagnosis. A needle technique can usually be performed under local anaesthetic. Ultra-sound or CT can be used to obtain better local-ization of pleural plaque for sampling. In difficult cases, an open biopsy at thoracoscopy or thoracotomy is necessary. Surgical biopsy has the advantage of yielding a larger specimen for histological analysis, drainage of pleural fluid and even simultaneous talc pleurodesis.

Ultrasound of thorax

This is a useful investigation for localizing the best place to perform a percutaneous pleural biopsy or aspiration of a loculated pleural effusion.

CT scan of thorax and abdomen

This is much better than plain radiographs for demonstrating pleural plaques (Fig. 7.13) and assessing the degree of local invasion. It can be useful for localizing a suitable site for needle biopsy. It is also useful in excluding gross involvement of the peritoneum.

Staging

There is no formal staging system in widespread clinical use. The modified Butchart staging clas-sification shown below is an example:

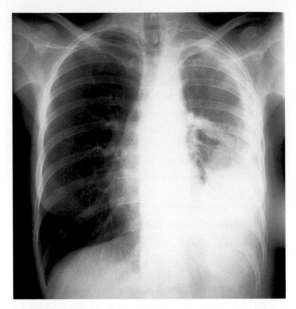

Figure 7.12 Mesothelioma. Chest radiograph showing encasement of the left lung. There is an associated pleural effusion.

- Stage I – disease confined within the cap-sule of the parietal pleura: ipsilateral pleura, lung, pericardium, and diaphragm
- Stage II – all of stage I with positive intrathoracic (N1 or N2) lymph nodes
- Stage III – local extension of disease into the following: chest wall or mediastinum; heart or through the diaphragm, peri-toneum; with or without extrathoracic or contralateral (N3) lymph node involve-ment
- Stage IV – distant metastatic disease.

Treatment

Comparative studies show a survival advantage for active treatment versus observation only. Very few patients are suitable for radical surgical resection. Pleuropneumonectomy (excision of lung, pleura, hemidiaphragm and ipsilateral half of pericardium) followed by high-dose hemitho-racic radiotherapy in selected patients has shown promising results but is yet to be tested in a ran-domized trial. Mortality (20–30 per cent) and morbidity is high. The less radical procedure of pleurectomy (mortality 2 per cent) may palliate

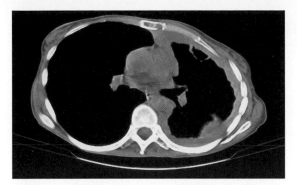

Figure 7.13 Mesothelioma. CT image of the patient in Figure 7.11 after drainage of the pleural effusion. Note the confluent plaque of tumour surrounding the lung.

selected patients with severe, recurrent pleural effusions. Patients can derive much symptomatic relief from simple drainage of a pleural effusion. Radiotherapy is of value in palliating chest pain. Treatment is usually given to the involved hemithorax. Two-thirds of patients will respond symptomatically, although it is difficult to demonstrate any objective tumour response to the moderate doses used. Cisplatin is an active drug in this disease. It can be combined with premetrexed (Alimta®). Vinorebine has also shown promising activity either as a single agent or in combination with cisplatin.

Tumour-related complications

Many patients succumb to respiratory failure from uncontrolled local disease. Pericardial constriction can occur owing to extrinsic tumour pressure, and malignant pericarditis can cause atrial fibrillation. Direct invasion of the myocardium can also compromise cardiac function. Mediastinal compression can lead to dysphagia and superior vena cava obstruction. Seeding of tumour cells along the path of an intercostal needle is common and can lead to subcutaneous and skin nodules. Peritoneal involvement can lead to intestinal obstruction and ascites. Non-metastatic manifestations include hypercoagulability of the blood, autoimmune haemolytic anaemia, phlebitis, hypoglycaemia and the syndrome of inappropriate ADH secretion leading to hyponatraemia.

Treatment-related complications

Pleuropneumonectomy has a mortality of approximately 20 per cent. Treatment of the whole hemithorax with radiotherapy can lead to oesophagitis, nausea owing to irradiation of the stomach and/or liver, and pneumonitis owing to the large volume of lung irradiated.

Prognosis

The disease runs a variable natural history, and therefore prognosis is unpredictable. In retrospective series of pleural mesothelioma patients, important prognostic factors have been found to be stage, age, performance status and histology. Epithelial variants have a better prognosis than sarcomatoid ones. For patients treated with aggressive surgical approaches, factors associated with improved long-term survival include: epithelial histology, negative lymph nodes and negative surgical margins. Prognosis is usually very poor with a mean survival of 9 months, only 30 per cent surviving to 1 year, falling to <5 per cent at 2 years.

Screening/prevention

The dangers of asbestos exposure are now appreciated. Asbestos is used much more sparingly in industry. Care must still be taken when older buildings are renovated, with careful isolation of the working area and use of respirators. High-risk individuals should be offered regular chest radiographs.

FURTHER READING

Baldi A. *Mesothelioma from Bench Side to Clinic*. Novo Science, Hauppauge, New York, 2008

Lorigan P. *Lung Cancer*. Mosby Elsevier, Edinburgh, 2007

O'Byrne K, Rusch V. *Malignant Pleural Mesothelioma*. Oxford University Press, Oxford, 2006

Raez LE, Silva OE. *Lung Cancer*. Saunders, Edinburgh, 2008

Roth JA, Cox JD, Hong WK. *Lung Cancer*. Blackwell, Oxford, 2008

Syringos KN, Nutting CM, Roussos C. *Tumours of the Chest*. Springer, Berlin, 2006

SELF-ASSESSMENT QUESTIONS

1. Which three of the following statements are true about the epidemiology of lung cancer?
   a. It is the second commonest cancer in the UK
   b. It is far less common in women
   c. Might be caused by asbestos exposure
   d. Might be caused by alcohol consumption
   e. Not proven to be caused by smoking tobacco
   f. Associated with a high fat diet
   g. Might be caused by environmental radiation exposure

2. Which one of the following statements is true about the pathology of lung cancer?
   a. Most are adenocarcinomas
   b. Adenocarcinomas tend to be fast growing
   c. Small cell carcinoma rarely spreads outside the lung
   d. Brain metastases are common at presentation
   e. Adrenal metastases are characteristic

3. Which three of the following statements are true about the presentation of lung cancer?
   a. Usually diagnosed on a routine chest X-ray in asymptomatic individuals
   b. Usually presents with symptoms of metastatic disease
   c. Palpable lymph nodes are usually present at diagnosis
   d. Cough is a common symptom
   e. Might present with recurrent chest infections
   f. Haemoptysis is rare
   g. Dyspnoea implies locally advanced disease

4. Which one of the following statements is true about the staging of lung cancer?
   a. Staging is only undertaken in those being considered for surgery
   b. Pulmonary angiography should be performed in all cases
   c. Bone marrow trephines are routinely performed

   d. PET imaging is of value in those being considered for curative surgery
   e. CT imaging is performed in selected cases

5. Which three of the following statements are true about the treatment of lung cancer?
   a. Adriamycin is the most active chemotherapy agent
   b. An attempt at curative surgery will be undertaken in the minority
   c. Small cell lung cancer is best treated with chemotherapy
   d. Radiotherapy is more effective for small cell carcinoma than non-small cell carcinoma
   e. Women have a higher response rate to chemotherapy than men
   f. Trastuzumab is an active agent
   g. Cranial radiotherapy is useful for early stages of small cell lung cancer

6. Which one of the following statements is true about the prognosis of lung cancer?
   a. 10–20 per cent will be cured
   b. Non-small cell lung cancer cannot be cured by radiotherapy
   c. Small cell histology is a poor prognostic factor
   d. The median survival of untreated small cell lung cancer is 12 months
   e. Adenocarcinomas have a particularly poor prognosis

7. Which three of the following statements are true about mesothelioma?
   a. There is an association with asbestos exposure
   b. Most cases are not caused by smoking
   c. Presents with haemoptysis
   d. Most patients will be considered for surgery
   e. Chemotherapy is the mainstay of treatment
   f. Distant metastases are uncommon
   g. Prophylactic cranial radiotherapy may be considered

8 BREAST CANCER

- Epidemiology — 89
- Aetiology — 90
- Pathology — 91
- Natural history — 92
- Symptoms — 95
- Signs — 95
- Differential diagnosis — 96
- Investigations — 97
- Staging — 100
- Treatment — 100
- Prognosis — 113
- Screening — 114
- Prevention — 115
- Further reading — 115
- Self-assessment questions — 116

The breasts are hormonally responsive organs. Their only purpose is to produce milk (lactation) in women. In men, they are vestigial, serving as a remnant of the common embryological development of males and females.

EPIDEMIOLOGY

Each year in the UK there are 45 000 cases of breast cancer, 325 cases arising in men, making it the commonest form of cancer, accounting for 16 per cent of all cancer cases and leading to a total of 12 000 deaths per annum. It is the most common malignancy in females, the average middle-aged woman having approximately a 1 in 10 chance of developing the disease at some point during her lifetime (see Table 8.1). Left sided cancers are slightly more common than right sided ones (relative risk 1.05). The peak age incidence is 50–70 years and only 0.5–1 per cent of cases arise in men. It is a disease of the Western world being much less prevalent in the Far East, particularly Japan. There is an increased incidence in higher socioeconomic groups.

TABLE 8.1 Probability of developing breast cancer according to age and life expectancy*

Age Free of breast cancer	Absolute risk by time interval (%)			
	+10 years	+20 years	+30 years	Lifetime
30 years	0.4	1.9	4.6	13.5 (1 in 7)
40 years	1.5	4.2	7.5	13.2 (1 in 7)
50 years	2.8	6.3	9.7	12.2 (1 in 8)
60 years	3.7	7.4	9.5	10.0 (1 in 10)

* (US population – adapted from SEER data 1997–1999).

AETIOLOGY

The majority of cases are therefore sporadic although hormonal influences are well recognized.

Breast cancer is more common in women with an early menarche or a late menopause. Use of the combined oral contraceptive pill is associated with a relative risk of around 1.25 for around 10 years after its cessation. Hormone replacement therapy (HRT) is also associated with an increased risk of breast cancer:

- 14 in 1000 women aged 50–64 not taking HRT develop breast cancer over 5 years.
- For those taking oestrogen-only HRT for 5 years, an extra 1.5 per 1000 will develop breast cancer.
- For those taking combined (oestrogen/progestogen) HRT for 5 years, an extra 6 per 1000 will develop breast cancer.
- 31 in 1000 women aged 50–79 not taking HRT develop breast cancer over 5 years.
- For those taking oestrogen only HRT for 5 years, no extra cases are observed.
- For those taking combined (oestrogen/progestogen) HRT for 5 years, an extra 4 per 1000 will develop breast cancer.

An artificial menopause (surgical oophorectomy or radiation ovarian ablation) before the age of 35 years, increasing parity, young age (<30 years) at first pregnancy and breastfeeding are protective. Obesity is associated with an increased risk of breast cancer, with weight >82 kg associated with a relative risk of 3 compared with those weighing <59 kg. Regular strenuous exercise is protective. The relative risk for women consuming 4 alcoholic drinks per day compared with non-drinkers is 1.3, increasing according to the amount of alcohol consumed.

Japanese women have a low risk of developing breast cancer. Japanese migrants to the US eventually acquire the risk of the indigenous population, suggesting that there is an unknown environmental cofactor involved.

An increased incidence of breast cancer has been reported in atomic bomb survivors, women treated with radiotherapy for postpartum mastitis, Hodgkin's disease or ankylosing spondylitis, and women who underwent regular chest fluoroscopies to monitor the progress of iatrogenic pneumothorax as treatment for tuberculosis. The carcinogenic effect of radiation on the breast varies inversely with age at the time of exposure and is dependent on radiation dose.

Historically, Bittner demonstrated that a virus transmitted via breast milk in mice led to the development of mammary tumours. A viral cause has not been demonstrated in humans with breast cancer.

Common benign lumps such as fibroadenomata do not progress to carcinoma, but atypical ductal hyperplasia confers an increased risk of breast cancer and such patients should be kept under regular surveillence. Ductal carcinoma in situ (DCIS) and lobular carcinoma in situ (LCIS) are both precursors to invasive malignancy (see below) and therefore their presence in a breast biopsy is a significant risk factor.

Only as few as 5 per cent of cases are due to inheritable genetic abnormalities (e.g. BRCA gene mutations). The relative risk (RR) of breast cancer is significantly increased when first-degree relatives have previously been affected:

- one first-degree relative (RR 2)
- first-degree relative diagnosed at <40 years (RR 3)
- two first-degree relatives (RR 4)
- bilateral breast cancer (RR 4).

Inheritance of mutated BRCA genes confers an 80–90 per cent lifetime risk of breast cancer. The chance of a woman without a history of breast/ovarian cancer carrying such a mutation is 1 in 500 (0.2 per cent), rising to 1 in 50 (2 per cent) if she has a history of breast cancer and 1 in 11 (9 per cent) if this was diagnosed at <40 years of age.

Some familial cases have been found to have a mutated BRCA1 gene located on chromosome 17 (17q12–21). BRCA1 carriers are more likely to develop the uncommon 'medullary' histological subtype of breast cancer and exhibit less in situ disease. Many BRCA1 tumours are derived from the basal epithelial layer of cells of the normal mammary gland, which characteristically exhibit high-grade features, areas of necrosis, are typically oestrogen receptor-negative, HER2-negative, and stain positive for cytokeratins 5/6, 14, or 17, which are markers of basal epithelium. *BRCA1* mutation carriers also have an increased risk of developing early onset carcinoma of the ovary and fallopian tube.

Female and male breast cancer may also be associated with another breast cancer gene – *BRCA2* on chromosome 13. *BRCA2* gene mutations also lead to an increased risk of pancreatic cancer, testicular cancer and early onset prostate cancer.

Two specific *BRCA1* mutations (185delAG and 5382insC) and a *BRCA2* mutation (6174delT) have been reported to be common in families of Ashkenazi Jewish descent. Other genetic abnormalities associated with familial breast cancer include:

- *TP53* mutations in Li–Fraumeni families (associated with leukaemia, gliomas, adrenocortical carcinomas and soft tissue sarcomas)
- *PTEN* mutation in Cowden's disease (macrocephaly, mucocutaneous hamartomas, thyroid disease)
- *STK11* in Peutz–Jeghers' syndrome
- Heterozygotes for the ataxia telangiectasia gene.

PATHOLOGY

Macroscopically, most carcinomas arise in the upper outer quadrant of the breast and are usually solitary, although multifocal tumours can occur in the same or opposite breast. The tumour can be well circumscribed or diffusely infiltrating. The cut surface and texture will vary depending on the tumour type. For example, a scirrhous tumour will have a gritty texture and grey/white cut surface, while a colloid carcinoma will have a more gelatinous texture. Conversely, a diffusely infiltrating lobular cancer might be invisible to the naked eye.

Microscopically, breast cancers are classified as 'lobular', arising in the lobules at the termination of the duct system of the breast, or 'ductal' arising from the extralobular ducts themselves. In situ carcinoma is diagnosed when all the malignant cells are confined to the lumen of the duct or lobule and do not breach the basement membrane. This contrasts with invasive carcinoma where malignant cells breach the basement membrane. The vast majority are ductal carcinomas but there are a number of variants including papillary, scirrhous, colloid, medullary and comedo carcinomas. Oestrogen and progesterone receptors are detectable, usually reaching high levels in well-differentiated tumours.

Variants worthy of special mention include the following.

Ductal carcinoma in situ (DCIS)

This is more common than lobular carcinoma in situ with a peak incidence 5–10 years later; 70–80 per cent are symptomatic with a lump palpable in 60 per cent; 10 per cent present with nipple discharge, usually blood stained. Central necrosis leads to calcium deposition and therefore 50 per cent can be detected by mammography. Two per cent of surgically staged patients have spread to the axilla owing to areas of unrecognized invasive carcinoma, and 40 per cent will progress to invasive carcinoma after biopsy alone.

Lobular carcinoma in situ (LCIS)

This could be an incidental finding in a biopsy performed for benign breast disease or associated with an invasive cancer; 70 per cent of cases arise in premenopausal women and it is frequently bilateral. It is usually undetectable clinically and might not be seen on a mammogram owing to the lack of necrosis (and therefore calcification) in the lesion. It is a marker of a high probability of subsequent invasive cancer. About one-third will develop invasive cancer in the same or contralateral breast within 20 years of diagnosis. The rate of progression to carcinoma after biopsy alone is approximately 1 per cent per annum.

Inflammatory carcinoma

This comprises only 2 per cent of all cases of breast cancers. Clinically there is ill-defined

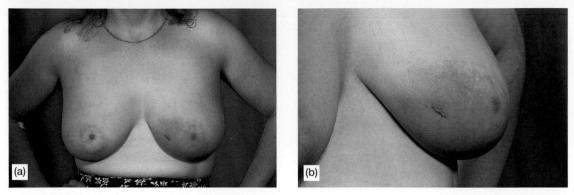

Figure 8.1 (a) Inflammatory breast cancer. (b) Note the small skin biopsy scar. The tissue removed confirmed dermal lymphatic invasion by carcinoma cells. This type of breast cancer can be confused with an infective process, particularly in lactating women.

erythema, tenderness, induration, and oedema (Fig. 8.1). It may be misdiagnosed as a breast abscess. Microscopically there is invasion of dermal lymphatics by tumour cells. It behaves aggressively with a high rate of local recurrence and distant metastases.

Paget's disease of the breast

This is a premalignant condition affecting the nipple and areola and arises in older women. Clinically there is erythema, dryness and fissuring of the nipple, sometimes with exudation of fluid, resembling eczema (Fig. 8.2). Unlike eczema, it is very rarely bilateral; it is confined to the nipple/areola, less itchy and not associated with vesicle formation. It is microscopically characterized by large, pale Paget cells within the epidermis, which do not invade the dermis. All patients have an associated ductal carcinoma. Half have an associated lump, more than 90 per cent of which are invasive carcinomas. If no lump is palpable, 30 per cent will have an underlying invasive carcinoma and 70 per cent ductal carcinoma in situ.

Bilateral breast cancer

This is more common in those with a strong family history of breast cancer and those diagnosed at an early age. Synchronous primaries (i.e. two tumours occurring simultaneously) are rare, occurring in <1 per cent of cases, while a metachronous primary (i.e. diagnosed 6 months or more after the original tumour) has an incidence of 1–2 per cent per year on follow-up. A second primary tumour is suggested by its being of a different histological type and differentiation to the original tumour with surrounding in situ changes.

'Basal' cancers

These are usually ductal carcinomas that are 'triple negative', i.e. hormone (oestrogen/progesterone) receptor- and HER2-negative. In younger women they may suggest an increased probability of an underlying genetic predisposition.

Male breast cancer

This is rare. There is an association with inherited *BRCA2* gene mutations. The tumours are morphologically the same as those seen in women and have a similar natural history. There is a high incidence of oestrogen receptor positivity. The management is largely comparable to that in female breast cancer.

NATURAL HISTORY

The primary tumour enlarges and invades adjacent breast tissue, eventually leading to fixation to the pectoral fascia, serratus anterior muscle

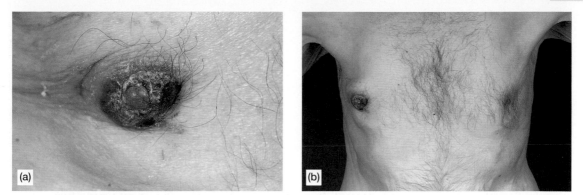

Figure 8.2 (a) Paget's disease of the nipple (male patient). Note the resemblance to eczema. (b) Note the large breast mass in the same patient suggestive of the underlying carcinoma.

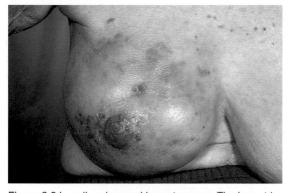

Figure 8.3 Locally advanced breast cancer. The breast is diffusely infiltrated by tumour. Multiple nodules are erupting over the surface of the breast.

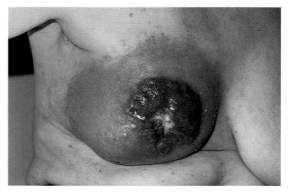

Figure 8.4 Locally advanced breast cancer. There is ulceration of the overlying skin. There are inflammatory changes in the surrounding skin suggesting invasion of the dermal lymphatics.

and ribs. The parietal pleura might be breached in neglected cases leading to transcoelomic spread within the pleural cavity. The dermal lymphatics can be invaded leading to 'peau d'orange' or satellite lesions. The dermis and epidermis can become infiltrated directly leading to nodules (Fig. 8.3), plaques, ulceration or inflammatory changes (Fig. 8.4). In neglected cases, the whole breast can be replaced by tumour with tumour growing externally as an exophytic mass (Figs 8.5 and 8.6). In exceptional cases, the breast can even be consumed by the cancer process (Fig. 8.7).

The likelihood of lymphatic involvement increases with increasing tumour size, decreasing tumour differentiation and lymphatic channel invasion within the primary tumour.

Approximately one-third will have macroscopic or microscopic spread to the axillary nodes at the time of diagnosis. Involvement of the supraclavicular nodes is of particularly poor prognostic significance and is classified as a distant metastasis in the TNM staging. Medial tumours can involve the internal mammary nodes in the parasternal region (Fig. 8.8), particularly if large and if the axillary lymph nodes are involved.

The most common site for distant metastases is the skeleton. Other sites include liver, lung, brain and skin. Bone metastases may be predominantly lytic (Fig. 8.9), sclerotic (Fig. 8.10, page 97) or a mixture of the two types. The disease can remain confined to the skeleton for much of its natural history and the burden of

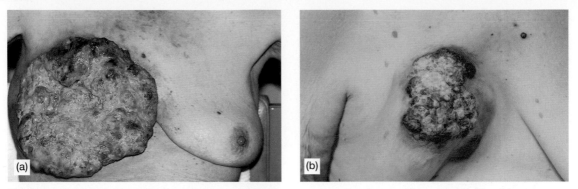

Figure 8.5 Examples of fungating breast cancer. (a) An enormous fungating tumour. This patient suffered from schizophrenia, which contributed to the late presentation. (b) Vascular tumour mass.

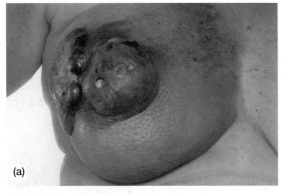

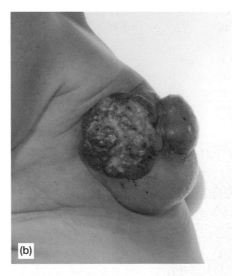

Figure 8.6 Another example of a locally advanced cancer with fungation. (a) Frontal view. Note the florid peau d'orange. (b) Side view.

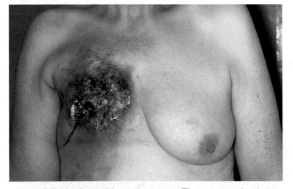

Figure 8.7 Neglected breast cancer. The woman had not undergone mastectomy – the breast has been consumed by the malignant process over years.

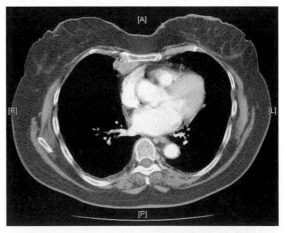

Figure 8.8 Internal mammary lymph node recurrence. CT image of the thorax. There is an expansile mass in the right parasternal region.

skeletal disease considerable (Fig. 8.11, page 98). Some patients present years after their original breast cancer diagnosis with respiratory symptoms from pleural disease (Fig. 8.12, page 98). Breast cancer occasionally spreads to both ovaries, giving rise to 'Krukenberg tumours', a phenomenon also seen in stomach cancer. Lobular cancers have a particular propensity for gastrointestinal and genitourinary involvement.

SYMPTOMS

The majority present with a painless breast lump or distortion of the breast, which might be associated with a blood-stained nipple discharge. Patients detected by screening are likely to be asymptomatic. Less frequently the presentation is with diffuse enlargement or reddening of the breast, and occasionally lymphadenopathy or symptoms from distant metastases.

SIGNS

The lump is usually non-tender, well defined and most likely to be located in the upper outer quadrant, which contains the majority of the breast tissue. Breast discomfort is occasionally a presenting symptom. In advanced cases, the overlying skin can be dimpled or frankly invaded by tumour leading to reddening, induration and nodular irregularity. Fixation to the skin or chest wall will limit mobility of the lump, and this should be sought by the clinician during physical examination. A very large lump will lead to obvious asymmetry of the breasts. There may be enlargement of the ipsilateral axillary lymph nodes, the mobility of which should be assessed as part of the clinical staging, and less frequently enlargement of the supraclavicular lymph nodes. Hepatomegaly could suggest metastatic infiltration while intrathoracic signs of collapse, consolidation or pleural

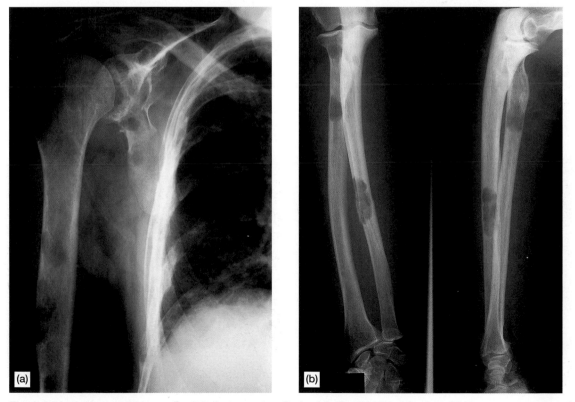

Figure 8.9 Lytic bone metastases. Such lesions are at particular risk of pathological fracture. (a) Humerus, scapula and clavicle. (b) AP and lateral views of forearm. *continued*

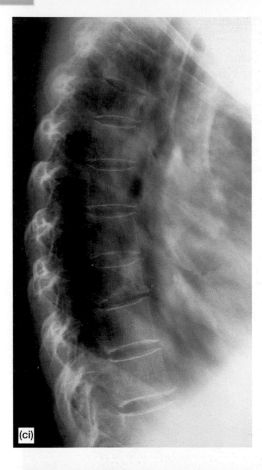

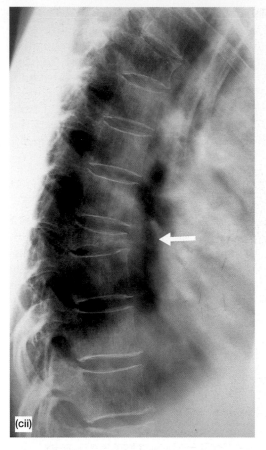

Figure 8.9 (c) i and ii: Vertebrae. Sequential lateral radiographs of the thoracic spine taken nearly 2 months apart showing development of a wedge collapse. (d) Skull.

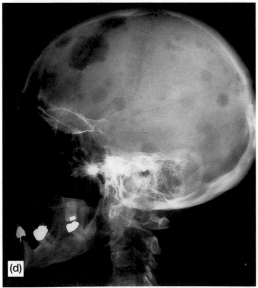

effusion could suggest pulmonary or pleural metastases. Bone metastases are most frequent in the thoracic and lumbar spine and can lead to tenderness when pressure is applied to the affected vertebrae.

DIFFERENTIAL DIAGNOSIS

A number of benign breast lumps are clinically indistinguishable from carcinoma including fibroadenoma, duct papilloma, breast abscess, fat necrosis, haematoma and galactocoele. Many

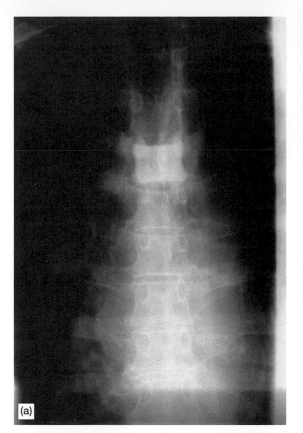

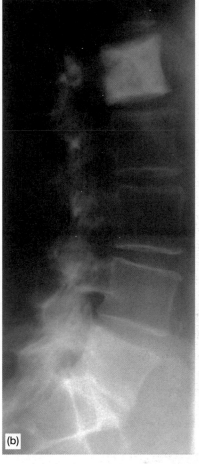

Figure 8.10 (a) Plain radiograph of the thoracic spine showing a sclerotic metastasis from breast cancer. (b) Lateral view of lumbar spine.

such cases will be diagnosed as non-malignant during preoperative investigations. Rarer malignant tumours of the breast may occasionally cause confusion ('rare tumours').

INVESTIGATIONS

'Triple assessment' comprises physical examination, mammography and ultrasonography.

Mammography

This comprises radiographic examination of the breasts using low energy X-rays to allow definition of the soft tissue detail and breast architecture. Two views are taken of each breast, usually in craniocaudal and oblique projections. These may substantiate the clinical diagnosis of carcinoma, detect ductal carcinoma in situ in both the affected and contralateral breast, and localize the tumour, to assist the planning of a biopsy or definitive surgical procedure. Carcinoma is suggested by an irregular mass lesion containing areas of microcalcification, sometimes with distortion of the surrounding breast architecture (Fig. 8.13).

Breast ultrasound

This enables the radiologist to determine whether a lump is solid or cystic, the former being more likely to be malignant, and facilitates fine needle aspiration or needle biopsy of small lumps under direct vision, reducing the risk of a geographical miss and thereby increasing the sensitivity of the procedure. It provides images that are complementary to those obtained by mammography (Fig. 8.14).

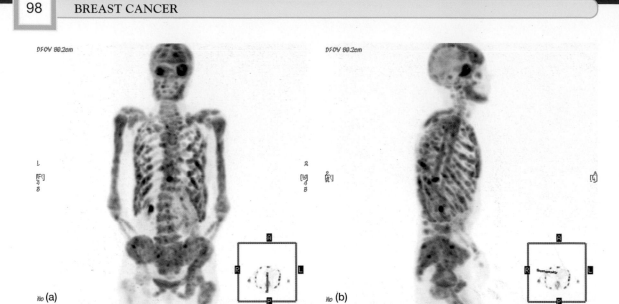

Figure 8.11 Widespread bone metastases. Whole body PET survey. (a) Coronal view. (b) Lateral view.

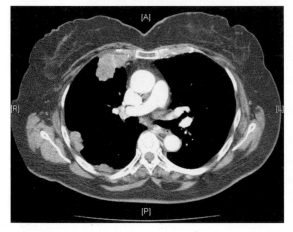

Figure 8.12 Pleural spread. CT image of the thorax. There is nodular involvement of the pleura on the right side.

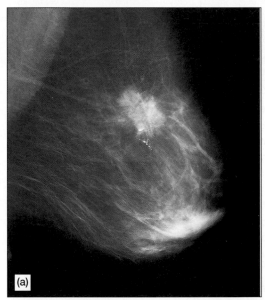

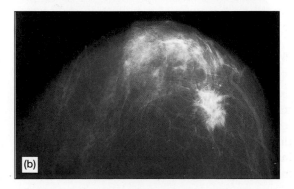

Figure 8.13 Two-view mammogram. There is a spiculate density with flecks of microcalcification typical of carcinoma. (a) Oblique view. (b) Craniocaudal view.

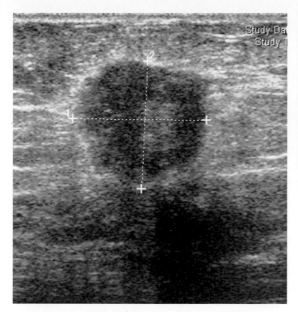

Figure 8.14 Ultrasound image of a breast cancer. The lesion is a sonographically rounded mass with complex echoes within it and a transmission void beyond the main mass.

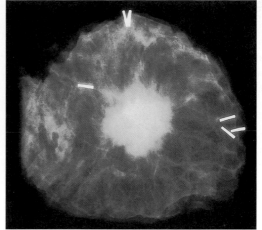

Figure 8.15 Specimen radiograph showing the tumour excised with a good margin of clearance all round. The radio-opaque markers allow the pathologist to orientate the specimen.

Magnetic resonance imaging

This is reserved for the investigation of more difficult cases, e.g. a suspicious lump arising in a breast augmented with a tissue expander or silicon implant, where mammography can be impractical. It is also useful in excluding multifocal disease in mammographically dense breasts and in excluding occult contralateral breast cancer in those with invasive lobular carcinoma.

Fine needle aspiration (FNA) cytology

This is a rapid, safe, relatively non-traumatic procedure which can be performed at an outpatient consultation and can provide a tissue diagnosis within hours. It should be performed whenever a palpable lump or suspicious area of induration is found, and is applicable to the primary tumour, regional lymph nodes or suspicious skin lesions. Small, impalpable lesions might have to be localized by stereotactic mammogram or ultrasound. It cannot, however, distinguish a focus of in situ carcinoma from invasive carcinoma, and does not allow accurate grading of the tumour.

Needle biopsy

This is performed under local anaesthetic and is a little more traumatic than FNA but gives a core(s) of tissue for histological analysis. This may allow a preoperative diagnosis of in situ versus invasive carcinoma, a preliminary grading and determination of hormone receptor status.

Nipple discharge cytology

This is useful in women presenting with a bloody nipple discharge in the absence of a palpable lump.

Excision biopsy

An excision biopsy is mandatory when it is not possible to obtain a tissue diagnosis by FNA or core biopsy. The procedure is usually performed under general anaesthetic and the specimen can be sent for instant frozen section so that, if a more radical operation is deemed necessary, it can be performed immediately. Small, impalpable lesions are first localized with a 'guidewire' under radiological control, which can be used to determine which piece of tissue should be excised. A specimen radiograph (Fig. 8.15) is useful to confirm peroperatively that the area under suspicion has been fully excised.

Exclusion of metastatic disease

The results of these investigations may influence the treatment planned, offer useful prognostic information and provide a valuable baseline assessment, which may be of assistance in the future care of the patient.

- CT scan of the brain, thorax, abdomen and pelvis
- isotope bone scan
- serum CA 15-3 breast cancer tumour marker assay. A very high preoperative level or persistently high level after surgery may suggest distant metastatic disease.

There is, however, little evidence that routinely performing such screening investigations in asymptomatic patients is either clinically useful or cost effective, but they should be performed if there is any clinical suspicion of metastases at these sites and should be considered in high-risk individuals (e.g. T3/T4 cancers, or those with four or more axillary lymph nodes).

STAGING

The TNM staging is the most frequently used and can be used as a guide to management and prognosis:

- T0 – No evidence of primary tumour
- .TX – Primary tumour cannot be assessed
- Tis – Carcinoma in situ
- T1 – 2 cm or less in greatest dimension
  - 1a – 0.5 cm or less in greatest dimension
  - 1b – >0.5 cm but not >1 cm in greatest dimension
  - 1c – >1 cm but not >2 cm in greatest dimension
- T2 – >2 cm but not >5 cm in greatest dimension
- T3 – >5 cm in greatest dimension
- T4 – Tumour of any size with extension to chest wall and/or skin
  - 4a – Invasion of chest wall (ribs, serratus anterior, intercostal muscles)
  - 4b – Oedema/'peau d'orange', ulceration, satellite nodules confined to same breast

- 4c – Both 4a and 4b
- 4d – Inflammatory carcinoma
- N0 – No lymphadenopathy
- N1 – Ipsilateral mobile axillary nodes
- N2 – Ipsilateral axillary nodes fixed to one another or to adjacent structures
- N3 – Ipsilateral internal mammary node metastases
- M1 – Involvement of supraclavicular nodes or distant metastases.

TREATMENT

The aims of treatment are:

- locoregional control with optimal cosmesis
- reduction of risk of developing distant metastatic disease
- minimization of short- and long-term treatment-related morbidity

The treatment of breast cancer for an individual depends on the clinical stage of the disease, menopausal state and performance status of the patient. Ideally, the patient should be assessed in a multidisciplinary breast clinic by both the surgeon and the oncologist prior to any definitive treatment so that the optimum treatment can be instituted at the outset.

Treatment of local disease

Ductal carcinoma in situ (DCIS)

DCIS is curable in the vast majority of patients. However, local treatment must ensure that it is eradicated as there is a high risk of local recurrence, which may be invasive in potential. Traditionally, simple mastectomy was the treatment of choice, and this is still the case for multifocal disease or when clear surgical margins cannot be attained. However, in recent years, the experience of breast conservation for invasive cancers has been extrapolated to DCIS. Whilst small foci of low/intermediate grade DCIS can be treated with excision alone, if adequate margins of clearance are attained, local excision and adjuvant radiotherapy to the breast alone is now standard treatment in many centres for unifocal DCIS that has been completely excised. Tamoxifen may further reduce

CASE HISTORY: BREAST CANCER 1

A 43-year-old premenopausal women presents with a 6 cm diameter lump arising within a small breast with no axillary lymph node enlargement. Mammography and ultrasound are suspicious for carcinoma. Fine needle aspiration confirms malignant cells and a core biopsy indicates a Grade 3 invasive ductal carcinoma, which is hormone receptor negative. Staging investigations indicate no evidence of metastatic disease. The tumour is therefore staged as T3N0M0. The only surgical option is mastectomy. The patient will require chemotherapy after mastectomy so opts to receive it as neoadjuvant (i.e. preoperative) treatment. A radio-opaque marker is inserted under ultrasound guidance to mark the site of the tumour radiologically. After three cycles of chemotherapy using doxorubicin and cyclophosphamide (60 mg/m^2 and 600 mg/m^2 repeated every 21 days), the lump clinically measures 2 cm in diameter. By six cycles, it is almost impalpable clinically but still visible on mammography. A breast-conserving operation is now feasible and she undergoes a wire localized excision of the residual disease and axillary lymph node dissection. Histopathological examination confirms a 1 cm diameter area of residual Grade 2 ductal carcinoma and DCIS, representing tumour that has been downgraded by chemotherapy. Two of 12 axillary lymph nodes sampled are involved. The tumour is confirmed as negative for oestrogen receptors, progesterone receptors and HER-2. Postoperative radiotherapy is delivered to the breast alone. No further adjuvant therapy is given as hormone manipulation will confer no advantage.

The woman remains well for 9 months after completing her treatment but then presents with a persistent aching pain in the right upper quadrant of the abdomen. Examination reveals tenderness and fullness in the right subcostal region. Liver function tests indicate a γ glutaryltransferase (GGT) of 470 U/L (normal <42) and alkaline phosphatase (ALP) of 350 U/L (normal range 38–126). The CA15-3 breast cancer marker is also elevated at 400 U/mL (normal range <50). Preliminary liver ultrasound confirms multiple hypo-echoic lesions suggestive of metastases. CT scan of the thorax/abdomen and isotope bone scan are undertaken as staging investigations. These confirm multiple metastases throughout both lobes of the liver but no disease elsewhere. In view of a relapse occurring within less than 1 year after treatment with an anthracycline, chemotherapy is recommended using a taxane (docetaxel 100 mg/m^2 every 21 days). Three cycles are given with resolution of the woman's presenting symptoms. Repeat examination is normal and CT of the liver shows a partial response. The CA15-3 is 75 U/mL and there has been more than 50 per cent decrease in GGT and ALP. A further three cycles of docetaxel are given with further clinical, biochemical and radiological response. CA15-3 falls to 40 U/mL by the end of chemotherapy and a baseline scan 6 weeks after the last cycle shows a further response compared with the previous one.

Six months later, she presents with increasing dyspnoea on exertion. Clinically, there are no signs of note. Chest X-ray shows bilateral perihilar opacification suggestive of lymphangitis. CT scan confirms military-type metastases throughout both lung fields and a further increase in the number and size of liver metastases. Further chemotherapy is delivered using vinorelbine 25 mg/m^2 on days 1 and 8 of a 21-day cycle. G-CSF growth factor support is necessary because of significant myelotoxicity. An interval scan after three cycles shows no response. It is decided that further active oncological treatment is inappropriate and that symptom control should be the priority. The woman dies approximately 2 years after presentation.

the risk of local recurrence within the breast after breast-conserving treatment if, as is usually the case, the DCIS is oestrogen receptor-positive. Pure DCIS should not spread to regional lymph nodes and therefore no axillary surgery is necessary. Similarly, DCIS has no potential for systemic spread, and therefore there is no role for chemotherapy in the management of DCIS.

Invasive cancer

Surgery

Surgery facilitates total clearance of the primary tumour and pathological examination of the primary tumour and regional lymph nodes. The operation used will depend on the size of the lump, its location within the breast, the size of the breast, the presence of multifocal disease or extensive carcinoma in situ in the surrounding breast tissue, and the surgeon's own practice and prejudices. Options for treating the primary tumour include:

- wide local excision
- simple mastectomy
- modified radical mastectomy
- radical mastectomy (rarely performed these days).

With *lumpectomy/wide local excision*, the tumour is excised with a small (approx. 1 cm) margin of apparently uninvolved surrounding breast tissue. This gives an excellent cosmetic result as it preserves the bulk of the breast and nipple/areola complex, even in women with small breasts. It is unsuitable for very large tumours (>5 cm in maximum dimension), particularly if located centrally, although with successful preoperative chemotherapy it could become a viable proposition. Inflammatory carcinomas are never treated with breast-conserving surgery. Even if the excision margins are clear after microscopic examination of the specimen, there is a risk of local recurrence in the order of 30 per cent without further local treatment.

Simple mastectomy involves complete removal of the involved breast. The pectoral muscles are preserved. The procedure is often combined with a breast reconstruction using either a tissue expander (Becker implant) or latissimus dorsi (LD) muscle transposition flap. If reconstruction is not undertaken, the physical appearance of the chest wall will be far superior to that after a more radical mastectomy.

Modified radical (Patey) mastectomy comprises a simple mastectomy and axillary lymph node dissection. *Radical (Halstead) mastectomy* involves en bloc removal of the breast, pectoralis major and minor muscles, and the axillary contents. It is rarely performed in the current era unless the tumour is directly invading the underlying pectoral muscle to a significant degree.

In recent decades, there has been an increasing trend towards a philosophy of breast conservation attributable to an improvement in the techniques of postoperative radiotherapy and an appreciation of its complementary role in the management of breast cancer. Mastectomy is still the treatment of choice in certain situations:

- when the patient wishes to have the breast removed
- extensive ductal carcinoma in situ
- Paget's disease of the nipple with an occult primary
- multifocal primaries
- inflammatory carcinoma
- treatment of malignant phylloides tumour or sarcoma
- a very large tumour in a small breast, particularly if centrally located
- salvage treatment after failure of conservative therapy
- as a toilet procedure for a fungating tumour.

The psychosexual trauma and disturbance of body image that breast surgery can inflict should be considered. Patients for whom a mastectomy is planned should have the opportunity to see a trained breast care nurse counsellor prior to their surgery so that the implications of the operation can be sympathetically and skilfully discussed. Patients may wish to be fitted with a prosthesis to maintain their chest contour or undergo immediate/subsequent surgical reconstruction of the breast using either a tissue

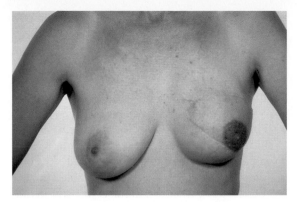

Figure 8.16 Reconstruction of the left breast using a latissimus dorsi (LD) flap. Note the nipple reconstruction.

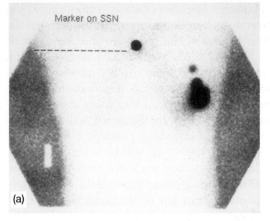

(a)

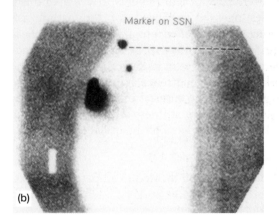

(b)

Figure 8.17 Sentinel lymph node scintigram. Radioactive technetium has been infiltrated around the breast cancer. The sentinel lymph node is shown (the midline spot is a sternal notch reference marker). (a) Front view. (b) Lateral view.

expander or autologous muscle flap transposition (Fig. 8.16). Patients undergoing conservative treatment should also be offered counselling, as studies suggest these patients experience psychological trauma similar to that of mastectomy patients.

The axilla is frequently a site for lymph node metastases, which in many cases cannot be detected clinically. The risk increases with increasing tumour size and grade, and the presence of lymphovascular invasion. The presence of lymph node metastases is a valuable prognostic factor, and correlates with the risk of the patient subsequently developing distant metastases. A surgical procedure to obtain lymph nodes for pathological analysis is therefore important in determining the need for adjuvant systemic therapy. An axillary procedure should be performed in all breast cancer cases as the results will help determine the optimal adjuvant therapy strategy. There are three possible procedures:

- sentinel lymph node mapping
- axillary sampling
- axillary dissection.

Sentinel lymph node mapping is being increasingly used in breast cancer patients. This entails preoperative injection of a vital dye and/or radiolabelled technetium colloid around the tumour. These visual and radioactive markers are then taken up by the regional lymphatic vessels and concentrated initially within the sentinel lymph node(s) (Fig. 8.17). The rationale is that, if this node(s) is removed alone and found histologically not to contain malignant cells, it is highly (>95 per cent) likely that no other regional lymph nodes are involved and therefore no further surgery is necessary. This procedure has the advantage of being a far less traumatic form of lymph node surgery and is therefore associated with a faster recovery and less compromise of the shoulder, arm and hand. Conversely, involvement of the sentinel lymph node(s) suggests that full axillary clearance is necessary.

Axillary sampling entails removal of the lower lymph node group up to the level of the lower border of the pectoralis minor muscle. It has largely been superseded by sentinel lymph node retrieval. At least four nodes should be obtained for histological examination. If these nodes are not involved by cancer, it is unlikely that nodes higher in the axilla will be either. Conversely, if a node is positive, a full axillary lymph node dissection will be necessary.

Axillary dissection is a more extensive surgical procedure comprising removal of the axillary contents at least up to the level of the upper border of the pectoralis minor muscle (level 2) or even axillary vein (level 3). Twenty to thirty nodes may be retrieved for the pathologist, giving more detailed prognostic information. It also has the advantage of being a one-stop thera-peutic manoeuvre in its own right, lessening the risk of axillary recurrence. It has the disadvantage of increasing the surgical morbidity, resulting in local sensory loss, stiffness of the shoulder and a risk of lymphoedema of the ipsilateral arm.

Radiotherapy

Radiotherapy is indicated in all patients treated by breast-conserving surgery. Such an approach produces long-term survival equivalent to that of mastectomy. External beam radiotherapy to the breast alone typically comprises a 5-week course of treatment to the whole breast to reflect the increased risk of recurrence at the site of the original primary but also the possibil-ity of recurrence elsewhere within the breast owing to occult foci of DCIS and LCIS. An extra 'boost' can be delivered specifically to the tumour bed when the margins of excision are narrow or focally involved, and is recom-mended in all women under 50 years of age. Despite data from studies initiated prior to 1975 indicating an excess risk of cardiovascular death for women treated with radiotherapy, this has not been shown to be the case for more recent studies, presumably reflecting more care-ful planning to exclude the myocardium and a lower dose per fraction. Many centres now use CT planning for breast cancer patients as this gives a greater appreciation of the relations of the breast to the other anatomical structures

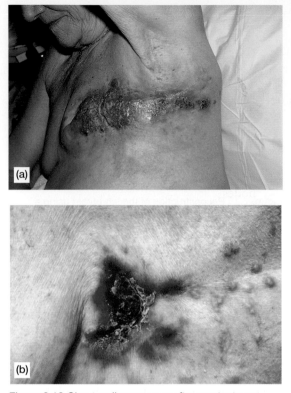

Figure 8.18 Chest wall recurrence after mastectomy. (a) Diffuse infiltrative change. (b) Nodular change with satellite lymphatic spread.

(especially the myocardium for left-sided can-cers), and also for very large breasted women where it allows more sophisticated treatment methods such as modulation of the beams to deliver a more homogeneous dose distribution. External beam partial breast radiotherapy is undergoing comparative evaluation against whole breast irradiation in the hope that the long-term cosmesis will be improved, but not at the expense of long-term local tumour control. Similarly, advances in brachytherapy hardware have led to the development of machines dedi-cated to the delivery of high doses of radiation to a small zone in and around the site of tumour excision. Again, long-term outcomes from this technological advance are uncertain and the subject of ongoing clinical trials.

Simple mastectomy alone is associated with a local recurrence rate of 5–10 per cent.

Radiotherapy reduces the risk of chest wall recurrence (Fig. 8.18) but is used more selectively for those at particularly high risk of chest wall relapse.

The following are recognized risk factors for local recurrence after mastectomy:

- T3 and T4 tumours
- poorly differentiated tumours
- lymphovascular invasion
- involved axillary lymph nodes, particularly in those with four or more involved lymph nodes
- incomplete microscopic excision, usually at the deep margin.

The axilla should not be routinely irradiated after axillary dissection irrespective of node status as there will be a considerable risk of lymphoedema of the arm and stiffness of the shoulder, which in some cases will be incapacitating. External beam radiotherapy may rarely be given to the axilla in those patients who have not undergone axillary surgery and in whom the risk of lymph node involvement is significant:

- primary tumour 20 mm or more
- any poorly differentiated tumour
- evidence of lymphovascular permeation.

The supraclavicular fossa can be irradiated after a significantly positive (four or more involved nodes) axillary node dissection.

Chemotherapy/hormone manipulation as initial treatment for locally advanced disease

Inoperable tumours are initially treated with systemic therapy. Chemotherapy (termed 'neoadjuvant' or 'primary') is the treatment of choice for most women. Those unfit or unsuitable for chemotherapy will be considered for hormone therapy alone providing the tumour has been confirmed as oestrogen receptor positive. Once maximal response to systemic therapy has been attained, the breast can be treated by appropriate surgery and followed by radiotherapy as appropriate. Preoperative systemic therapy has been established as a means of decreasing the mastectomy rate, although it has no significant survival advantage over postoperative chemotherapy.

Adjuvant systemic therapy

Adjuvant systemic therapy complements the role of radiotherapy or surgery to the breast. The former acts upon cancer cells that have already metastasized outside the breast and its regional lymphatics, while the latter reduces the local relapse rate. It is now widely accepted that adjuvant systemic therapy is of proven benefit in reducing the risk of distant relapse owing to metastatic spread, and that this translates into a significant benefit in disease-free and overall survival. Breast cancer is statistically an important cancer accounting for much morbidity and mortality among women, and so only a small increase in these parameters will be worthwhile. There are two main types of adjuvant systemic therapy.

Hormone therapies

Adjuvant hormone therapy can reduce the risk of distant metastatic relapse. Tamoxifen is an antioestrogen, which acts by blocking the action of oestradiol on its receptors. The dose is 20 mg once daily. There is no evidence that a higher dose is any more effective. In women with oestrogen receptor-positive tumours, 5 years of tamoxifen reduces:

- the odds of recurrence by approximately 40 per cent, an absolute reduction of approximately 13 per cent by 15 years of follow-up
- the odds of dying from breast cancer by approximately 30 per cent, an absolute reduction of approximately 9 per cent by 15 years of follow-up.

In the same group of patients, the addition of chemotherapy to tamoxifen produces a further benefit in terms of recurrences and deaths from breast cancer versus tamoxifen alone. These benefits are also independent of age and lymph node status. Tamoxifen also halves the risk of developing a contralateral primary breast cancer over the 5 years it is taken and for up to 5 years afterwards. All patients should be prescribed tamoxifen for 5 years. Uncertainty exists as to whether more than 5 years of tamoxifen confers additional benefits.

The aromatase inhibitors anastrozole and letrozole are at least equally effective. Their integration into the adjuvant setting has been shown to improve disease-free survival. They can be used in several ways:

- as sole endocrine treatment taken for 5 years
- used after 2 years of tamoxifen to complete the 5 years of endocrine blockade
- used for an additional 5 years after 5 years of tamoxifen in high-risk individuals.

Chemotherapy

The criteria used to determine whether a patient should receive adjuvant chemotherapy vary from centre to centre and should be considered flexible rather than rigid. A typical set of criteria are presented, any one of which would be sufficient to recommend chemotherapy as standard treatment:

- Premenopausal women:
  - age <35 years
  - tumour 20 mm or greater in maximum microscopic diameter
  - poorly differentiated (grade 3) tumour of any size
  - axillary lymph node involvement
  - oestrogen receptor negativity
- Postmenopausal women 50–69 years:
  - axillary lymph node involvement
  - poorly differentiated tumours >20 mm
  - oestrogen receptor negativity
- For women <50 years of age, adjuvant chemotherapy has been proven to reduce:
  - the odds of recurrence by approximately 35–40 per cent, an absolute reduction of approximately 11 per cent by 15 years of follow-up
  - the odds of dying (breast cancer and other causes) by approximately 25–30 per cent, an absolute reduction of approximately 5 per cent for node-negative cases and 11 per cent for node-positive cases by 15 years of follow-up
- For women 50–69 years of age, adjuvant chemotherapy has been proven to reduce:
  - the odds of recurrence by approximately 20 per cent, an absolute reduction of

approximately 5 per cent by 15 years of follow-up
  - the odds of dying from breast cancer by approximately 10 per cent, an absolute reduction of approximately 2–4 per cent by 15 years of follow-up.

Adjuvant chemotherapy therefore confers greater benefit to younger patients. Its effect is independent of hormone receptor status. There are comparatively few data available for the use of adjuvant chemotherapy is the >70-year age group. Women of this age group should be considered for chemotherapy only if their cancer is hormonally insensitive and very adverse risk factors are present e.g. four or more involved axillary lymph nodes.

There is still no consensus as to what should be considered as the optimum chemotherapy regime. There is evidence that 6 months of chemotherapy using a combination of at least two drugs is to be preferred. The most tried and tested regimen is 'classical' CMF comprising:

- cyclophosphamide 100 mg/m^2 p.o. day 1 to day 14
- methotrexate 40 mg/m^2 i.v. day 1 and day 8
- 5-fluorouracil 600 mg/m^2 i.v. day 1 and day 8
- repeat cycle 4 weekly for 6 cycles.

CMF has now been superseded, although it is still used after epirubicin in the sequential hybrid regiman E/CMF (see below). The pooled results from randomized trials suggest that an anthracycline (doxorubicin or epirubicin)-containing regimen may yield an extra 4–5 per cent absolute survival advantage after 10 years of follow-up compared with CMF. Anthracycline-containing combinations include AC and FEC.

- AC:
  - Adriamycin (doxorubicin) 60 mg/m^2 i.v. day 1
  - cyclophosphamide 600 mg/m^2 i.v. day 1
  repeat cycle 3 weekly for 4 cycles
- FEC:
  - fluorouracil 600 mg/m^2 i.v. day 1
  - epirubicin 50–100 mg/m^2 i.v. day 1
  - cyclophosphamide 600 mg/m^2 i.v. day 1
  - repeat cycle 3 weekly for 6 cycles.

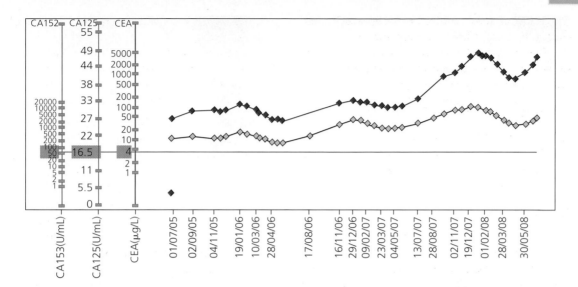

Figure 8.19 Graph of tumour marker measurements versus time (CA153 – green, CEA – red). The rises and falls correspond to clinically apparent relapses and remissions over a period of 3 years.

In high-risk individuals, a hybrid regimen of two different forms of chemotherapy has been shown to be advantageous e.g. E/CMF:

- epirubicin 100 mg/m² i.v. day 1
- repeat cycle 3 weekly for 4 cycles followed by 4 cycles of CMF as above.

Recent studies have also shown superiority for taxanes versus non-taxane drug combinations when used as adjuvant therapy. An example is TAC:

- taxotere 75 mg/m² i.v. day 1
- Adriamycin 50 mg/m² i.v. day 1
- cyclophosphamide 500 mg/m² i.v. day 1
- repeat cycle 3 weekly for 6 cycles.

Immunotherapy

Approximately 15 per cent of women with early breast cancer will have tumours that test positive for human epidermal growth factor receptor 2 (HER2) oncogene overexpression. The monoclonal antibody trastuzumab (Herceptin®) has revolutionized the treatment of breast cancer. Trastuzumab is a humanized murine antibody that specifically targets the HER2-positive cells. Randomized trials in women with early breast cancer have confirmed that, when it is used in combination with chemotherapy, trastuzumab given for 1 year halves recurrence and breast cancer mortality by one-third compared with the same chemotherapy used alone. The only significant toxicity is a small risk of reducing left ventricular ejection fraction of the heart leading to a risk of congestive cardiac failure in susceptible individuals.

Treatment of metastatic disease

The disease is incurable at this stage, and treatment is aimed to palliate symptoms and maintain the patient as active as possible with minimal side-effects and the least inconvenience. As for other solid tumours, active treatment will have a superior outcome to best supportive care. The serum tumour markers (e.g. CA 15-3) are surrogates for the whole body breast cancer activity for a given individual, and can be useful in assessing response to treatment, providing information complementary to that available from imaging (Fig. 8.19).

Surgery

There is no role for breast surgery in the patient with metastatic disease provided a tissue

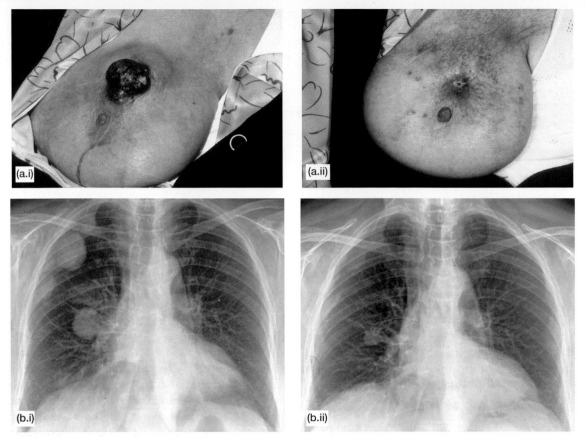

Figure 8.20 Examples of dramatic responses to endocrine therapy alone. (a) i: Locally advanced disease at presentation. (a) ii: After 6 months' endocrine therapy. (b) i: Chest radiograph. Lung metastases at presentation. (b) ii: After 4 months' endocrine therapy.

diagnosis has already been obtained and satisfactory local control of the breast tumour can be achieved by other treatment modalities. Toilet mastectomy is occasionally performed for symptomatic locally uncontrollable disease. Thoracoscopic talc pleurodesis is sometimes of value in the treatment of recurrent malignant pleural effusions, and internal fixation is indicated if fracture of a weight-bearing bone has occurred or is imminent. In highly selected patients who are fit, with a long disease interval and a solitary cerebral metastasis as sole site of disease, craniotomy, excision and postoperative radiotherapy should be considered

Radiotherapy

The natural history of breast cancer dictates that most patients with metastatic breast cancer will have symptomatic bone metastases leading up to the terminal phase of the disease, although some will also be troubled by brain, cutaneous or choroidal metastases. Radiotherapy is the treatment of choice for metastases causing local symptoms.

Hormone therapy

Tamoxifen is the agent of first choice in women who are not taking it as adjuvant therapy. The response rate is greatest in those with high levels of oestrogen receptor, usually those with well-differentiated tumours, and the elderly, with an objective response in 40 per cent of oestrogen receptor-positive tumours and 10 per cent of oestrogen receptor-negative ones (Fig. 8.20). Median duration of response is 10 months. Unless already performed as adjuvant therapy, premenopausal women with metastatic disease should undergo some form of artificial menopause (surgical oophorectomy or regular treatment with a gonadotrophin-releasing hormone analogue).

Other options include:

- an aromatase inhibitor such as anastrozole, letrozole or exemestane. These are only suitable for postmenopausal women. Preliminary data from a large trial comparing tamoxifen with anastrozole have shown anastrozole to be at least as effective as tamoxifen as first-line treatment of metastatic disease but with a lower incidence of side-effects
- a progestogen such as megestrol acetate 80 mg bd or medroxyprogesterone acetate 400 mg bd.

There is good evidence that for postmenopausal women, aromatase inhibitors are superior to progestogens with respect to duration of response and survival. There is emerging evidence of an advantage in their use as first-line agents in the treatment of metastatic disease. Responses to second-line hormone therapy are more likely in those who have responded convincingly to first-line hormone therapy.

Chemotherapy

Chemotherapy is effective against soft tissue metastases but is less effective than radiotherapy for palliating bone metastases. The choice of first-line metastatic regimen will depend on that used for adjuvant therapy (if any). At least six cycles are administered unless chemoresistence is demonstrated by progression during treatment. After six cycles the treatment can be continued for as long as some objective response is obtained, unless toxicity is so severe as to compromise the patient's quality of life and warrant termination of treatment.

- Those patients failing CMF can be treated with an anthracycline regime:
  - doxorubicin 75 mg/m^2 repeated every 21 days
  - epirubicin 90 mg/m^2 repeated every 21 days.

- For anthracycline refractory patients, a taxane should be considered:
  - paclitaxel 175 mg/m^2 repeated every 21 days, or 80 mg/m^2 repeated weekly
  - docetaxel 100 mg/m^2 repeated every 21 days, or 35 mg/m^2 repeated weekly.
- Other options include:
  - vinorelbine 25 mg/m^2 days 1 and 8 of a 21-day cycle
  - capecitabine 2500mg/m^2 divided into two oral doses per day for days 1 to 14 of a 21-day cycle
  - carboplatin (AUC 6) repeated every 21 days
  - methotrexate 35 mg/m^2 and mitozantrone 11 mg/m^2 (MM) repeated every 21 days.

Biological therapies

Approximately 25 per cent of those individuals developing metastatic disease will have tumours that overexpress HER2. In combination with certain cytotoxic agents such as paclitaxel, docetaxel, capecitabine, vinorelbine and carboplatin, trastuzumab increases overall response rates and leads to a significant improvement in median survivals without any significant increase in toxicity. In those who respond to treatment, trastuzumab is continued after chemotherapy until proven disease progression. In certain circumstances, chemotherapy may be deemed inappropriate for a woman with HER2-positive metastatic breast cancer and if so, trastuzumab can be used alone to good effect (Fig. 8.21). Women on long-term trastuzumab are at significantly increased risk of developing brain metastases.

In those patients who have progressed on herceptin, the dual (HER1 and HER2) kinase inhibitor lapatinib (Tyverb®) can be used in combination with capecitabine. These are both orally delivered. Being a relatively small molecule, lapatinib has the advantage over trastuzumab of crossing the blood–brain barrier. Diarrhoea is the prime toxicity of this combination.

Recent trials have indicated that the addition of the vascular endothelial growth factor (VEGF) receptor inhibitor bevacizumab (Avastin®) to weekly paclitaxel increases

CASE HISTORY: BREAST CANCER 2

A 54-year-old postmenopausal women presents with a painless lump in the left breast. Clinical examination, mammography and ultrasonography suggest a malignant tumour approximately 2.5 cm in diameter. She proceeds to core biopsy, which indicates a Grade 2 invasive ductal carcinoma that is oestrogen receptor strongly positive and HER2 positive (3+) on immunohistochemistry. She undergoes wide local excision and sentinel lymph node biopsy. Definitive histology confirms a 3 cm maximum diameter Grade 3 invasive ductal carcinoma. The sentinel lymph node contains a macrometastasis 5 mm in diameter. A level 2 axillary dissection is performed yielding one further involved lymph node out of the 15 removed. She receives three cycles of FEC chemotherapy (fluorouracil 500 mg/m^2, epirubicin 100 mg/m^2, cyclophosphamide 500 mg/m^2 repeated every 21 days) followed by three cycles of docetaxel (100 mg/m^2 repeated every 21 days). This is immediately followed by a 6-week course of radiotherapy to the breast alone using CT planning to avoid the myocardium. After a baseline DEXA scan she starts endocrine therapy with letrozole. During radiotherapy a MUGA cardiac scan confirms a left ventricular ejection fraction of 63%. She receives a loading dose of trastuzumab (8 mg/kg) followed by 17 maintainence doses (6 mg/kg) over a period of 12 months to complete her adjuvant therapy.

She remains well over the next 4 years, having 2-yearly DEXA scans to confirm preservation of bone mineral density. She then presents with increasing pain arising from the mid-thoracic spine. A plain radiograph confirms collapse of the 7th thoracic vertebra. An isotope bone scan confirms isolated uptake in T7. In order to confirm the diagnosis a magnetic resonance scan is performed, which in fact confirms bone metastases at T7 and at other levels in the spine. A vertebroplasty is performed and leads to immediate pain relief. She is commenced on a high potency bisphosphonate and switches over to tamoxifen. Six months later, despite an initial fall in the CA15-3 breast cancer serum marker protein, the CA15-3 begins to rise, doubling over a 3-month period of observation. Repeat staging confirms metastases in both lobes of the liver and progression in the skeleton. She receives six cycles of docetaxel chemotherapy once again in combination with trastuzumab, followed by maintence doses of trastuzumab every 3 weeks. GCSF support is necessary to sustain the neutrophil count to facilitate treatment every 21 days. Despite an initial response, 6 months after stopping docetaxel there is further evidence of progressive disease in the liver. She therefore receives the orally delivered chemotherapy agent capecitabine (2000 mg/m^2/day for 14 out of every 21 days) in combination with the dual kinase inhibitor lapatinib (1250 mg/day continuously). She remains on this for 6 months before a further rise in Ca15-3 indicates disease progression. Despite further treatment with vinorelbine (25 mg/m^2 day 1 and day 8 every 21 days) and carboplatin (AUC 6 every 21 days), she dies from progressive visceral metastatic disease.

response rates and time to progression compared with the same chemotherapy used alone.

Other drugs

High potency modern generation bisphosphonates such as zoledronic acid and ibandronic acid have a role in those with skeletal metastatic disease. Regular administration of such bisphosphonates may reduce:

- risk of bone pain
- risk of hypercalcaemia
- risk of pathological fracture
- need for palliative radiotherapy
- tumour-related complications.

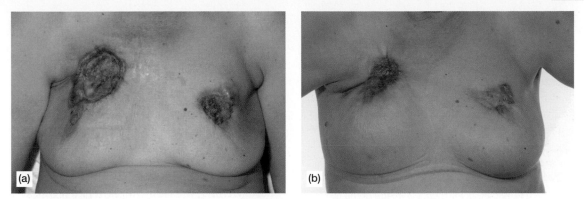

Figure 8.21 Response to single agent trastuzumab (Herceptin®). (a) Locally advanced bilateral breast cancer at presentation. (b) After 6 months' treatment. Both tumours were HER-2 positive.

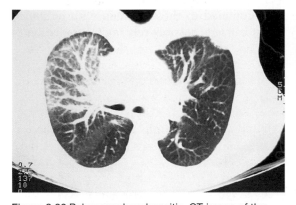

Figure 8.22 Pulmonary lymphangitis. CT image of the thorax. Note the widened lymphatic channels emanating from the hila bilaterally.

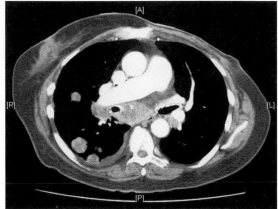

Figure 8.23 Mediastinal lymphadenopathy. CT image of the thorax. There is a mass of bulky lymph nodes compressing the oesophagus posteriorly. Note also the lung metastases and right pleural effusion.

Fungating tumours can become infected causing an offensive discharge or lead to chronic blood loss. Uncontrolled disease in the axilla can lead to brachial plexopathy and/or lymphoedema of the arm. Hypercalcaemia, spinal cord compression and pathological fracture are seen in patients with widespread skeletal metastases (see Chapter 22). Pulmonary spread can lead to nodules, pleural effusion and lymphangitis (Fig. 8.22). Mediastinal lymph node spread can lead to local complications such as superior vena cava obstruction, oesophageal compression or recurrent laryngeal nerve palsy (Fig. 8.23). Occasionally, pericardial invasion will lead to a pericardial effusion, which may in turn lead to cardiac tamponade

(Fig 8.24). Disseminated intravascular coagulation is a rare complication of advanced disease when the tumour burden is high and usually heralds the terminal phase of the disease. Mucin production by the tumour can activate the clotting cascade causing uncontrolled coagulation coupled with a physiological thrombolysis leading to occlusion of both small and large blood vessels. Consumption of clotting factors deranges thrombin time and activated partial thromboplastin time resulting in a bleeding tendency, while platelet consumption leads to

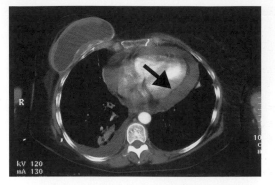

Figure 8.24 Pericardial effusion. CT image of the thorax showing a thick layer of fluid around the myocardium.

thrombocytopenia manifested as epistaxis, petechiae and bruising. Fibrin degradation products are elevated.

Treatment-related complications

Radiotherapy

Breast radiotherapy leads to breast erythema, swelling, skin irritation and tenderness, which settle within 4 to 8 weeks of completing treatment. The skin may temporarily break down in areas subject to friction such as the inframammary fold. Late complications of radiotherapy are uncommon and include chronic breast/chest wall discomfort, breast shrinkage, breast swelling, breast firmness, telangiectasia of the skin, rib fractures, radiation costochondritis and pulmonary fibrosis. Data from randomized trials initiated prior to 1975 have suggested an increased risk of death from cardiovascular disease, confined to those women with left-sided breast cancers, possibly relating to irradiation of

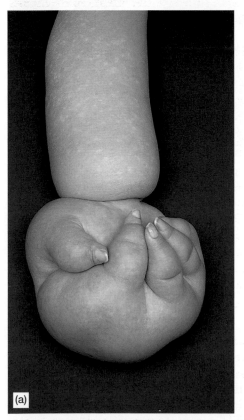

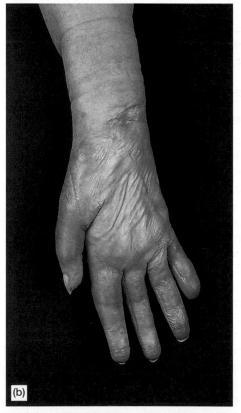

Figure 8.25 Massive lymphoedema of the arm. This woman had a full axillary dissection followed by radiotherapy to the axilla 20 years earlier. The brachial plexus was damaged so there is no motor function in the arm or hand.
(a) Before treatment. (b) After an intensive course of compression bandaging and manual lymphatic drainage. The arm is still non-functional but lighter to carry and less disfiguring.

the coronary arteries rather than the myocardium itself. Axillary irradiation (and surgery) is associated with late morbidity such as lymphoedema of the arm (Fig. 8.25), stiffness of the shoulder, radiation injury to the brachial plexus and radionecrosis of the irradiated skeleton, although with current techniques the incidence is very low.

Chemotherapy

Infertility, as evidenced by amenorrhoea, is a frequent complication of chemotherapy. This will be permanent and associated with menopausal symptoms in many. The age at receiving chemotherapy is the most important factor for predicting the chance of spontaneous recovery of the menstrual cycle. Many studies with long-term follow-up have suggested an increased risk of leukaemia and myelodysplasia in long-term survivors who have received chemotherapy. Anthracyclines such as epirubicin and doxorubicin can cause a reduction in left ventricular function. This is more likely to become manifest in those with severe hypertension or co-existing cardiac conditions, and leads to an increased risk of congestive cardiac failure later in life.

Hormone therapy

Menopausal symptoms, particularly vasomotor symptoms such as hot flushes, are the main problems with endocrine therapies. Vasomotor symptoms are particularly difficult to treat. Many oncologists remain reluctant to prescribe hormone replacement therapy, although there is no direct evidence of it being detrimental. Megestrol acetate at low doses of 40 mg daily is a useful treatment. Some SSRI antidepressants also have activity. Acupuncture is also worthwhile for some patients.

Tamoxifen is associated with a three- to fourfold increase in the risk of thromboembolic phenomena (deep vein thrombosis, pulmonary embolism) and endometrial cancer in postmenopausal women. The aromatase inhibitor drugs (anastrozole, letrozole and exemestane) are associated with a risk of osteoporosis and an assessment of bone mineral density is advisable in those on these as adjuvant treatment. They are also associated with troublesome muscu-loskeletal symptoms such as joint stiffness and sexual dysfunction (vaginal dryness, loss of libido).

Immunotherapy

Trastuzumab can cause allergic reactions at the time of infusion and potentially reversible declines in baseline cardiac contractility. Lapatinib can cause diarrhoea, rashes and pneumonitis. Bevacizumab can cause hypertension, proteinuria and abnormalities in blood clotting.

PROGNOSIS

The prognosis from breast cancer has improved significantly in a stepwise manner decade on decade. Breast cancer is a good example of how cancer outcomes can be substantially improved by adding together a number of small advantages from a variety of treatment improvements over the years. Approximately one in three women diagnosed with breast cancer would die from their disease if no adjuvant therapy were administered. The addition of radiotherapy and systemic therapies will lead to a significant improvement in survival by independently contributing additional odds reductions in recurrence and in turn mortality. The following should be considered adverse prognostic factors:

- young age (<35 years) at diagnosis
- increasing TNM stage
- poorly differentiated tumours
- lymphatic vessel and/or vascular channel invasion
- oestrogen and progesterone receptor negativity
- positivity for the *HER2* oncogene.

The best prognostic model to incorporate these prognostic factors is Adjuvant (www.adjuvantonline.com), which is widely used across the world to give a consistent guide to 10-year disease outcomes. Figure 8.26 illustrates its usefulness in providing an objective and evidence-based insight into 10-year outcomes. There is now increasing use of gene 'signature' profiling to aid in prognostication. At least two commercially available systems (Oncotype DX®, Mammaprint®) are being

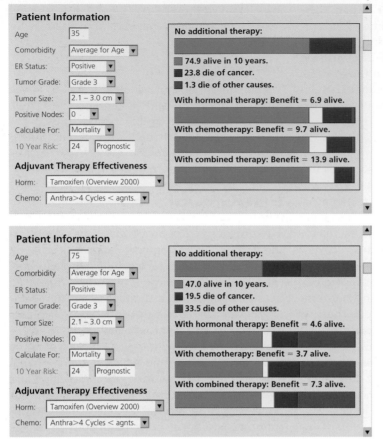

Figure 8.26 Examples of prognosis estimation using the Adjuvant software. (a) Example of a 35-year-old woman with a 2–3 cm Grade 3 node-negative oestrogen receptor-positive cancer, showing the relative and absolute advantages of hormone therapy alone, chemotherapy alone and combined treatment versus no treatment. (b) Same scenario but for a 75-year-old woman. Note the much higher risk of dying of other causes over the next 10 years. Note also the smaller absolute survival advantage for each treatment option.

used. This involves testing a sample of the primary cancer for a panel of genes, looking for a pattern of amplification or suppression that has been validated against known breast cancer outcomes. These tools are still in their infancy but could be useful in borderline cases where further information will help decide which individuals will benefit from chemotherapy, or conversely which individuals can be spared the rigours of chemotherapy.

SCREENING

Screening should permit the diagnosis of a higher proportion of early stages of the disease. As early stage at diagnosis is an important favourable prognostic factor, and breast cancer has a defined non-invasive phase that is readily detectable by imaging; this should translate into a reduction in mortality from invasive breast cancer.

Breast self-examination (BSE) should be routinely practised by women at the same time each month to take account of the variation in breast size and consistency with the menstrual cycle. However, to date BSE has not conclusively been shown to have decreased breast cancer mortality and there has been concern as to the stress of such a practice, together with the inevitably high false positive rate and false negative rate.

Mammography is a sensitive means of detecting carcinomas, often before the lump is palpable by the patient or clinician, thereby facilitating the detection of early breast cancers with a particularly good prognosis. In the United Kingdom the National Breast Screening Programme screens all women aged 50–70 with 3-yearly mammograms. This age range will be extended to 47–73 over the next few years. Women older than this can be screened on request. Such a programme should result in a mortality reduction of

20–30 per cent. There is at present no consensus as to what age premenopausal women should be included in a screening programme, as they tend to have dense breasts, which can obscure the radiological signs of early breast cancers; studies to date have indicated a much smaller impact on survival than in the >50 years age group. However, young women with a family history of breast cancer should be offered regular clinical assessments and mammographic screening at an earlier age. Digital mammography seems to lead to fewer false positive results that traditional film-based mammography and is superior for young women with dense breasts. Ultrasonography is a poor substitute for mammography. In younger women with dense breasts, particularly those with *BRCA* gene mutations, magnetic resonance mammography is the optimum screening modality.

PREVENTION

Patients with a strong family history of breast cancer should be referred to a specialist genetics clinic for risk assessment, counselling and identification of other susceptible family members. Those shown (by gene testing or by statistical modelling) to be *BRCA* gene mutation carriers are at sufficient lifetime risk of developing breast cancer to be considered for bilateral mastectomy, which very substantially reduces the risk, although it does not eliminate it completely.

Breast cancer is sufficiently common to make prevention a worthwhile exercise. Any method of prevention must be easy to comply with, free of short- and long-term adverse effects and be cost effective. The difference in dietary fat intake between the Western world and Africa and Asia contributes to the geographical variation in incidence. A reduction in the proportion of daily calories obtained from dietary fat could make a significant impact on the incidence of breast cancer. Dietary manipulation has the advantage of being inherently cost effective, and can reduce morbidity and mortality from cardiovascular and cerebrovascular disease and colorectal cancer. Uncertainty exists as to when such a dietary adjustment should be instituted and for how long, although its other advantages make it desirable to make it a lifelong commit-

ment. Reducing body mass index and alcohol consumption, and regular strenuous exercise may all help prevent breast cancer, although this is yet to be proven in prospective trials.

Breast cancer is one of the few malignant diseases for which a large randomized trial has shown that chemoprevention is not only feasible but also effective. Tamoxifen 20 mg daily as adjuvant therapy has been conclusively shown to decrease the risk of contralateral breast cancer. This observation has been extrapolated to the prevention setting where a large (15 000 women) placebo-controlled, double-blind, randomized trial has shown this regimen to significantly reduce the risk of developing DCIS and invasive breast cancer. There is an increased risk of thromboembolic disease and endometrial cancer in women receiving tamoxifen. Tamoxifen incidentally reduces cholesterol levels and helps maintain bone mineral density in postmenopausal women, and could therefore have additional health benefits. The osteoporosis-prevention drug raloxifene has also been shown to reduce substantially the risk of developing breast cancer, and has the advantage of not causing hyperstimulation of the endometrium. The aromatase inhibitor anastrozole also reduces the risk of contralateral breast cancer in women receiving the drug as treatment for metastatic breast cancer. Anastrozole could therefore be a promising prevention strategy for postmenopausal women.

FURTHER READING

Buzdar A. *Endocrine Therapies in Breast Cancer.* Oxford University Press, Oxford, 2007

Dixon M. *ABC of Breast Diseases.* BMJ books, London, 2005

Harris JR, Lippman ME. *Diseases of the Breast.* Lippincott Williams and Wilkins, Philadelphia, 2004

Hunt KK, Robb GL, Mendelsohn J, Strom EA. *Breast Cancer.* MD Anderson Cancer Care Series, Texas, 2008

Piccart M, Wood WC. *Breast Cancer Management and Molecular Medicine.* Springer, Berlin, 2007

Skarin AT, Wardley AM, Chen WY. *Breast Cancer.* Elsevier Mosby, Edinburgh, 2007

Winchester DJ, Winchester DP, Hudis C, Norton L. *Breast Cancer.* BC Decker, Hamilton, Ontario, 2006

SELF-ASSESSMENT QUESTIONS

1. Which three of the following statements are true about the epidemiology of breast cancer?
   a. It is the third commonest cancer in the UK
   b. 1 in 1000 cases will arise in men
   c. Environmental factors are important causes
   d. Genetic predisposition is an uncommon causative factor
   e. There is no association with smoking tobacco
   f. Hormonal influences are important causes
   g. Radiation exposure does not cause breast cancer

2. Which one of the following statements is true about the pathology of breast cancer?
   a. Lobular carcinomas are more common than ductal
   b. Paget's disease of the nipple is always associated with an underlying cancer
   c. Most are squamous carcinomas
   d. LCIS is frequently detected by a mammogram
   e. Inflammatory cancers account for 10 per cent of cases

3. Which three of the following factors are associated with an increased probability of lymph node spread?
   a. Increasing tumour size
   b. Tumours arising in men
   c. Lymphovascular invasion in and around the primary tumour
   d. Medial quadrant breast cancers
   e. Screen-detected cancers
   f. High-grade cancers
   g. Cancers arising close to the nipple

4. Which one of the following statements is untrue about the patterns of spread of breast cancer?
   a. Distant relapses can occur more than 10 years after presentation
   b. The skeleton is the commonest site for metastatic spread
   c. Bone metastases may be lytic or sclerotic
   d. Lobular cancer is more likely to spread to the lymph nodes
   e. Ovarian metastases are uncommon

5. Which three of the following statements are true about the presentation of breast cancer?
   a. There will always be a palpable lump
   b. A breast lump in a woman will usually be malignant
   c. Most cases will present with palpable lymph nodes
   d. The cancer is usually painful
   e. The supraclavicular lymph nodes could be enlarged
   f. Can cause a blood-stained nipple discharge
   g. There might be distant metastases at diagnosis

6. Which one of the following is true about the use of trastuzumab in breast cancer?
   a. Most patients benefit from it
   b. Heart toxicity is common
   c. It is only used in advanced forms of the disease
   d. Brain metastases are a particular problem
   e. Cannot be used concurrently with chemotherapy

SELF-ASSESSMENT QUESTIONS

7. Which three of the following statements are true about hormone treatments for breast cancer?
   a. Progesterone is contraindicated in women with a history of breast cancer
   b. Letrozole and exemestane are both aromatase inhibitors
   c. Adjuvant hormone therapy reduces the risk of distant metastatic relapse
   d. Aromatase inhibitors cause endometrial cancer
   e. Tamoxifen is associated with an increased risk of ovarian cancer
   f. Hormone therapy is not usually necessary if the patient receives chemotherapy
   g. Tamoxifen reduces the risk of contralateral breast cancers

8. Which one of the following is not an important prognostic factor?
   a. Tumour size
   b. Histological grade
   c. Centrally located tumour
   d. TNM stage
   e. Age at diagnosis

GASTROINTESTINAL CANCER

9

■ Carcinoma of the oesophagus   118
■ Carcinoma of the stomach   124
■ Carcinoma of the pancreas   130
■ Hepatocellular cancer   135
■ Cholangiocarcinoma   139
■ Carcinoma of the gallbladder   141

■ Carcinoma of the colon and rectum   142
■ Carcinoma of the anus   152
■ Tumours of the peritoneum   156
■ Further reading   157
■ Self-assessment questions   158

CARCINOMA OF THE OESOPHAGUS

Epidemiology

Each year in the UK there are 7600 cases of oesophageal cancer, 4900 cases in men and 2700 cases in women, accounting for 2.7 per cent of all cancer cases and leading to a total of 7400 deaths per annum. Tumours of the upper third are much more common in females. The peak incidence is at 60–70 years. The highest incidence is found in Russia, Turkey, China, Iran and Southern Africa.

Aetiology

Tobacco smoking is a strong risk factor for oesophageal cancer. The regular consumption of alcoholic spirits predisposes to cancer from chronic irritation of the mucosa. Carcinogenic contaminants of alcoholic drinks have also been implicated in some cases, e.g. the home-made beer consumed by the Xhosa people in Transkei. In achalasia there is chronic stasis and pooling of food and secretions in a dilated oesophagus, owing to a loss of oesophageal motility. The increased risk of cancer is due to prolonged contact of the mucosa with carcinogens within the food or produced from food by the action of bacteria. Patterson–Brown-Kelly syndrome (Plummer–Vinson syndrome) is characterized by koilonychia, iron-deficiency anaemia, the presence of an 'oesophageal web' in the upper third of the oesophagus on barium swallow and is usually seen in women. It leads to a carcinoma of the upper third of the oesophagus typically in the postcricoid region. Tylosis is a very rare, dominantly inherited condition characterized by palmar and plantar hyperkeratosis and a strong predisposition to oesophageal carcinoma. Barrett's oesophagus is characterized by glandular metaplasia of the squamous epithelium of the lower third of the oesophagus, usually in response to chronic gastro-oesophageal reflux from a hiatus hernia. Patients are at risk of developing an adenocarcinoma of the oesophagus. A high body mass index is also associated with an increased risk of adenocarcinoma.

Pathology

Approximately 40–50 per cent arise in the middle third of the oesophagus, 40–50 per cent in the lower third, and less than 10 per cent in the upper third, the tumour appearing nodular, ulcerating or diffusely infiltrative. If there is oesophageal obstruction, the proximal oesophagus is frequently dilated and contains food debris. A fistula can exist between the oesophagus and trachea or bronchial tree, and there may be evidence of an aspiration pneumonia particularly in the lower lobes of the lungs. Cancers of the upper two-thirds of the oesophagus are invariably squamous cell carcinomas. Those in the lower third are most commonly squamous but one-third are adenocarcinomas, which may have arisen in an area of metaplasia such as Barrett's oesophagus. These must be distinguished from adenocarcinoma of the proximal stomach that has infiltrated the oesophagus. The histological spectrum of oesophageal cancer is changing with an increasing proportion being classified as adenocarcinomas.

Natural history

The tumour will spread within the oesophagus both longitudinally and circumferentially, eventually resulting in complete oesophageal obstruction. Invasion through the deeper layers of the oesophageal wall will result in spread to the surrounding mediastinal structures such as the trachea, main bronchi (especially left), pleura, lung, vertebrae and great vessels. Insidious spread along the submucosa is common and can lead to skip lesions some distance from the main tumour. The pattern of lymphatic involvement reflects the complex blood supply to the oesophagus. Tumours of the upper third will spread to the deep cervical and supraclavicular nodes, those of the middle third to the mediastinal, paratracheal and subcarinal nodes, and those of the lower third to the nodes of the coeliac axis below the diaphragm. The venous drainage of parts of the oesophagus is into the portal circulation and so the liver is the most common site of distant metastases, although the lungs and skeleton may also be involved.

Symptoms

Dysphagia is the most common presenting symptom. A middle-aged or elderly patient complaining of this symptom should be considered to have oesophageal cancer until proven otherwise and referral to a gastroenterologist is mandatory. The symptom begins insidiously as a sensation of food sticking, usually when solids such as meat have been eaten, progresses so that there is difficulty with softer foods/liquids, and can be associated with retrosternal discomfort owing to stretching of the oesophagus and increased peristalsis. Regurgitation usually accompanies severe dysphagia. Retrosternal discomfort is followed by effortless regurgitation of the oesophageal contents. These do not taste sour as they have not entered the stomach. This contrasts with gastro-oesophageal reflux where there will be a strong taste of acid. Weight loss is due to both reduced caloric intake owing to dysphagia and/or regurgitation, and the non-specific effects of malignancy. Recurrent aspiration is a problem in patients with proximal tumours leading to overflow into the upper respiratory tract or with a fistula connecting the oesophagus to the lower respiratory tract. The patient experiences a severe bout of coughing within a short time of swallowing, and may expectorate solid material from the food bolus. Both predispose to recurrent chest infections that can be fatal.

Signs

There is often evidence of malnutrition, the degree of which is dependent on the duration and severity of dysphagia and whether there has been a history of alcoholism. In cases of oesophageal obstruction the patient could even be dehydrated owing to poor fluid intake. Women with Plummer–Vinson syndrome can appear anaemic and have koilonychia, while alcoholics may have stigmata of chronic liver disease. There is usually no palpable evidence of disease although an epigastric mass is sometimes palpable in tumours of the lower third of the oesophagus and if there are large intra-abdominal lymph nodes. The cervical and supraclavicular lymph nodes should be palpated carefully. Hepatomegaly suggests metastatic disease but also fatty infiltration or cirrhosis in heavy drinkers.

Differential diagnosis

Care has to be taken not to confuse a tumour arising from the oesophageal mucosa with a tumour arising from an adjacent structure and invading into the oesophagus, e.g. carcinoma of the left main bronchus (most often squamous or small cell carcinoma), carcinoma of the fundus of the stomach or gastro-oesophageal junction (adenocarcinoma). Other differential diagnoses include a benign oesophageal stricture owing to chronic gastro-oesophageal reflux, achalasia, and hysteria, although this is a diagnosis only made after excluding all other possible causes.

Investigations

Serum alkaline phosphatase, γ-glutamyl transferase and a liver ultrasound should be performed in all cases to screen for liver metastases, and a chest X-ray performed to exclude lung metastases and mediastinal lymphadenopathy.

Barium swallow and meal

A barium swallow will outline the whole oesophageal lumen, a carcinoma appearing as a stricture, filling defect or abnormal flow of barium (Fig. 9.1). It might also suggest the presence of a fistula connecting the oesophagus to the bronchial tree, although the radiologist should be warned if this is thought to be likely at the time of requesting the examination. This investigation will not give a tissue diagnosis and all patients should proceed to endoscopy.

Endoscopy

This is the investigation of choice. The oesophagus starts at the lower border of the cricoid cartilage at the level of the 6th cervical vertebra, approximately 15 cm from the incisor teeth. It is 25 cm in length, entering the stomach at the level of the 10th thoracic vertebra (i.e. approximately 40 cm from the incisors). Endoscopy allows a thorough assessment of the whole

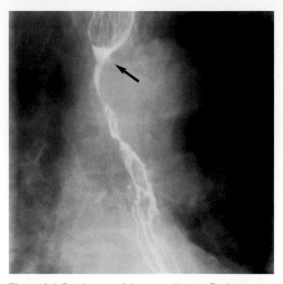

Figure 9.1 Carcinoma of the oesophagus. Barium swallow showing an irregular, malignant stricture of the middle third of the oesophagus. Note the small pool of barium at the top of the stricture (arrowed).

oesophagus. The tumour can be visualized directly, a biopsy taken for histology and brushings for cytology. It also allows a thorough evaluation of the stomach, which is particularly important in tumours of the lower third of the oesophagus, and is the most sensitive means of detecting small primary tumours and skip lesions. Endoscopic ultrasound is also a useful tool, permitting direct imaging of the tumour. It is particularly sensitive for determining the depth of invasion and involvement of first station lymph node groups.

Computed tomography (CT) of the thorax and upper abdomen

This provides information on the local extent of the disease with respect to invasion beyond the oesophagus and is of value in planning radiotherapy or surgery because it will also allow an assessment of the regional lymph nodes, liver, lungs and adrenals.

MRI of the thorax and upper abdomen

This will be useful in the preoperative assessment of candidates for radical surgery. The improvement in soft tissue contrast will aid in patient selection and surgical planning.

Positron emission tomography (PET)

This is now routinely performed to complete whole body staging prior to curative surgery. It has the advantage of disclosing the presence of metastatic disease at occult sites in the body (e.g. adrenal glands, perigastric, mediastinal and coeliac lymph nodes) and can show foci of active cancer in other areas where CT can be equivocal (e.g. liver).

Bronchoscopy

This could be necessary to exclude direct invasion of the posterior tracheal wall and left main bronchus when the operability of a tumour of the upper or middle third is being considered.

Staging

The TNM staging system is most frequently used:

- Tis – Carcinoma in situ
- T0 – No evidence of primary
- TX – Primary cannot be assessed
- T1 – Involving lamina propria/submucosa
- T2 – Involving muscularis propria
- T3 – Involving adventitia
- T4 – Involving adjacent structures
- N0 – No regional lymphadenopathy
- N1 – Regional lymph node involvement
- M0 – No distant metastases
- M1 – Distant metastases.

Treatment

Many patients will be poorly nourished, which lessens their tolerance of radical treatment and therefore referral to a dietitian is advisable in all cases. A liquidizer may help the patient to continue eating food prepared at home. It may be necessary for the patient to be given liquid dietary supplements to maintain calorie intake, and enteral feeding via a nasogastric tube or via a percutaneous gastrostomy catheter might be the only means of maintaining nutrition.

Radical treatment

Surgery

Surgery is a potentially curative treatment modality and is the treatment of choice for localized lower third tumours as th[...] surgically accessible part of the oe[...]

Contraindications to surgery inc[...]

- poor performance status
- severe malnutrition
- vocal cord palsy, indicating infiltration/pressure on the recurrent laryngeal nerve, suggesting spread beyond the oesophagus
- broncho-oesophageal fistula
- invasion of great vessels (aorta, superior vena cava), pericardium
- cervical/coeliac node involvement clinically or radiologically
- distant metastases.

Tumours of the middle third have historically been treated by an Ivor Lewis two-stage oesophagectomy. The stomach is mobilized via upper abdominal incision, the oesophagus approached via the right 5th intercostal space, the tumour resected allowing a 5 cm margin of macroscopically normal oesophagus, and the oesophagus then reanastomosed. The operative mortality is high depending on patient selection and the surgeon's skill. For tumours of the lower third, a left thoracoabdominal incision is made, the tumour mobilized via a trans-hiatal approach and resected with re-anastomosis of the transected oesophagus. In experienced hands and with appropriate patient selection, the operative mortality will be <5 per cent. Advances in laparoscopic surgery significantly hasten recovery and thereby reduce the duration of postoperative care in hospital, particularly when there is a combined thoracoscopic–laparoscopic approach.

Radiotherapy

Radiotherapy is the treatment of choice for tumours of the upper third, where surgery would be difficult, but can also be used for tumours elsewhere that are not amenable to surgery. The treatment-related mortality is much lower than radical surgery. Although distant metastases are a contraindication to radical radiotherapy, extra-oesophageal invasion can still be encompassed within the radiation high-dose zone. Treatment is given daily over 5–6 weeks.

Neoadjuvant chemotherapy is increasingly used and is the subject of ongoing clinical trials.

This typically involves the use of 5FU and either cisplatin or mitomycin C, yielding objective response rates of 30–60 per cent. As with other tumour sites, most published experience has been with its use in squamous carcinomas. The combination of epirubicin, cisplatin and protracted venous infusion of 5FU is more useful for adenocarcinomas. Whilst there appears to be a prolongation of disease-free survival, no benefit in overall survival has been established.

In recent years, there has also been increasing interest in synchronous chemoradiotherapy (CRT), particularly for squamous carcinomas and inoperable tumours. The advantage of upfront chemotherapy and radiotherapy is that there could be synergy between the two treatments, leading to the maximum probability of preoperative downstaging. This may in turn facilitate curative surgery for some individuals or maximize non-surgical treatment for those who remain inoperable. To date, the few randomized trials of CRT versus radiotherapy alone have shown a promising improvement in median and overall survivals for the CRT group, with 3-year survivals of 20–30 per cent. Similar trials of preoperative CRT and surgery versus surgery alone have shown pathological complete response rates of 20–30 per cent and 3-year survival rates similar in magnitude. This is clearly an advance on historical controls and is therefore a promising approach that deserves further study.

Chemotherapy

Apart from synchronous CRT (see above), there is no defined role for chemotherapy in the curative treatment of oesophageal cancer. Adjuvant chemotherapy is less established as a valid approach compared with other forms of cancer.

Palliative treatment

Dysphagia and regurgitation are the symptoms most often requiring treatment. Both are extremely distressing and can erode the quality of life significantly.

Radiotherapy

A short course of radiotherapy will relieve dysphagia in most patients with acceptable short-term morbidity and can usually be repeated if necessary. This may be given as a course of external beam irradiation or intraluminal brachytherapy whereby a high-activity radiation source is inserted directly into the oesophagus via a nasogastric tube.

Chemotherapy

5FU and cisplatin combinations have a role in the palliative treatment of oesophageal cancer. One such regimen of particular value, particularly in adenocarcinomas, is ECF:

- epirubicin 60 mg/m^2 i.v. day 1
- cisplatin 60 mg/m^2 i.v. day 1 with full pre- and posthydration
- 5 FU 200 mg/m^2 i.v. daily by protracted venous infusion (PVI)
- repeat bolus chemotherapy 3 weekly for 6 cycles

For squamous and undifferentiated cancers there is evidence to suggest that the PVI 5FU can be replaced by the orally delivered drug capecitabine (Xeloda®) – ECX regimen. Similarly, outcomes can be further improved by using ECX and substituting cisplatin with oxaliplatin – EOX. This is now the standard of care for locally advanced and metastatic oesophageal cancer.

Other treatments

Fibreoptic endoscopy permits a number of procedures to be performed under direct vision. Dilatation using metal bougies allows a stricture to be stretched and relieves dysphagia to some degree in the majority, although the procedure might need to be repeated a number of times during the patient's remaining lifetime. Alternatively, an endoprosthesis such as a rigid Atkinson tube can be inserted to maintain oesophageal patency and is particularly useful in relieving recurrent aspiration owing to a fistula. Laser therapy can be given to coagulate a bleeding tumour or to unblock an obstructed oesophagus. Administration of laser light-sensitizing agents can be used as part of a course of 'photodynamic therapy' to kill tumour cells more selectively.

CASE HISTORY: OESOPHAGEAL CANCER

A 60-year-old man with a history of chronic bronchitis develops dysphagia. He experiences retrosternal discomfort when he swallows solid foodstuffs, e.g.meat, bread. He has a long history of gastro-oesophageal reflux and had a barium swallow some years earlier which confirmed a hiatus hernia. He initially self-medicates himself with a proton pump inhibitor in addition to a mucosal surface protectant. His discomfort temporarily improves but then worsens and is accompanied by regurgitation of food.

He is referred to a gastroenterologist. Endoscopy reveals a polypoid tumour at 32–36 cm obstructing the lumen of the oesophagus with no extension into the stomach. Biopsy confirms a poorly differentiated adenocarcinoma with some evidence of an underlying Barrett's oesophagus and chronic oesophagitis. CT scan shows no evidence of mediastinal or abdominal lymphadenopathy and no evidence of liver metastases.

He is initially treated with chemoradiation over a 5-week period during which time his symptoms improve significantly. Repeat endoscopy 6 weeks later reveals no obvious mucosal abnormality and random biopsies show chronic inflammatory cells alone. At this time, his shortness of breath is worse than usual and he has a dry cough. Chest X-ray confirms opacification corresponding to the radiation fields suggesting a degree of radiation pneumonitis. In view of an apparent pathological complete response, and his respiratory compromise, he is not deemed a suitable candidate for major surgery.

Eighteen months later, he presents with recurrent dysphagia. He is referred to a dietician for dietary advice. Endoscopy confirms a recurrence at the same level as previously, which is dilated. Adenocarcinoma is confirmed histologically; 6 weeks later, his symptoms have recurred. An oesophageal stent is inserted that provides good symptom control for 3 months. He then develops right upper quadrant pain and anorexia. Liver ultrasound confirms hepatic metastases. He declines further chemotherapy. There is a symptomatic improvement with dexamethasone but he dies of his disease 4 weeks later.

Tumour-related complications

Malnutrition can be caused by chronic dysphagia. Invasion of tumour into the adjacent main bronchi sometimes leads to a broncho-oesophageal fistula (Fig. 9.2). Aspiration of food into the respiratory tract will lead to pneumonia, which may be further complicated by lung abscess and empyema. Haemorrhage is a rare but potentially fatal local tumour complication.

Treatment-related complications

Surgery

Loss of oesophageal integrity after surgical resection can lead to a fistula or mediastinitis which sometimes is fatal, while pneumothorax, pulmonary collapse and pneumonia can complicate a thoracotomy.

Radiotherapy

During treatment, it is inevitable that the patient will experience some worsening of dysphagia owing to a radiation oesophagitis. This can be minimized by avoidance of very hot or cold food/fluids, and relieved by Mucaine 10 mL tds sipped slowly. Anorexia and nausea/vomiting are likely if stomach and/or liver is included in the radiation fields, and will be helped by a regular anti-emetic. Radiation pneumonitis is uncommon and usually subclinical, although it can cause a dry cough, fever and dyspnoea. Oesophageal stricture can occur from 6 months after radiotherapy giving rise to dysphagia, and needs to be distinguished from recurrent tumour, preferably by endoscopy so that a dilatation can be performed simultaneously.

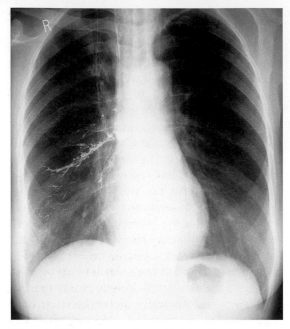

Figure 9.2 Broncho-oesophageal fistula. Chest radiograph taken after a gastrograffin swallow. Contrast has leaked into the right side of the bronchial tree.

Chemotherapy

Apart from drug-specific toxicity, combined modality treatment with chemotherapy and radiotherapy leads to a severe acute oesophageal reaction, which can compromise nutrition and require supportive therapy.

Prognosis

Overall 5-year survival is only 5–10 per cent and is usually due to many cases having occult lymph node or distant metastases at presentation. For the subgroup undergoing potentially curative surgery, the 5-year survival rate is 20 per cent or more depending on selection criteria.

Screening/prevention

In the UK, patients with a Barrett's oesophagus and achalasia should be offered annual endoscopic examination because of their high risk of developing carcinoma. Routine endoscopic screening of a population is not a proven strat-

egy, and is associated with risks of the procedure such as perforation, aspiration, vasovagal events and bleeding.

Informing the public of the risks of tobacco and alcohol could reduce the incidence of oesophageal cancer. Other factors associated with reducing the risk of oesophageal cancer include a diet rich in green vegetables and long-term use of non-steroidal anti-inflammatory drugs.

Rare tumours

Adenoid cystic carcinoma

This is a tumour arising from the mucous glands of the mucosa and is of the same type as those arising in the parotid salivary gland and elsewhere.

Small cell carcinoma

Although infiltration from an underlying lung primary should be considered, a primary tumour of this type has been described.

Melanoma

This is a rare site for mucosal melanoma. Prognosis will be very poor owing to advanced stage at presentation.

Carcinoid

This is an uncommon site for this rare tumour. It should be treated as elsewhere by surgical resection.

Leiomyosarcoma

This tumour arises from the smooth muscle fibres of the oesophageal wall. It is best treated by radical surgery combined with radiotherapy.

CARCINOMA OF THE STOMACH

Epidemiology

Each year in the UK there are 8200 cases of stomach cancer, 5200 cases in men and 3000 cases in women, accounting for 2.9 per cent of all cancer cases and leading to a total of 5300 deaths per annum. There is a peak incidence at 50–70 years. Blood group O confers some protection against developing stomach cancer while blood group A is associated with a higher incidence of the diffuse form of stomach cancer. The incidence is very high in Japan and Chile, and increased in lower socioeconomic groups.

Aetiology

The stomach is exposed to a variety of carcinogens both ingested and produced from the action of bacteria within the stomach. Nitrosamines have been implicated in stomach cancer, as has a diet rich in smoked foodstuffs. Excessive dietary salt has been implicated. Atrophic gastritis and achlorhydria both increase the risk of developing stomach cancer, in the case of pernicious anaemia by five-fold. This could be related to bacterial overgrowth and increased production of endogenous carcinogens. Infection with *Helicobacter pylori* is associated with increased risk of stomach cancer. A partial gastrectomy or gastroenterostomy is also associated with an increased cancer risk, probably owing to a chronic reflux of bile salts into the stomach. An adenoma–carcinoma sequence has been seen but is much rarer than in the large bowel.

Pathology

Stomach cancers usually form discrete ulcerating lesions, but can be nodular or polypoid. They are occasionally diffusely infiltrating leading to obliteration of the stomach lumen. Fifty per cent arise in the pyloric region while, of those arising in the body, most are found along the lesser curvature; 95 per cent are adenocarcinomas, and 5 per cent squamous carcinoma or adenoacanthoma (adenocarcinoma with areas of squamous metaplasia). There is sometimes evidence of prior intestinal metaplasia and carcinoma in situ in the surrounding mucosa.

Natural history

Cancers spread longitudinally and circumferentially within the stomach and, as with carcinoma of the oesophagus, insidious submucosal spread is frequent. Occasionally, this leads to diffuse infiltration of the whole stomach with luminal narrowing and rigidity of the stomach wall, and a picture known as 'linitis plastica'. Progressive invasion into the muscle layer of the stomach wall eventually leads to invasion of the serosa and in turn invasion of adjacent viscera, such as the omentum, pancreas, spleen, left kidney and adrenal. Invasion superiorly by a tumour of the fundus can result in occlusion of the lower third of the oesophagus leading to dysphagia and regurgitation. There is a propensity for transcoelomic spread with diffuse peritoneal seeding leading to ascites (Fig. 9.3) and ovarian deposits (Krukenberg tumours – Fig. 9.4), particularly with the signet ring variant. Spread to the regional lymph nodes (gastric, gastroduodenal, splenic and coeliac groups) occurs early in the natural history, and Virchow's node in the left supraclavicular fossa can be involved (Troisier's sign). Distant spread occurs in the liver via the portal venous circulation, lung, bone, brain and skin.

Symptoms

The patient frequently presents with non-specific gastrointestinal symptoms such as epigastric discomfort, anorexia, nausea, vomiting and weight loss, which are frequently confused with a benign condition such as peptic ulceration or gastritis, and can even be relieved by the antacids, H2-antagonists or proton pump inhibitors prescribed for these conditions. Others present with the symptoms of an iron-deficiency anaemia, and stomach cancer should always be considered in the assessment of such patients. A more acute presentation occurs with stomach perforation, haematemesis and/or melaena.

Signs

At presentation, many will have been losing weight, and cachexia is a frequent finding. An epigastric mass might be palpable as can be lymph nodes in the left supraclavicular fossa. The liver is sometimes enlarged, tender and

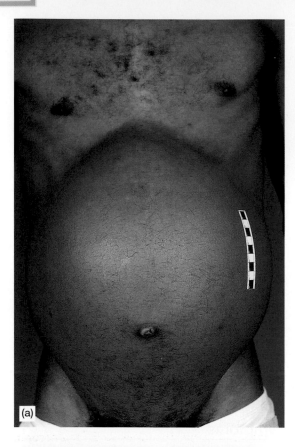

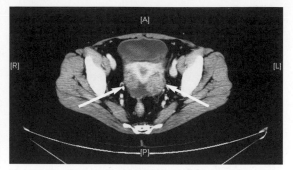

Figure 9.4 Krukenberg tumours. CT image of the pelvis. There are bilateral ovarian masses representing metastatic spread from gastric cancer.

Differential diagnosis

This includes:

- inflammatory conditions, e.g. peptic ulcer
- other malignant gastric tumours, e.g. lymphoma, leiomyosarcoma
- benign gastric tumours, e.g. leiomyoma, carcinoid.

Investigations

Barium meal

Double contrast barium meal will outline the gastric mucosa and is a sensitive investigation for detecting mucosal abnormalities. Although carcinomas often have a characteristic appearance, they can be confused with benign peptic ulcers and therefore further investigation to obtain a tissue diagnosis is mandatory.

Fibreoptic endoscopy

This allows direct visualization of the gastric mucosa with a more accurate assessment of the macroscopic appearances of an abnormality. It also allows biopsy and brushings for cytology to give a tissue diagnosis.

CT scan of the abdomen

This will provide the surgeon with information regarding invasion beyond the stomach and whether the regional lymph nodes are enlarged, and thereby help determine whether the tumour is operable (also see below).

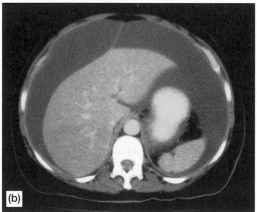

Figure 9.3 Massive ascites. (a) Frontal view of abdomen. (b) Transverse CT image of abdomen.

knobbly, suggesting metastatic infiltration, and there may be ascites. Non-metastatic manifestations such as dermatomyositis and acanthosis nigricans might also be seen.

Laparoscopy

This facilitates direct visualization of the stomach, regional lymph nodes, liver and peritoneal surfaces. It is complementary to high quality cross-sectional imaging and is important in a condition with a high rate of lymphatic involvement and transcoelomic spread. The revelation of an otherwise occult disease might in turn spare the patient unnecessary surgery.

Tests to exclude metastatic disease

These include:

- Baseline liver function tests
- CT scan of the brain, thorax, abdomen and pelvis to stage locoregional disease and exclude hepatic and/or pulmonary metastases
- carcinoembryonic antigen, which may be elevated reflecting tumour burden but is not routinely of value. It sometimes permits early diagnosis of distant and/or local relapse after curative treatment.

Staging

The TNM system is widely used:

- Tis – Carcinoma in situ
- T0 – No evidence of primary
- TX – Primary cannot be assessed
- T1 – Involving lamina propria/submucosa
- T2 – Involving muscularis propria/subserosa
- T3 – Penetrates serosa
- T4 – Involving adjacent structures
- N0 – No regional lymphadenopathy
- N1 – 1 to 6 regional lymph nodes involved
- N2 – 7 to 15 regional lymph nodes involved
- N3 – >15 regional lymph nodes involved
- M0 – No distant metastases
- M1 – Distant metastases.

Treatment

Radical treatment

Surgery

This is the only potentially curative treatment but only two-thirds of patients are deemed operable after full staging investigations and a further two-thirds of these will be found to be inoperable, meaning that overall only 1 in 5 patients stand any chance of being cured. The extent of surgical resection remains an area of controversy. A partial or total gastrectomy is performed in operable cases depending on the size and site of the tumour. Total gastrectomy in smaller tumours will have the advantage in surgically clearing occult mucosal spread and synchronous second primary cancers. A D1 resection involves removal of the first echelon perigastric lymph nodes, whilst a D2 resection will remove the second echelon nodes and invariably is a more substantial surgical procedure, requiring greater expertise and a higher operative mortality. Despite this, evidence is emerging particularly from Japan of the superiority of a D2 lymphadenectomy particularly for larger, more deeply penetrating tumours. There is no evidence to support routine removal of the spleen.

Recent advances in laparoscopic surgery are being applied to gastric cancer. This may involve a small incision to allow passage of digits (laparoscopically assisted digital gastrectomy) or a hand (hand-assisted laparoscopic gastrectomy). If there are perioperative complications, conversion to an open procedure is usual. There are fewer cases of ileus and postoperative chest infections after laparoscopic surgery but it might result in fewer lymph nodes being removed. Long-term outcomes are therefore awaited.

Radiotherapy

Radiotherapy has no curative role in treatment owing to the dose-limiting toxicity induced in the stomach and adjacent structures such as the small bowel and transverse colon when a high dose of radiation is administered. Adjuvant postoperative radiotherapy does not significantly improve survival but does reduce the risk of local recurrence approximately three-fold. A recent, large, randomized trial indicated that postoperative chemoradiation (CRT) substantially improved overall survival in high-risk completely resected locally advanced adenocarcinoma of the stomach and gastroesophageal junction. In the United States, this CRT regimen is becoming the standard of care.

Chemotherapy

Recent randomized trials of preoperative and perioperative chemotherapy have helped define the role of chemotherapy in this disease which hitherto had been treated exclusively by surgery or a palliative care approach. Preoperative/perioperative chemotherapy using cisplatin and 5FU with or without epirubicin increases the rate of subsequent curative surgery and yields a 5-year improvement in overall survival of 10–15 per cent.

Palliative treatment

Surgery

Intestinal bypass surgery (e.g. gastrojejunostomy) is effective in relieving gastric outflow obstruction while gastrectomy may be justified in the presence of metastatic disease when massive bleeding cannot be controlled by less invasive methods.

Radiotherapy

Radiotherapy is valuable in relieving the local symptoms of inoperable disease such as dysphagia, haemorrhage or pain owing to retroperitoneal infiltration.

Chemotherapy

As with other solid tumours, there is some evidence suggesting that immediate chemotherapy confers a survival advantage compared with best supportive care. This could be of value in relieving symptoms from metastatic disease, particularly for lung and liver metastases. The most active single agent is 5FU, which may be used in combination with other drugs such as Adriamycin and mitomycin C (FAM)/methotrexate (FAMtx) or epirubicin and cisplatin (ECF). Response rates of 30–40 per cent have been reported with median survivals in the region of 6–12 months. As gastric cancer has some analogies with colorectal cancer with respect to 5FU being the agent with the greatest track record, it is not surprising that drugs such as irinotecan are also being tested. Building on their success at other sites, the taxanes are also the subject of further study in this disease.

Endoscopic procedures

Laser therapy is particularly useful for the photocoagulation of a persistently bleeding tumour or debulking of a large tumour that is narrowing the oesophageal lumen. An oesophageal endoprosthesis is occasionally of benefit for a tumour of the upper stomach occluding the oesophagus from below.

Tumour-related complications

Haemorrhage can be life threatening if a major gastric vessel is eroded, while chronic blood loss will lead to an iron-deficiency anaemia with a reduced serum ferritin. Invasion through the stomach wall into the peritoneal cavity sometimes leads to leakage of gastric contents and an acute peritonitis. Pyloric stenosis can lead to gastric outflow obstruction, eventually leading to episodes of projectile vomiting, visible peristalsis, a 'succussion splash' and obstruction. Mucin secretion by the tumour might rarely result in activation of the plasmin/plasminogen cascade, leading to a disseminated intravascular coagulation manifested by abnormal clotting, thrombocytopenia and raised fibrin degradation products (see Chapter 8).

Treatment-related complications

Surgery

Loss of stomach volume will lead to a feeling of fullness after small portions of food, while loss of gastric acidity can predispose to iron deficiency. Impaired intrinsic factor production will lead to vitamin B12 deficiency secondary to impaired absorption at the terminal ileum resulting in a macrocytic anaemia, while impaired digestion can result in malabsorption and a 'dumping syndrome' owing to hypoglycaemia. Sternal ulceration and ultimately a second malignancy might occur.

Radiotherapy

During treatment the patient will experience some degree of anorexia, nausea and vomiting.

High doses of radiation to the stomach can result in a chronic gastritis. The left kidney might receive a dose sufficient to impair its function permanently, which will be relevant if the right kidney function is subnormal. Radiation enteritis is also a recognized complication.

Prognosis

The median survival for patients with unresectable disease is about 4 months and the 5-year survival is <10 per cent overall, rising to 15–20 per cent in those undergoing successful surgical resection. Early gastric cancer has a good 5-year survival of 70 per cent or more. In stage TisN0M0 disease confined to the mucosa, results from radical surgery are excellent with 5-year survivals of 90 per cent or more. Adverse prognostic factors include increasing tumour stage at presentation, unresectable disease, diffuse morphology and poor tumour differentiation.

Screening/prevention

A screening programme of double contrast barium examination of the stomach and gastroscopy has been successfully implemented in Japan. This has led to a greater proportion of early cancers being detected, resulting in a decline in mortality. The efficacy of screening in Western populations is yet to be proven. Logic would suggest that treatment of *Helicobacter pylori* and adoption of a healthy diet rich in vegetables and low in salt should decrease the incidence of gastric cancer but this is yet to be proven.

Rare tumours

Gastrointestinal stromal tumour (GIST)

GISTs are mesenchymal neoplasms occurring in later life: 70 per cent arise in the stomach, 25 per cent in the small intestine. They express a growth factor receptor with tyrosine kinase activity (c-kit) which can be detected with CD117 immunohistochemistry. Their uncontrolled cell proliferation makes them highly malignant tumours that are relatively resistant to conventional treatments and invariably fatal.

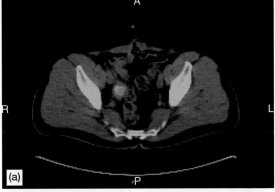
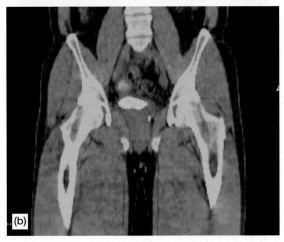

Figure 9.5 GIST tumour. PET scan showing high glucose metabolism within a GIST tumour arising just above the bladder superimposed on the CT anatomy for spatial reference. (a) Transverse view. (b) Coronal view.

They typically take up glucose avidly and therefore PET imaging is a sensitive way of visualizing them (Fig. 9.5). However, significant responses and long-term survivors have been seen with the antibody imatinib (Glivec®) which targets c-kit. Consideration should therefore be given to identifying such tumours when usual sites/histological patterns of gastrointestinal malignancy are diagnosed, so that the few individuals with this disease can be identified and treated appropriately.

Leiomyoma

This is a benign tumour arising from smooth muscle of the stomach wall, often found incidentally during investigation of the upper gastrointestinal tract but it may ulcerate leading to haematemesis.

Carcinoid

The stomach is a very uncommon site for carcinoid tumours, which are best treated surgically (see Chapter 14).

Lymphoma

The stomach is a common site for extranodal lymphoma – usually a low-grade tumour mucosal associated lymphoid tissue (MALToma).

CARCINOMA OF THE PANCREAS

Epidemiology

Each year in the UK there are 7400 cases of pancreatic cancer, 3600 cases in men and 3800 cases in women, accounting for 2.6 per cent of all cancer cases and leading to a total of 7300 deaths per annum. Most patients are over 50 years at diagnosis, the peak incidence being at 60–80 years. It is a disease of industrialized countries.

Aetiology

Pancreatic cancer has been associated with:

- smoking tobacco
- high dietary fat and meat consumption
- high coffee and/or alcohol consumption
- diabetes mellitus
- chronic pancreatitis
- previous surgery for peptic ulcer disease
- industrial exposure to the insecticide DDT
- familial cancer syndromes, e.g. multiple endocrine neoplasia type 1, von Hippel–Lindau syndrome, ataxia telangiectasia.

Pathology

The tumour is well circumscribed or diffusely infiltrating the pancreas; 30 per cent arise in the head and are often associated with a dilated common bile duct, and 20 per cent in the body or tail, the remainder being more diffuse in origin. Carcinoma arises from the ducts (90 per cent) and glandular elements (10 per cent) rather than the hormone-producing cells and is invariably a mucin-producing adenocarcinoma. There might be evidence of a chronic pancreatitis distal to any blocked pancreatic ducts and the majority stain for carcinoembryonic antigen (CEA).

Natural history

The tumour infiltrates diffusely through the gland, or might grow along the pancreatic duct system, eventually reaching the common bile duct and ampulla of Vater. The capsule can be breached leading to invasion of the stomach, duodenum, spleen, aorta and retroperitoneal tissues, and transcoelomic spread can occur with diffuse peritoneal involvement and ascites. Regional lymph nodes are frequently involved and include the pancreaticoduodenal, gastroduodenal, hepatic, superior mesenteric and coeliac groups. The majority have distant metastases by the time of diagnosis at sites including the liver, lung, skin and brain.

Symptoms

Pancreatic cancer is notorious for presenting late in the natural history of the disease, reflecting the deep-seated anatomical position of the pancreas and high prevalence of non-specific upper gastrointestinal symptoms in the population. Tumours of the head of the pancreas most frequently present with obstructive jaundice (progressive jaundice, dark urine, pale stools, itching) owing to occlusion of the common bile duct. Tumours of the body and tail of the pancreas are more likely to present with pain, usually epigastric with radiation to the back. Extensive pancreatic infiltration or blockage of the major ducts will lead to malabsorption owing to exocrine dysfunction, which will result in pale, fatty, offensive stools (steatorrhoea) which float on water and are difficult to flush down the lavatory pan. Pancreatic endocrine dysfunction will lead to impaired glucose tolerance or diabetes mellitus in 20 per cent, causing thirst, polyuria, nocturia and weight loss.

Signs

The patient often has jaundice, and the gall-bladder may be palpable in the right upper quadrant of the abdomen, suggesting extrahepatic biliary obstruction that is not due to chronic gallstone disease (positive Courvoisier's sign). There will be pale stools on rectal examination and dark urine. Scratch marks on the trunk are a sign of pruritus owing to bile salt retention. A mass might be palpable in the epigastrium, fixed owing to its retroperitoneal location. Weight loss is common and can lead to profound cachexia. The liver might be enlarged and knobbly, consistent with metastatic infiltration. Petechiae, purpura and bruising are seen in advanced disease from disseminated intravascular coagulation (DIC).

Differential diagnosis

Gallstones are a common cause of obstructive jaundice and abdominal pain, although they are not commonly associated with systemic symptoms and are not a cause of glucose intolerance. Benign tumours such as a glucagonoma, gastrinoma or VIPoma should also be considered.

Investigations

Liver function tests

These will demonstrate the degree of obstructive jaundice, characterized by raised total serum bilirubin, elevated alkaline phosphatase and γ-glutamyltransferase with normal or slightly elevated liver transferases (ALT).

Clotting profile

There will be derangement of vitamin K-dependent clotting factors. This is reflected in a prolongation of the international normalized ratio (INR), and will show clinically as bruising and a tendency to prolonged bleeding. A full blood count and clotting profile should always be per-formed prior to invasive investigations such as an ERCP or CT-guided biopsy, and serum collected for grouping so that fresh frozen plasma or blood can be given at short notice should there be a haemorrhage after biopsy. Patients suspected of having DIC should have blood sent to measure fibrin degradation products (FDPs).

CA 19-9 tumour marker assay

This is worth measuring as a baseline. It is a potentially useful response marker of disease activity.

Chest X-ray

A chest X-ray is indicated to exclude pulmonary metastases.

Computed tomography (CT) of the abdomen

This characteristically shows dilatation of the common bile duct associated with a mass lesion in the head of the pancreas, a discrete mass in the body or tail of the pancreas, or diffuse enlargement of the pancreas. All patients considered suitable for radical surgery should undergo this investigation as it is the best way of defining the extent of local invasion, presence of enlarged regional lymph nodes and liver metastases. It also facilitates a fine needle biopsy when a definitive diagnosis cannot be made by less invasive procedures.

Magnetic resonance imaging (MRI)

The superior soft tissue resolution of MRI is best exploited when curative surgery is contemplated. It is useful for clarifying the local extent of tumour infiltration with regard to adjacent anatomical structures that cannot be sacrificed, and may be of use in surgical planning.

Positron emission tomography (PET)

This is now routinely performed to complete whole body staging prior to curative surgery. Careful patient selection is vital for radical surgery where morbidity and mortality are very high. It has the advantage of disclosing the presence of metastatic disease at occult sites in the body (e.g. peritoneal cavity) and can show foci of active cancer in abdominal lymph where CT can be equivocal or negative.

Endoscopic retrograde cholepancreaticogram (ERCP)

A side-viewing endoscope is passed into the duodenum allowing cannulation of the ampullary duct under direct vision. With an image intensifier, a cannula is advanced into the main pancreatic duct and contrast injected to opacify the pancreatic duct system and extra-hepatic biliary tree. Gallstones will appear as filling defects in the ducts while pancreatic carcinoma will lead to distortion and obstruction of the pancreatic ducts and extrinsic compression of the common bile duct. Duodenal and pancreatic aspirates collected through the endoscope can be sent for cytology.

Percutaneous transhepatic cholangiography (PTC)

A needle is passed through the skin into a dilated extrahepatic bile duct under ultrasound control and a cholangiogram obtained by injecting contrast into the biliary tree. It will visualize any gallstones in the biliary tree, and in the case of carcinoma confirm blockage of the common bile duct by extrinsic compression at the level of the pancreas.

Laparotomy

Occasionally, it is not possible to make a diagnosis from less invasive investigations. If there are no metastases detected during staging and the tumour is otherwise operable, laparotomy is justified with a view to radical surgery if frozen section is positive for malignancy.

Staging

The TNM system is widely used:

- Tis – Carcinoma in situ
- T0 – No evidence of primary
- TX – Primary cannot be assessed
- T1 – Limited to pancreas, 2 cm or less in greatest dimension
- T2 – Limited to pancreas, >2 cm in greatest dimension

- T3 – Direct invasion involving any of duodenum, bile duct, peripancreatic tissues
- T4 – Direct invasion involving any of stomach, spleen, colon, adjacent large vessels
- N0 – No regional lymphadenopathy
- N1 – Regional lymph nodes involved
- M0 – No distant metastases
- M1 – Distant metastases.

Treatment

Radical treatment

Pancreatic cancer is a condition where more effective management strategies are required. Very few advances have been made over the last decade and the prognosis remains poor. Such patients should therefore be recruited to clinical trial protocols whenever possible.

Surgery

This is the only potentially curative option. Patients must be carefully selected for radical surgery as only 10–20 per cent will be suitable candidates. Improvements in imaging technology, including spiral CT, MRI, positron emission tomography (PET), endoscopic ultrasound examination and laparoscopic staging can aid in the diagnosis and the identification of patients with disease that is not amenable to resection. The operation of choice was originally described by Whipple and comprises a pancreaticoduodenectomy, although this is associated with significant operative morbidity and mortality, even in the hands of surgeons regularly performing the operation. Contemporary variants include pylorus-sparing pancreaticoduodenectomy. For those patients with localized disease and small cancers (<2 cm) with no lymph node metastases and no extension beyond the capsule of the pancreas, complete surgical resection can yield actuarial 5-year survival rates of approximately 20 per cent.

Radiotherapy

Carcinoma of the pancreas is incurable using current radiotherapy techniques and doses owing to the high incidence of metastases at diagnosis, and the proximity of radiation dose-limiting normal tissues such as the spinal cord, small bowel and kidneys. Some of these issues can be overcome by delivering radiotherapy intraoperatively but even this has not made a significant impact on curability and survival. Newer radiotherapy techniques such as intensity-modulated radiotherapy (IMRT) could allow a higher dose delivery in the future. For the present, local recurrence remains a major problem with recurrence rates varying between 50 and 80 per cent. The only treatment that has been shown to reduce this is postoperative chemoradiotherapy (CRT) using 5FU, which is more effective than radiotherapy alone, but the problem of occult liver metastases is not adequately addressed with this approach and the start of treatment is invariably delayed by the recovery period after surgery. Preoperative CRT has the advantage of starting immediately following diagnosis and allowing greater selection for surgery pending the results of restaging of the local disease and liver after CRT. The optimum use of multimodality treatment is still a matter of debate and controversy.

Chemotherapy

Adjuvant chemotherapy using gemcitabine after potentially curative surgical resection nearly doubles the median disease-free survival to 13 months compared with 7 months for observation alone. Although there is only a small overall median survival advantage of 3 months, it is estimated that this may double 5-year survival to 21 per cent for gemcitabine-treated patients compared with 9 per cent for observation alone.

Palliative treatment

Surgery

Many patients are found at laparotomy to be inoperable. Rather than going on to perform an operation that stands no chance of prolonging the patient's survival, if the patient has obstructive jaundice or is at risk of developing it in the near future, surgeons should consider a bypass procedure (choledochojejunostomy) to allow free drainage of bile. Gastroenterostomy will relieve duodenal obstruction by a large peri-ampullary carcinoma.

Radiotherapy

This is of value for relieving pain from retroperitoneal tumour extension, but is not a satisfactory treatment for the relief of obstructive jaundice.

Chemotherapy

It may not be justified to treat patients with pancreatic carcinoma with chemotherapy as most patients will already have systemic symptoms, an impaired performance status and short life expectancy. The FAM (5FU, Adriamycin, mitomycin C) combination has been historically favoured. This was then superseded by single-agent gemcitabine. Recent data indicate that the combination of gemcitabine and capecitabine is superior to gemcitabine alone with a 1-year survival advantage of around 7 per cent (26 per cent versus 19 per cent). This is now considered to be a reasonable standard of care.

Hormone therapy

Initial in vitro experiments suggested the possible usefulness of hormone therapies. This stimulated clinical trials of tamoxifen. No significant advantage was proven with this approach.

Biological therapy

The orally delivered tyrosine kinase inhibitor erlotinib (Tarceva®) inhibits the intracellular pathways involved in cell signalling and, when combined with gemcitabine chemotherapy, yields a 7 per cent 1-year survival advantage in those with locally advanced or metastatic disease.

Medical treatment

Endoscopic placement of a bile duct stent helps to relieve obstructive jaundice. Cholestyramine can relieve the pruritus of intractable obstructive jaundice, while pancreatic enzyme supplements will relieve the steatorrhoea associated with the malabsorption of fats. Vitamin K administered intravenously is indicated if there is a symptomatic coagulopathy related to a deficiency of the vitamin K-dependent clotting factors. Coeliac axis nerve blocks can alleviate intractable pain.

CASE HISTORY: PANCREATIC CANCER

A previously fit 55-year-old man presents with dark urine, pale stools and jaundice. Liver function tests indicate a γ-glutamyl-transferase (GGT) of 670 U/L (normal <42) and alkaline phosphatase (ALP) of 725 U/L (normal range 38–126). The bilirubin is elevated at 90 µmol/L (normal range <17). Liver ultrasound suggests dilatation of the extrahepatic biliary tree, with enlargement of the head of the pancreas. An ERCP is performed and washings from the pancreatic duct confirm adenocarcinoma cells. CT imaging confirms a mass in the head of the pancreas with no evidence of metastatic disease elsewhere. This is confirmed by PET imaging. The CA19-9 is not elevated. He is referred to a hepatobiliary surgeon and undergoes a radical pancreatico-duodenectomy. Pathological examination of the surgical specimen confirms complete excision of a pancreatic adenocarcinoma. He is started on insulin for iatrogenic diabetes mellitus and pancreatic enzyme supplements. He expresses a wish to be treated as actively as possible so receives six cycles of postoperative adjuvant chemotherapy using single agent gemcitabine.

Two years later, he develops pain in the right upper quadrant of the abdomen. Liver ultrasound confirms multiple liver metastases. During this time, he develops swelling of the left leg and a Doppler ultrasound confirms a deep vein thrombosis. Despite anticoagulation with warfarin, 2 weeks later the toes on the right foot become painful, cold and discoloured. Arteriography confirms a popliteal artery thrombosis. This is managed conservatively; 24 hours later, before he can be considered for salvage chemotherapy, he dies of a sudden, massive pulmonary embolus from the coagulopathy induced by his cancer.

Tumour-related complications

There are a number of recognized vascular complications:

- renal vein thrombosis
- portal vein thrombosis
- splenic vein thrombosis
- thrombophlebitis migrans
- disseminated intravascular coagulation.

Renal vein thrombosis results in renal congestion and a nephrotic syndrome. Portal vein thrombosis leads to a Budd–Chiari syndrome, characterized by the rapid accumulation of ascites and hepatic congestion, while splenic vein thrombosis leads to portal hypertension and oesophageal varices. Thrombophlebitis migrans is characterized by intermittent bouts of tenderness, erythema and induration of superficial veins. Disseminated intravascular coagulation is due to mucin production by the tumour, which leads to an inappropriate activation of the clotting cascade (see Chapter 8).

Non-metastatic manifestations include:

- profound depression
- migratory thrombophlebitis
- hypercalcaemia (production of parathyroid hormone-like peptides)
- Cushing's syndrome (ACTH production)
- carcinoid syndrome (5-HT production)
- murantic endocarditis
- syndrome of metastatic fat necrosis.

Treatment-related complications

Surgery

Radical pancreaticoduodenectomy has an extremely high operative morbidity and mortality. The loss of exocrine and endocrine pancreatic secretions will lead to permanent diabetes mellitus requiring insulin and malabsorption of fat requiring enzyme supplements with each meal.

Radiotherapy

Radiotherapy to the pancreatic bed will result in temporary anorexia, nausea, vomiting, gastritis, colic and diarrhoea. Late complications are infrequently encountered owing to the extremely poor prognosis of the disease.

Prognosis

The outlook is extremely poor with a 5-year survival of less than 5 per cent. Of those undergoing radical surgery, there is a 5-year survival of about 10–20 per cent.

Rare tumours

Gastroenteropancreatic (GEP) neuroendocrine tumours

These comprise:

- carcinoid
- gastrinoma
- insulinoma
- glucagonoma
- VIPoma.

The pancreas is a rare site for *carcinoid* (see Chapter 14). Partial pancreatectomy will be curative unless there has been metastasis to the liver.

Gastrinoma is a gastrin-secreting tumour which leads to the Zollinger–Ellison syndrome, characterized by hypersecretion of acid in the stomach leading to intractable peptic ulceration. An elevated serum gastrin level is diagnostic and about two-thirds are malignant. It is sometimes associated with adenomata of the pituitary and parathyroid as part of multiple endocrine neoplasia type 1 (MEN 1). After detailed staging with a CT scan and selective venous angiography, the treatment of choice is a partial pancreatectomy.

Insulinoma arises from the beta cells of the islets and secretes insulin, leading to fasting hypoglycaemia. There is an association with MEN 1. Ninety per cent are benign and 10 per cent multiple. Treatment is surgical as for gastrinoma. Historically, diazoxide (a beta cell toxin) has been used to relieve the unremitting hypoglycaemia of advanced disease.

Glucagonoma from the alpha cells of the pancreas secretes glucagon, leading to a syndrome of diabetes mellitus, a migratory necrolytic erythema of the skin and stomatitis. Approximately half are malignant with metastases in the liver. Surgery is the treatment of choice.

VIPoma leads to Werner–Morrison syndrome characterized by severe watery diarrhoea and hypokalaemia. The majority are benign.

The somatostatin analogue octreotide can be radiolabelled and used as a useful tracer for whole body imaging. It therefore contributes to staging and predicts for response to octreotide when used therapeutically. Octreotide has shown considerable activity in GEP tumours and therefore has an important role in symptom relief and disease stabilization in advanced stages of disease.

HEPATOCELLULAR CANCER

This is synonymous with hepatoma.

Epidemiology

This is one of the most common tumours worldwide, but is comparatively rare in the UK. Each year in the UK there are 2900 cases of liver cancer, 1700 cases in men and 1200 cases in women, accounting for 1 per cent of all cancer cases and leading to a total of 3100 deaths per annum. It should be noted that worldwide, it is the fourth commonest cancer. The peak incidence in the developed countries is at 40–60 years compared with 20–40 years in endemic areas. There is a very high incidence in areas where hepatitis B is endemic such as West Africa and China.

Aetiology

The hepatitis B and C viruses are implicated, an observation supported by the geographical variation of hepatoma following that of areas where hepatitis B and C are endemic in the population. Hepatitis A and G are not implicated in the causation of hepatoma. Hepatoma often arises in a cirrhotic liver although the aetiological agent (e.g. alcohol, iron in haemochromatosis, autoantibodies in chronic active hepatitis) responsible for the cirrhosis is unimportant. Macronodular cirrhosis is a greater risk factor than micronodular, and males greatly outnumber females with this complication. Aflatoxin is a mycotoxin produced by the fungus *Aspergillus flavus*, which is found in stored cereals and is a hepatic carcinogen when ingested. Thorotrast was used historically as a radiographic contrast agent and contains a high level of the radioactive isotope thorium, which emits alpha particles, leading to intense irradiation of the liver which in turn may lead to hepatoma. Hepatoma has also been described in men following use of androgenic anabolic steroids for body building.

Pathology

The tumour grows rapidly, is usually large, arises from the liver parenchyma or a cirrhotic nodule and may be multifocal. In cut section there is bile staining, haemorrhage and necrosis. It invades through the liver capsule, along the hepatic ducts and blood vessels. Intrahepatic ducts proximal to the tumour will be obstructed and therefore dilated. The tumour is composed of hepatocytes which have lost the characteristic architecture of the portal tracts and frequently stain for α-fetoprotein (AFP).

Natural history

The tumour may remain confined to the liver, invading along the intrahepatic bile ducts and hepatic veins, or breach the liver capsule, leading to invasion of adjacent structures such as the hepatic veins, portal vein, inferior vena cava, right hemidiaphragm, right kidney, right adrenal, stomach and transverse colon. The hilar lymph nodes at the base of the liver and portal nodes are frequently involved.

The lungs are the most common site of distant metastases, although bone, skin and brain can also be involved. Spread beyond the liver capsule sometimes leads to diffuse peritoneal involvement which in turn can cause malignant ascites.

Symptoms

There is often a long history of increasing ill-health with hepatic pain owing to distension of the liver capsule which contains many stretch receptors. The onset of pain can be acute and severe if precipitated by a sudden haemorrhage into the tumour, which leads to its rapid enlargement. Swollen legs are a common complaint in advanced cases owing to a combination of hypoalbuminaemia and compression of the inferior vena cava. Systemic symptoms such as anorexia, nausea, weight loss, fever and malaise are frequent.

Signs

There might be evidence of an underlying cirrhosis such as clubbing, leukonychia, palmar erythema, jaundice, spider naevi, gynaecomastia, testicular atrophy, ascites, ankle oedema, dilated superficial abdominal wall veins and splenomegaly. Signs of hepatic encephalopathy are rare. The liver can be diffusely enlarged owing to cirrhosis, focally enlarged owing to the hepatoma or both. An arterial bruit and hepatic rub might be heard over the tumour owing to its rich vascular supply and capsular invasion, respectively.

Differential diagnosis

A poorly differentiated hepatoma can cause confusion with a carcinoma of unknown primary metastasizing to the liver. A high serum AFP or positive staining for AFP within a biopsy supports the diagnosis of hepatoma.

Investigations

Liver function tests, clotting parameters

Liver function derangement is common but more likely to be due to an underlying cirrhosis rather than the hepatoma itself. Assessment of clotting is necessary prior to liver biopsy or any invasive procedure.

Hepatitis serology

Serology for types A,B,C and D should be performed.

Serum α-fetoprotein

This is elevated in 90 per cent of cases. It is a useful diagnostic test, of value in monitoring response to therapy (especially surgery) and in predicting relapse.

Chest X-ray

This is mandatory prior to surgery to exclude pulmonary metastases, with a CT scan of the thorax if there is any suggestion of metastases from the plain radiographs.

Liver ultrasound and percutaneous biopsy

This localizes and measures the tumour, assesses the inferior vena cava and other large blood vessels for obstruction, and allows percutaneous biopsy under direct vision. A random biopsy of the contralateral lobe is desirable in patients for whom resection is planned.

Computed tomography (CT) of the liver and upper abdomen

This complements information obtained from abdominal ultrasound and facilitates percutaneous biopsy when the tumour is not adequately localized by ultrasound. Typically, it demonstrates a large necrotic filling defect in the liver (Fig. 9.6). It is also very useful for excluding invasion of the portal vein and/or hepatic veins. It is mandatory if surgery or radiotherapy is planned.

Magnetic resonance imaging (MRI) of liver

This can provide additional information for the surgeon regarding the tumour extent within the liver and thereby determine operability.

Laparoscopic biopsy

This is indicated if multiple percutaneous biopsies have failed to give a result.

Angiography

This will define the tumour precisely in terms of its size, position and vascular supply, and is mandatory prior to surgical resection or embolization. CT or MRI angiography is desirable.

Staging

The TNM system is widely used:

- Tis – Carcinoma in situ
- T0 – No evidence of primary
- TX – Primary cannot be assessed
- T1 – Solitary tumour 2 cm or less in greatest dimension without vascular invasion
- T2 – Solitary tumour 2 cm or less in greatest dimension with vascular invasion; or multiple tumours limited to one lobe, none >2 cm without vascular invasion; or solitary tumour >2 cm without vascular invasion
- T3 – Solitary tumour >2 cm in greatest dimension with vascular invasion; or multiple tumours limited to one lobe, none >2 cm with vascular invasion; or multiple tumours limited to one lobe, any >2 cm with or without vascular invasion
- T4 – Multiple tumours in more than one lobe; or tumour(s) involving a major branch of the portal or hepatic vein(s); or tumour(s) with direct invasion of adjacent organs other than gallbladder; or tumour(s) with perforation of visceral peritoneum
- N0 – No regional lymphadenopathy
- N1 – Regional lymph nodes involved
- M0 – No distant metastases
- M1 – Distant metastases.

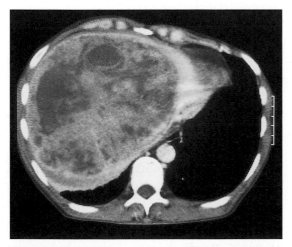

Figure 9.6 Hepatocellular carcinoma. CT image of the upper abdomen showing a very large, round, necrotic tumour arising from the substance of the liver.

Treatment

Radical treatment

Surgery

Up to 90 per cent of the liver can be resected as the remaining portion has a remarkable capacity for regeneration. Patients requiring very extensive surgery or those with cirrhosis could be considered for hepatectomy and liver transplantation. Meticulous preoperative staging is required whenever such surgery is planned.

Radiotherapy

High-dose radiotherapy with curative intent is impractical at this anatomical site and hepatoma is a tumour type that is relatively resistant to radiation.

Palliative treatment

Surgery

Hepatomas derive their blood supply from the hepatic artery and ligation of this vessel close to the liver can palliate local symptoms, particularly pain. The portal vein must be patent to prevent ischaemic necrosis of the liver and a cholecystectomy must be performed lest there be necrosis of the gallbladder. Mortality from this procedure is less than 5 per cent, but the response is short-lived owing to development of a collateral tumour circulation.

Radiotherapy

Low doses of radiation can be given with the expectation of relieving hepatic pain.

Radiofrequency ablation

This is a minimally invasive technique whereby the tumour is thermally ablated by alternating current radiofrequency using a probe implanted directly into the tumour. It is best suited to small, unifocal tumours. It may be preferred to surgery in those with severe background cirrhosis.

Chemotherapy

Adriamycin, 5FU and cisplatin are the most active agents. The advent of other drugs effective in the management of other gastrointestinal malignancies has increased the treatment options although response rates remain low (typically <25 per cent). Regional chemotherapy delivered via the hepatic artery, either as infusions of drugs or as embolism microspheres, is used in some specialist centres.

Biological therapies

Sorafenib (Nexavar®) is a multikinase inhibitor, which decreases cell growth and angiogenesis. It increases median survival to 11 months compared with 8 months for those treated by placebo. The commonest side-effects are diarrhoea, hand–foot syndrome and fatigue.

Hepatic artery embolization

This is less invasive than ligation of the artery, and has a longer symptomatic response, as the collateral circulation develops more slowly, and it is also anatomically more selective. Unlike ligation, it can be repeated when symptoms recur. Responses of up to 50 per cent are seen.

Percutaneous ethanol injection (PEI)

This is an effective chemical means of inducing tumour necrosis in small tumours. It is relatively free of serious toxicity.

Tumour-related complications

A number of non-metastatic manifestations are recognized including:

- hypoglycaemia (insulin-like peptides)
- polycythaemia (erythropoietin-like peptides)
- hypercalcaemia (parathyroid hormone-like peptides)
- feminization (oestrogens)
- pyrexia of unknown origin (pyrogens)
- porphyria cutanea tarda (porphyrins).

Portal vein thrombosis will lead to splenomegaly, ascites and oesophageal varices, while hepatic vein thrombosis will lead to a Budd–Chiari syndrome with ascites, hepatomegaly and leg oedema. Inferior vena cava obstruction will lead to oedema below the umbilicus. Sudden haemorrhage can occur into the tumour causing acute right upper abdominal pain, or into the abdomen causing abdominal pain and distension, which may lead to death.

Treatment-related complications

Surgery

Partial hepatectomy can lead to hepatic decompensation if the function of the remaining liver is poor. Transplant patients will also have the problems of rejection and chronic immunosuppression to overcome.

Radiotherapy

Hepatic irradiation invariably causes anorexia, nausea and vomiting during treatment, and radiation hepatitis can result when a large volume of liver has been irradiated.

Hepatic artery embolization

Ectopic embolic phenomena can lead to infarction of other abdominal viscera.

Prognosis

Untreated, median survival is around 8 months. Surgery is the only potentially curative treatment and even after liver transplantation for carefully selected patients, less than 20 per cent will have long-term disease-free survival. Sorafenib is the only systemic therapy thus far to improve survival.

Prevention

Vaccination against hepatitis B is a sensible strategy. Health education and improved food storage to avoid contamination with aflatoxin might decrease the incidence of hepatoma in endemic areas.

Screening

Measurements of α-fetoprotein and liver ultrasound are probably the most sensitive investigations for screening and detecting hepatoma while it is operable. High-risk populations would include hepatitis B surface antigen-positive individuals with cirrhosis or other conditions where the risk of hepatoma is very high (e.g. haemochromatosis).

Rare tumours

Angiosarcoma

This is very rare and associated with medical exposure to thorotrast and industrial exposure to vinyl chloride monomer.

CHOLANGIOCARCINOMA

This is a malignant tumour arising from the epithelium lining the extrahepatic biliary tract.

Epidemiology

This is rare in developed countries. For example, in the UK there are fewer than 1000 new cases and 300 deaths registered per annum. It is about half as common as carcinoma of the gallbladder. The peak age incidence is 50–70 years and there is a slight female predominance. It is more common in areas where liver flukes are endemic, e.g. South East Asia.

Aetiology

Recognized associations include:

- liver flukes, e.g. *Clonorchis sinensis*
- primary sclerosing cholangitis – a rare complication of chronic ulcerative colitis
- chronic infective cholangitis secondary to gallstones
- radiation – previous use of thorotrast contrast medium (of historical significance only)
- congenital biliary abnormalities, e.g. choledochal cyst.

Pathology

Tumours of the upper third of the extrahepatic biliary tree tend to be diffusely sclerosing leading to a malignant stricture. Tumours in the middle third tend to be nodular while those in the lower third tend to be papillary. The tumour is usually a well-differentiated mucin-secreting adenocarcinoma with about half staining for carcinoembryonic antigen (CEA).

Natural history

Tumours of the upper third can infiltrate the liver, while those of the lower third can infiltrate the duodenum and pancreas. Tumours also spread to the hilar, superior mesenteric and coeliac lymph nodes. The liver is the most common site of distant metastases, although lung and bone may also be involved.

Symptoms

The most common presentation is with obstructive jaundice, pruritus, dark urine and pale stools. Recurrent cholangitis from subacute biliary tract obstruction also occurs.

Signs

The patient will be jaundiced, the gallbladder may be palpable (positive Courvoisier's sign) and the liver congested and therefore smoothly enlarged.

Differential diagnosis

Other causes of obstructive jaundice include:

- gallstones
- carcinoma of the head of the pancreas
- carcinoma of the ampulla of Vater
- benign biliary tract stricture following surgical trauma
- sclerosing cholangitis
- lymph node metastases at the porta hepatis.

Investigations

Endoscopic retrograde cholepancreaticogram (ERCP)

This is the investigation of choice as it will allow an accurate anatomical localization of the tumour, brushings and biliary aspirates for cytology, and therapeutic manoeuvres such as passage of a stent to relieve jaundice.

Percutaneous transhepatic cholangiogram (PTC)

This is indicated when ERCP has failed to opacify the biliary tree or adequately display the tumour owing to its position.

CT scan of the upper abdomen

This will show the degree of local invasion, any enlarged regional lymph nodes and exclude liver metastases.

Staging

The TNM staging is used for tumours of the extrahepatic ducts:

- Tis – Carcinoma in situ
- T0 – No evidence of primary tumour
- TX – Primary tumour cannot be assessed
- T1 – Tumour invades subepithelial connective tissue or fibromuscular layer
  - T1a – Tumour invades subepithelial connective tissue
  - T1b – Tumour invades fibromuscular layer
- T2 – Tumour invades perifibromuscular connective tissue
- T3 – Tumour invades adjacent structures: liver, pancreas, duodenum, gallbladder, colon, stomach
- NX – Regional lymph nodes cannot be assessed
- N0 – No regional lymph node metastasis
- N1 – Metastasis in cystic duct, pericholedochal and/or hilar lymph nodes (i.e. in the hepatoduodenal ligament)
- N2 – Metastasis in peripancreatic (head only), periduodenal, periportal, coeliac, and/or superior mesenteric and/or posterior pancreaticoduodenal lymph nodes
- MX – Presence of distant metastasis cannot be assessed
- M0 – No distant metastasis
- M1 – Distant metastasis.

Treatment

Radical treatment

As this is a very rare tumour, the optimum management with surgery and/or radiotherapy is undetermined.

Surgery

This offers the best chance of cure although only 10–20 per cent will be resectable. The optimum surgical procedure for carcinoma of the extrahepatic bile duct will vary according to its location along the biliary tree, the extent of hepatic parenchymal involvement, and the proximity of the tumour to major blood vessels in this region. Distal tumours are more likely to be resectable than proximal ones. Tumours of the lower third require pancreaticoduodenectomy, while those with more proximal lesions may be carefully staged and selected for hepatic lobectomy or liver transplantation.

Radiotherapy

This tumour is rarely cured by radiotherapy. The difficulties of giving high-dose irradiation to this region are lessened by the use of interstitial brachytherapy for localized strictures. A nasobiliary tube is inserted at ERCP or a percutaneous tube inserted under ultrasound control, and an iridium-192 source is passed down this conduit using either a wire straddling the tumour for 5–7 days or a high-dose rate afterloading technique fractionated over several treatments. Tumours with extraductal invasion are best treated with external beam irradiation and a brachytherapy boost.

Palliative treatment

Surgery

Choledochojejunostomy will relieve obstructive jaundice in cases not amenable to endoscopic or percutaneous stenting. Cholecystectomy should be considered to prevent the possibility of an acute cholecystitis.

Radiotherapy

This is best reserved for palliating pain from local infiltration.

Chemotherapy

This can be considered only within clinical trial protocols. Cisplatin and 5FU are the most active agents tested. Bearing in mind the success of chemoradiotherapy at other gastro-intestinal sites, this is an option that deserves further study.

Tumour-related complications

These include:

- acute cholangitis, which presents with fever, rigors and right upper abdominal pain and usually responds to broad-spectrum antibiotics
- secondary biliary cirrhosis, which is caused by chronic cholestasis.

Treatment-related complications

Surgery

The bile duct is a delicate structure prone to stricturing after handling. Biliary fistulae are also a problem after anastomosis.

Radiotherapy

Insertion of a nasobiliary tube and the iridium wire carries a high risk of cholangitis. External beam irradiation carries the same morbidity as outlined for stomach cancer.

Prognosis

The mean survival in untreated cases is only 3 months. Palliative biliary drainage increases this to 9 months while radical radiotherapy gives 2-year survivals of 10–20 per cent.

CARCINOMA OF THE GALLBLADDER

This is the commonest biliary tract tumour but a rare tumour in developed countries. Each year in the UK there are 600 cases of gallbladder cancer, 400 cases in women and 200 cases in men, accounting for 0.2 per cent of all cancer cases and leading to a total of 400 deaths per annum. In developed countries it has a peak age incidence of 60–80 years. Aetiological factors include:

- gallstones – 0.5–1 per cent of cholecystectomies performed for cholelithiasis will yield an occult carcinoma of the gallbladder
- typhoid carriage – there is a greatly increased risk owing to carriage of the

Salmonella typhi bacterium in the gallbladder, which in turn leads to a chronic cholecystitis
- working in rubber plants
- large gallbladder polyps
- choledochal cysts and other biliary tract anatomical anomalies.

Many patients are diagnosed incidentally at cholecystectomy and are asymptomatic with no physical signs. Otherwise the presentation resembles benign gallbladder disease with bouts of acute cholecystitis or more chronic and less severe right upper abdominal pain where a mass could be palpable. Eighty per cent arise at the fundus or neck of the gallbladder and 90 per cent are adenocarcinomas. The adjacent liver capsule and parenchyma are involved early and there can be lymphatic spread to the hilar nodes around the liver. The liver and lungs are the most common sites for blood-borne metastases.

Staging investigations include liver function tests, chest X-ray, liver ultrasound and a CT/MRI scan of the upper abdomen.

Treatment comprises cholecystectomy with a wide excision of the surrounding liver, excision of the extrahepatic bile duct and regional lymph node dissection. Low-dose radiotherapy can be of value in relieving pain from local infiltration, and a biliary drainage procedure will palliate biliary obstruction. In those with superficial involvement of the mucosa, the disease might be cured with cholecystectomy alone. Of those with liver involvement, 50 per cent die within 3 months of diagnosis and less than 5 per cent survive 1 year. As one would expect for a rare tumour, chemotherapy and radiotherapy strategies are far less well developed. 5FU is the most established agent with activity in this disease.

CARCINOMA OF THE COLON AND RECTUM

The colon and rectum are parts of the large bowel located in the abdomen and pelvis and are in continuity with each other. The colon acts as a site of water absorption, turning the liquid effluent from the small bowel into solid stool. The more distal rectum acts as a reservoir for this stool prior to its evacuation through the anus.

Epidemiology

Each year in the UK there are 36 000 cases of colorectal cancer, 22 000 cases in men and 16 000 cases in women, making it the third commonest form of cancer; it accounts for 12.7 per cent of all cancer cases and leads to a total of 16 000 deaths per annum. Colon cancer accounts for 22 000 of these, with a male to female ratio of 1:1. Rectal cancer accounts for 14 000 of these, with a male to female ratio of 3:2. The vast majority occur in the over 50 age group, the peak age incidence being 60–80 years. There has been a recent trend towards more right colonic tumours, which could reflect surveillence programmes that have decreased the incidence of left-sided cancers. Colon cancer is commonest in social classes I and II. There is no social class trend for rectal cancer. It is predominantly a disease of the developed world, being most common in New Zealand, Canada, USA and UK while rare in Africa and Asia.

Aetiology

Diet could account for the marked geographical variation in incidence. This is presumed to be due to changes in the bowel flora, which produce carcinogens from ingested food, the effect being exacerbated by the slower bowel transit time seen in people taking a low-fibre diet. The incidence has increased in Japan as a Western style diet has been adopted, and Japanese migrants to the West have subsequently acquired the risk of the indigenous population. Important dietary factors include:

- high meat consumption
- high total fat consumption
- high calorific intake
- high alcohol intake.

Individuals with an affected first-degree relative have a 2–3 fold increased risk of developing colorectal cancer themselves, the lifetime risk rising from 4 to 9 per cent. Cancer develops around a decade earlier in such individuals. This risk is higher if the index case is diagnosed at under 45 years of age. If two first-degree relatives have had the disease, the risk rises 4–5-fold to 16 per cent.

Hereditary non-polyposis colon cancer (HNPCC) accounts for 20 per cent of cases and is synonymous with Lynch syndrome. This is a dominantly inherited condition, i.e. there is a 50 per cent chance of inheriting the mutated DNA mismatch repair gene from an affected parent. Such families often have three or more cases of colon cancer. Unlike familial adenomatous polyposis (FAP), there are no characteristic extracolonic physical signs and there is no propensity to develop a multitude of polyps. Colon cancer on average develops at 40 years of age. Cancers other than just colonic ones are associated. Families can be divided into syndromes I and II. In Lynch syndrome I, the cancers are mainly gastrointestinal. In Lynch syndrome II, endometrial and ovarian cancers may arise at a young age.

FAP is a rare, dominantly inherited condition, i.e. there is a 50 per cent chance of inheriting the mutated *APC* tumour-suppressor gene from an affected parent. The *APC* gene is located on chromosome 5q21. It has a prevalence of 1 in 10 000 births. There are characteristic physical signs to indicate a gene carrier, e.g. congenital hypertrophy of the retinal pigment epithelium (CHRPE), osteomas of the jaw, prepuberty epidermoid cysts. Affected individuals develop multiple (>100) benign polyps from a very young age (puberty). Inevitably, over the subsequent years, one or more of these polyps will transform into a cancer, usually during the third and fourth decades, 20–30 years before the general population. The risk for colorectal cancer is estimated at 90 per cent by age 45 years. Prophylactic surgical excision of the colon and rectum is advised in young adults. Upper gastrointestinal malignancy (usually duodenal) will also develop in 5 per cent and benign desmoid tumours in 10 per cent. The latter can arise within the abdomen and may prove fatal owing to relentless local spread.

Gardener's syndrome is similar to familial polyposis coli but characterized by skeletal and cutaneous abnormalities, e.g. osteomas of the mandible and skull, sebaceous cysts, dermoid cysts.

Peutz–Jeghers syndrome is dominantly inherited and caused by a mutation in the *STK11* tumour-suppressor gene located on chromosome 19p13. It is characterized by the development of multiple bowel hamartomas and an increased risk of colon cancer. The risk for colorectal cancer is estimated at 40 per cent by age 70 years.

Turcot's syndrome is associated with the development of multiple benign adenomas but to a lesser degree than FAP. It presents during childhood with brain tumours, usually astrocytomas. Such patients have a high incidence of leukaemia after radiotherapy. Cowden's syndrome is due to a mutated *PTEN* gene and is also an inherited risk factor for colorectal cancer. Chronic inflammation of the bowel is a rare cause. In the case of ulcerative colitis, the increased risk is related to both the extent and duration of the colitis. Those with disease extending beyond the splenic flexure and/or of more than 10 years' duration are at greatest risk. Chronic Crohn's colitis also confers an increased risk of colorectal cancer. Tobacco smoking is associated with an increased risk of polyps and increased rate of recurrence after excision of polyps. Interestingly, use of hormone replacement therapy appears protective for women.

Pathology

One-third arise in the rectum or rectosigmoid, one-quarter in the sigmoid colon and one-tenth at the caecum. The rest are evenly distributed along the large bowel, two-thirds arising on the left side. Most cancers represent malignant change in a benign adenomatous polyp (e.g. tubular, tubulovillous and villous), the highest risk being from villous adenomas, especially those greater than 2 cm. The tumour may be nodular, ulcerating or diffusely infiltrating, and multiple primaries are found in approximately 5 per cent. The vast majority are adenocarcinomas (85 per cent glandular, 15 per cent mucinous, 2 per cent signet ring), usually well differentiated, and may show evidence of a preceding benign adenomatous polyp. The tumour cells frequently stain for carcinoembryonic antigen (CEA) and CK20.

Natural history

The tumour spreads longitudinally and circumferentially along the mucosa, in some cases leading to obstruction of the bowel lumen, and invades deep to the mucosa to infiltrate the muscular wall of the bowel and serosa. Penetration of the serosa leads to direct infiltration of the surrounding abdominal and pelvic viscera, while submucosal spread in the lamina propria can lead to skip lesions well away from the primary tumour. Tumour cells have a propensity to seed in abdominal scars, perineal skin (Fig. 9.7), stomas and even anal fissures. Transcoelomic spread may lead to diffuse peritoneal involvement resulting in ascites and spread to the ovaries. The regional (mesenteric) lymph nodes can be involved, the likelihood of lymph node metastases increasing with the depth of bowel wall invasion. The tumour spreads to the liver (Fig. 9.8) via the portal circulation, and from there to the lungs, bone, brain and skin. Rectal cancer has a particular propensity for local recurrence and often this leads to a presacral mass (Fig. 9.9).

Symptoms

The tumour most commonly presents with symptoms referable to the large bowel, 20 per cent presenting as a surgical emergency with acute bowel obstruction or peritonitis owing to perforation. In the remainder there is usually a history of one or more of the following:

- change in bowel habit
- blood per rectum
- mucus per rectum
- tenesmus
- obstructive symptoms
- iron-deficiency anaemia.

A change in bowel habit is often the presenting symptom with an increase or decrease in

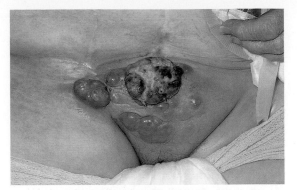

Figure 9.7 Perineal spread from rectal cancer.

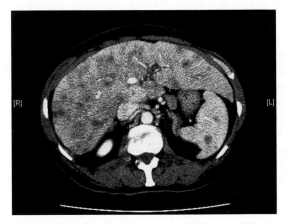

Figure 9.8 Multiple liver metastases. CT image of the upper abdomen in a patient with colon cancer showing multiple, well circumscribed, hypodense lesions in both lobes of the liver. Note that there is also spread to the spleen.

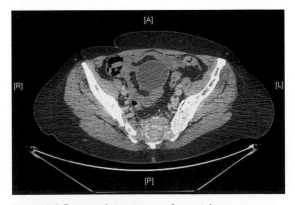

Figure 9.9 Presacral recurrence of a rectal cancer. Transverse pelvic CT image.

frequency of defaecation or a change in stool consistency. Alternating diarrhoea and constipation is highly suspicious of cancer. Blood per rectum is another symptom that leads patients to seek medical advice. It varies in quantity depending on degree of tumour ulceration and/or vascularity. The blood will be bright red and more likely streaked on the outside of the stool if the tumour arises in the rectum or sigmoid, or dark red and mixed in with the stool if the tumour arises more proximally in the colon. Mucus per rectum is more likely to be noticed with distal lesions, particularly those of a mucinous variety. Tenesmus is a frequent urge to defaecate but leading to the passage of a little stool on each occasion and lack of the feeling of complete rectal emptying. This is usually seen in rectal tumours, particularly if bulky or invading deeply. Obstructive symptoms can manifest as intermittent colicky abdominal pain. They are more common in tumours of the descending colon where the faeces are more solid compared with right colon tumours where the stool is more liquid. Chronic bleeding leads to iron deficiency and in turn anaemia. It is a particular feature of right-sided colonic tumours, which have few associated gastrointestinal symptoms.

Signs

The primary tumour may be palpable by digital examination of the rectum as a circumscribed area of mucosal induration, often with irregular heaped-up margins and a friable ulcer base, which bleeds on contact. Proximal tumours may be palpable in the pouch of Douglas per vaginam, and caecal tumours by abdominal examination. Signs indicative of spread outside the pelvis include:

- Troisier's sign owing to enlargement of Virchow's lymph node in the left supraclavicular fossa; this is uncommon at presentation and heralds a poor outcome from the disease
- ascites indicating peritoneal involvement
- hepatomegaly suggesting possible liver metastases.

Rarely, locally advanced disease in the pelvis can lead to formation of a fistula between the adjacent bladder (colovesical – suggested by faecal debris in the urine or pneumaturia) or vagina (colovaginal – suggested by leakage of faeces per vaginam).

Investigations

Digital examination of the rectum/vagina

This permits evaluation of the site, size and extent of local invasion of tumours of the rectum. A normal digital examination does not exclude the diagnosis of rectal cancer.

Proctoscopy and sigmoidoscopy

This is mandatory for tumours of the distal 25 cm of the large bowel, as it allows an accurate assessment of the tumour size, extent and distance from the anal verge and permits biopsy to obtain a tissue diagnosis.

Double contrast barium enema

This is a very sensitive and specific investigation which can detect tumours 1 cm or more and should be performed in all cases. It allows rapid assessment of the large bowel from the rectum to the caecum and can detect synchronous primaries or benign polyps elsewhere. Circumferential tumours give rise to a characteristic 'apple core' stricture.

Flexible sigmoidoscopy

This visualizes tumours of the distal 50–60 cm of the large bowel and is better tolerated than colonoscopy for biopsy of such lesions.

Colonoscopy

This facilitates a detailed survey of the whole large bowel, is more sensitive than a barium enema and is useful for biopsy of tumours of the transverse and ascending colon. It is the best way of excluding a synchronous primary cancer or polyp elsewhere in the large bowel.

Computed tomography (CT)

CT of the thorax/abdomen/pelvis is mandatory to delineate locoregional extent of tumour and exclude hepatic and/or pulmonary metastases.

Endorectal ultrasound or magnetic resonance imaging (MRI)

These are particularly useful for delineating the extent of a low rectal tumour in relation to the sphincters (Fig. 9.10) and aid surgical planning.

Staging

The clinicopathological staging according to Dukes is the best known staging system:

- Stage A – Confined to the bowel wall and has not penetrated its full thickness
- Stage B – Tumour has breached the bowel wall
- Stage C – Regional lymph node involvement
- Stage D – Distant metastases.

There are a number of variants in clinical use. An alternative is the TNM system:

- Tis – Carcinoma in situ
- T0 – No evidence of primary
- TX – Primary cannot be assessed
- T1 – Involving submucosa
- T2 – Involving muscularis propria
- T3 – Involving subserosa, non-peritonealized pericolic/perirectal tissues
- T4 – Other organs/structures/visceral peritoneum
- N0 – No regional lymphadenopathy
- N1 – 3 or fewer pericolic/perirectal lymph nodes
- N2 – >3 pericolic/perirectal lymph nodes
- N3 – Nodes on named vascular trunk/apical node(s)
- M0 – No distant metastases
- M1 – Distant metastases.

Management

Radical treatment

Surgery

This is the only curative treatment modality; 80 per cent of all tumours are resectable. Prior to resection of the primary tumour, a detailed inspection and palpation of the open abdomen and pelvis is performed to document the exact

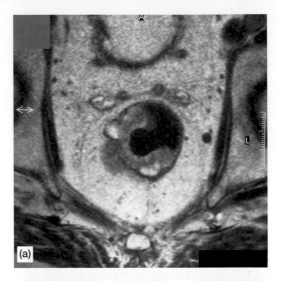

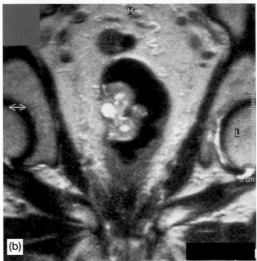

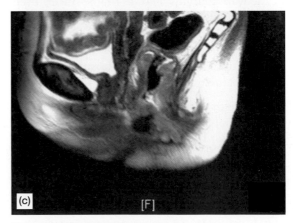

Figure 9.10 Rectal carcinoma. Staging MRIs. (a) Transverse view. (b) Coronal view. (c) Sagittal view.

extent of disease, with special reference to the liver, and suspicious tissues should be biopsied if not part of the main resection. The ovaries should be checked in women as they represent a potential site of spread.

Tumours of the colon are treated by hemicolectomy with either immediate reanastomosis (usual) or formation of a temporary colostomy, which can be closed at a later date. Some surgeons ligate the vascular pedicle prior to mobilization of the tumour to try to prevent vascular dissemination of tumour. Laparoscopic-assisted colectomy is associated with more rapid recovery and reduced hospital stays.

Rectal cancer surgery is difficult and technically challenging owing to the relative inaccessibility of the rectum. The usual operation is an anterior resection. This can be associated with a high risk of local recurrence of up to 30 per cent in some series, mainly owing to the problems involved in balancing morbidity from surgery against the need to attain an adequate cuff of normal tissue around the tumour-bearing tissue, and to some extent variations in surgical skill. In recent years, there has been much interest in the total mesorectal excision (TME). This involves a meticulous circumferential surgical excision down the avascular plane between the mesorectum and the pelvic side wall. In those patients where a clear circumferential resection margin (CRM) is attained following TME, the risk of local recurrence is far lower than when the CRM is involved:

- Dukes B CRM – : <5 per cent local recurrence at 5 years
- Dukes B CRM + : 60 per cent local recurrence at 5 years
- Dukes C CRM – : 25 per cent local recurrence at 5 years
- Dukes C CRM + : 85 per cent local recurrence at 5 years.

Abdominoperineal resection may be required for the lowest rectal tumours, but in many cases can be avoided with current surgical techniques. In each case, the mesentery containing the regional lymph nodes is also resected.

Advances in laparoscopic techniques and robotic surgery have made such refinements available to patients with colorectal cancer. Although more costly with prolonged operating times, they offer the advantage of less perioperative blood loss, reduced postoperative pain and ileus, and more rapid postoperative recovery times. The long-term surgical oncology outcomes are awaited.

Radiotherapy

Radiotherapy has little role in the curative treatment of colon cancer. This is due to:

- local recurrence not being a major cause of relapse
- the difficulty in accurately determining the volume to be irradiated
- the proximity of a number of organs at risk limits the dose of radiation that can be delivered.

Conversely, rectal cancer has a higher risk of recurrence owing to the technical difficulties and anatomical challenges faced by the surgeon. The volume to be irradiated is also far easier to define and there are fewer dose limiting organs at risk in the lower pelvis.

Preoperative radiotherapy might be of use in rectal cancer for converting an inoperable or partly fixed tumour to one that is operable, and thereby offer a chance of a curative approach to treatment. Despite the use of only moderate doses of radiation (e.g. 25 Gy in 5 fractions on consecutive days), and surgery within a short time after completing radiotherapy, there is a surprisingly large reduction in the odds of recurrence of rectal cancer (approximately 60 per cent), reducing the absolute risk of recurrence from 20 per cent down to less than 10 per cent. A meta-analysis of individual studies suggests a significant survival advantage with a reduction in the odds of dying of rectal cancer of approximately 20 per cent, equivalent approximately to 7 per cent in absolute survival benefit. Preoperative short course radiotherapy is thus considered by many to be the standard of care for all stages of disease. However, some of this benefit is offset by an increase in mortality from non-cancer causes within 1 year of receiving radiotherapy. It should also be noted that many of the trials of preoperative radiotherapy were conducted in an era before TME surgery was widely performed.

Postoperative radiotherapy to the region of the primary tumour decreases the odds of local recurrence in carcinoma of the rectum by approximately 40 per cent, reducing the absolute risk of recurrence by 5 per cent from 15–20 per cent to 10–15 per cent. There is, however, in contrast to preoperative radiotherapy, no statistically significant benefit in terms of a survival advantage. In practice, postoperative radiotherapy is reserved for those deemed to be at high risk for local recurrence e.g. T4 cancers with invasion of adjacent pelvic viscera, involved CRM. Evidence is emerging that synchronous chemoradiotherapy (CRT) may be of value in high-risk rectal cancers. Typically, radiotherapy is used synchronously with 5FU, applying a dose reduction during radiotherapy to limit additive toxicity.

Radiation given with curative intent in inoperable cases is limited by the close proximity to radiosensitive normal tissues, which makes it very difficult to give a tumoricidal dose and the fact that colorectal cancer is not particularly radiosensitive. There is also a high incidence of occult metastases in this group, which limits the treatment outcome.

Chemotherapy

Despite an 80 per cent resection rate, almost half Dukes C stage patients will have a relapse of their disease in the liver, usually within 2 years of surgery. Much effort has therefore been put into assessing the role of adjuvant chemotherapy to eradicate the micrometastases shed from the tumour prior to or during its resection. Chemotherapy has a role in the adjuvant therapy of both colonic and rectal cancers.

Historically, the most utilized chemotherapy agent in colorectal cancer is 5FU with response rates of 15–25 per cent in metastatic disease. Improved response rates can be seen when 5FU is 'modulated' by combining it with calcium leucovorin (folinic acid) which enhances the inhibition of the enzyme thymidylate synthetase required by the cancer cells to produce DNA. 5FU has therefore formed the backbone of adjuvant chemotherapy in the modern era.

Patients who have had surgery for Dukes C tumours benefit from 6 months' adjuvant therapy with 5FU/folinic acid chemotherapy. This strategy will yield an absolute reduction in mortality of approximately 6 per cent at 5 years. The issue of adjuvant chemotherapy for Dukes B disease is less clear. There is a significant survival benefit for Dukes B patients but it is smaller in magnitude than for Dukes C patients, perhaps amounting to a 2–3 per cent absolute survival benefit at 5 years. It is likely that recent trials have been underpowered to detect such an advantage owing to the small numbers of Dukes B patients included in clinical trials. It is standard practice to offer adjuvant chemotherapy to patients with Dukes C tumours and those with selected (higher risk) Dukes B tumours, e.g. those with T4 cancers, presentation with obstruction or perforation, venous invasion, inadequate lymph node sampling.

Bolus 5FU and folinic acid is a simple regime. Delivered weekly or 4 weekly for 6 months, it produces relatively little toxicity. The main side-effects are stomatitis, diarrhoea and myelosuppression. There is no evidence that high-dose folinic acid confers any advantage over a low dose, which is far more cost-effective. It is now common practice for capecitabine (Xeloda®) to be used as a substitute for 5FU, as it is orally administered thus lessening the burden on the patient as well as the oncology chemotherapy administration clinic. Capecitabine is at least as effective as 5FU/folinic acid with lower frequencies of alopecia, severe mucositis and neutropenia. In recent years, oxaliplatin (Eloxatin®) has been combined with 5FU/folinic acid at a dose of 85 mg/m² delivered every 2 weeks for 6 months as standard adjuvant therapy, as combination therapy has been shown to decrease the relapse rate, although the data are too immature to show a significant overall survival advantage. Peripheral neuropathy is the most siginificant toxicity.

Palliative treatment

Meta-analysis of the randomized trials addressing active treatment versus best supportive care shows an unequivocal advantage to a pro-active approach. Active treatment yields a 35 per cent mortality reduction, equivalent to a 16 per cent 1-year absolute improvement in survival, and improvement in median survival from 8 months for best supportive care to 12 months for active treatment. These benefits are independent of the age of the patient.

Surgery

If the tumour is inoperable, a bypass procedure or defunctioning colostomy may be of value in alleviating symptoms. In the case of those with liver metastases, it is well worth undertaking further investigations to assess the patient with respect to their suitability for partial hepatic resection. A CT or preferably PET scan should be undertaken to exclude local recurrence at the site of the original primary tumour and extrahepatic disease. The hepatic disease can be assessed by MRI and MR angiography. Preoperative laparoscopy will define a small group who will be inoperable owing to peritoneal dissemination not visualized by imaging. In those with inoperable isolated liver relapse, effort should be directed to downstaging hepatic metastatic disease with chemotherapy to make it potentially operable. Of those selected individuals undergoing potentially curative excisions of all tumour-bearing liver, approximately one in three will survive 5 years and one in four will survive 10 years. This contrasts with a 5-year survival of not more than 5 per cent for inoperable cases.

Radiotherapy

This is of benefit in inoperable disease, local recurrence after surgery and symptomatic metastases. It is very effective in relieving bleeding, mucorrhoea and local pain, with response rates of about 75 per cent. Symptomatic presacral recurrence is a particular problem after surgery and can be helped greatly by radiotherapy. In an era where more patients will have received preoperative radiotherapy, re-treatment of the pelvis poses a dilemma for the oncologist.

Chemotherapy

Those developing metastatic disease are best treated actively. Comparisons of best supportive care versus immediate 5FU chemotherapy indicate a doubling in survival for the more proactive approach.

For the palliation of metastatic disease, PVI 5FU produces superior response rates to bolus doses (23 versus 11 per cent). Addition of leucovorin to bolus 5FU also improves the response rate (23 versus 13 per cent). Addition of mitomycin C delivered 6 weekly also improves response rates of PVI 5FU. Another strategy is to 'chronomodulate' 5FU to exploit circadian variations in its metabolism. This entails infusing 5FU for 12 hours overnight. Meta-analysis of trials of hepatic arterial infusion (HAI) of 5FU versus bolus 5FU delivered into a peripheral vein indicates superior response rates for HAI (42 versus 14 per cent).

Despite these many strategies, one of the most favoured is the de Gramont regimen, which is a hybrid of infused and bolus 5FU with high-dose folinic acid modulation, combining all of these approaches and highly active in metastatic disease:

- 200 mg/m^2 folinic acid as a 2-hour infusion on days 1 and 2
- 5FU 400 mg/m^2 as i.v. bolus on days 1 and 2
- 5FU infusion 600 mg/m^2 over 22 hours on days 1 and 2
- repeated every 2 weeks.

Irinotecan (CPT 11) is an active agent and is combined with 5FU/folinic acid for the first-line treatment of metastatic colorectal cancer. It is also used as monotherapy for metastatic disease that has been proven to be refractory to 5FU. The recommended dose of irinotecan for first-line combination therapy is 180 mg/m^2 given once every 2 weeks as an intravenous infusion, administered over 30–90 minutes and followed by an infusion of 5FU/FA. For second-line monotherapy, the recommended dose is 350 mg/m^2 given every 3 weeks, administered over 30–90 minutes. The main toxicities are acute cholinergic symptoms, diarrhoea, alopecia and myelosuppression. The addition of irinotecan to 5FU increases response rates by about 20 per cent and improves median overall survival by 2–3 months compared with 5FU alone.

Oxaliplatin is a water-soluble platinum derivitive that prevents DNA replication, and hence cell division, by cross-linking DNA. It is highly active in colorectal cancer. The recommended dose for oxaliplatin is 85 mg/m^2 when given in combination with 5FU/FA. It is administered as an intravenous infusion over 2–6 hours every 2 weeks and followed by an infusion of 5FU/FA. Prime toxicities are peripheral neuropathy and myelosuppression, with fewer gastrointestinal side-effects than with irinotecan. The addition of oxaliplatin to 5FU increases response rates by about 30 per cent and improves median progression-free survival by 3 months compared with 5FU alone. Unlike the irinotecan experience, no overall survival advantage is gained with this approach.

Studies comparing these two combination regimens and their sequencing show little advantage with median survival consistently around 15 months. However, there is some evidence to suggest that the higher response rates from oxaliplatin/5FU may be more useful in downstaging hepatic disease to render it resectable.

Capecitabine is an oral formulation of a 5FU-like prodrug that is converted into the active cytotoxic agent by an enzyme (thymidine phosphorylase – TP) found at high concentration within malignant cells. It is given at a dose of 2500 mg/m^2 daily in two divided doses for 14 days followed by a 1-week period of rest before the next cycle begins. Apart from some potential therapeutic gain in sparing normal cells and being preferentially activated within tumour tissue, it has the convenience of being easy to administer. Preliminary data suggest superiority with standard 5FU (26 per cent response rate versus 17 per cent for 5FU) with lower rates of stomatitis and myelosuppression, the latter in turn leading to lower rates of neutropenic fever and sepsis. Capecitabine has therefore superseded 5FU in many centres.

Biological therapy

Cetuximab (Erbitux®) is a monoclonal antibody. It inhibits the epidermal growth factor receptor (EGFR) which is often overexpressed in colorectal cancer. The commonest side-effect is an acne-like rash. Cetuximab is given alone or in combination with irinotecan, although the response rate is doubled (to nearly 25 per cent, with a 2-month prolongation in median survival) with combination treatment even in those shown previously to be resistant to irinotecan. K-ras is involved in signal transduction 'downstream' from EGFR. Testing for mutations of the K-ras oncogene can be undertaken on tissue from diagnostic biopsy or definitive surgical specimen and this may predict those patients unlikely to respond to cetuximab.

Bevacizumab (Avastin®) is an inhibitor of vascular endothelial growth factor (VEGF), which is involved in tumour angiogenesis. When added to chemotherapy using leucovorin-modulated 5FU and irinotecan, it leads to improvements in duration of response, progression-free survival and a 4–5 month prolongation of median overall survival. Care has to be taken to avoid using bevacizumab in the immediate period after major surgery as it can lead to haemorrhage and bowel perforation.

Prognosis

Dukes staging and operability are the most important prognostic factors. The 5-year survivals are 90 per cent, 70 per cent and 40 per cent for Dukes A B and C tumours, respectively.

Unfavourable histopathological features include:

- increasing anatomical extent of tumour – depth of local invasion, lymph gland involvement (increasing number and proximal location are poor features) and distant metastases
- incomplete surgical excision of tumour, e.g. circumferential resection margin (CRM) positivity following total mesorectal excision (TME)
- infiltrative tumour margins rather than expansile
- no peritumoural lymphoid reaction at deepest point of invasion and absence of lymphoid aggregates in the surrounding tissue

CASE HISTORY: COLON CANCER

A 60-year-old man presents to his GP with a 6-week history of intermittent bright red blood per rectum noticed as smearing on the lavatory paper associated with some perianal irritation. His bowels are regular and he has no other symptoms of note. Visual inspection of the anal orifice shows a prolapsed haemorrhoid and digital examination of the rectum is declined as he has had similar symptoms over the preceding 5 years. A diagnosis of haemorrhoids is made and the symptoms settle by the time he returns for a prescription of antihypertensive medicines 2 weeks later.

Eight weeks later, he returns with a 4-week history of more frequent and profuse passage of fresh blood per rectum. This is associated with mucoid discharge per rectum and a feeling of incomplete rectal evacuation. Rectal examination is strongly suggested and this reveals an ulcerating tumour of the mid-rectum. He is referred to a colorectal surgeon for further investigation. Digital examination confirms a tumour distinct from the prostate with an impression of tethering laterally. Rigid sigmoidoscopy shows no other mucosal abnormality and biopsies confirm a moderately differentiated adenocarcinoma. Barium enema confirms no other mucosal abnormality elsewhere in the large bowel. Chest X-ray is normal. CT scan of the abdomen and pelvis shows no evidence of liver metastases, no pelvic lymphadenopathy and no evidence of direct invasion of the adjacent pelvic viscera. The serum CEA is twice the upper limit of normal (normal range <4 µg/L) and the liver function tests normal. After discussion at the multidisciplinary team meeting,

he is referred to a clinical oncologist and receives five fractions of preoperative radiotherapy using fields encompassing the rectum and immediate lymphatic drainage. One week later, he undergoes a total mesorectal excision with immediate re-anastomosis. Histopathological review confirms a moderate/poorly differentiated adenocarcinoma, which penetrates through the full thickness of the rectal wall but has a clear circumferential resection margin and clear margins of excision proximally and distally. There is no involvement of the perirectal or other pelvic lymph nodes but prominent venous invasion is noted. The CEA returns to normal during the immediate postoperative period. His tumour is therefore designated as Dukes B and he receives 6 months of adjuvant 5-FU/folinic acid chemotherapy because of the vascular invasion and poorly differentiated elements of the tumour.

He remains entirely well on routine follow-up until 18 months later when a routine pre-clinic CEA estimation is found to be 12 times the upper limit of normal at 48 µg/L. There are no adverse physical signs. This triggers re-staging investigations. CT reveals two metastases in the left lobe of the liver and no evidence of locoregional recurrence of the original primary tumour. The chest is clear. There is no radiological abnormality elsewhere. MRI of the liver confirms a smaller third metastasis in the left lobe close to the other two and no involvement of the major hepatic vessels. He is referred to a hepatobiliary surgeon and is deemed medically fit for salvage surgery. A segmental resection of the left lobe of the liver is performed. The CEA returns to normal postoperatively. He remains well and disease-free 4 years later.

- increasing tumour grade (decreasing differentiation)
- venous invasion
- lymphatic invasion
- perineural invasion
- signet-ring and small cell types
- preoperative CEA >5 mg/L.

Screening

For asymptomatic individuals, screening was previously thought to be expensive and unrewarding. However, it does allow diagnosis of colorectal cancer at an early stage, as evidenced by an increase in the proportion of Dukes A and

B tumours in the screened population. This in turn leads to an apparent survival advantage for the screened population.

Digital rectal examination (DRE) is cheap and simple to apply to a population. However, it is only going to screen the most distal large bowel. It has not been shown to be an effective screening strategy.

The most cost-effective and socially acceptable method of screening is faecal occult blood testing (FOBT). A tiny sample of stool is obtained non-invasively and chemically tested for the presence of blood. The specimen collection can be undertaken in the patient's own home and can be mailed back to the laboratory; 95 per cent will be negative at the first screen, whilst 3–4 per cent will be weakly positive. Most of these will re-test as negative after dietary restriction (no vitamin C, no iron supplements, no NSAIDs, no red meat, no fresh fruit). This leaves approximately 2 per cent with a positive FOBT who will require further investigation (e.g. colonoscopy, sigmoidoscopy/double contrast barium enema): less than 10 per cent of these individuals will be found to have a bowel cancer. As with any screening method, a very small proportion of patients will have a false negative result. It is estimated that FOBT screening reduces mortality from colorectal cancer by 15–30 per cent, a figure comparable to that attributed to mammographic screening for breast cancer. Specific gene mutations associated with polyps and cancer might be detected in cellular material shed into the stool and provide a complementary screening tool to FOBT in the future.

Double-contrast barium enema can be used for screening but is inferior to direct visualization of the bowel mucosa, which allows detection of flat, premalignant lesions and direct sampling of equivocal areas. High-risk groups require regular colonoscopy, in particular those with strong family histories of colon cancer or a long-standing history of extensive ulcerative colitis.

Recent advances in computed tomography have led to the concept of virtual colonoscopy whereby the large bowel can be reconstructed in three dimensions from a single high-resolution abdominopelvic scan. It is less invasive and aesthetically more acceptable but its sensitivity and specificity compared with traditional colonoscopy is yet to be defined.

Prevention

Dietary interventions such as increasing fibre and reducing consumption of meat and animal fats can be a useful strategy. There is evidence that non-steroidal anti-inflammatory drugs (e.g. sulindac) and COX-2 inhibitors (e.g. celecoxib, rofecoxib) reduce the odds of developing colorectal cancer by approximately half, particularly in women. Such drugs can lead to regression of adenomata in those with FAP. Hormone replacement therapy lessens the incidence of colorectal cancer by 20–30 per cent for postmenopausal women as one of its incidental advantages. Prompt diagnosis and excision of large bowel benign polyps, particularly villous adenomata, will prevent subsequent transformation into a cancer. In those with FAP, Lynch syndrome with proven large bowel polyposis and selected cases of chronic, extensive ulcerative colitis, risk-reducing colectomy is a very worthwhile strategy.

CARCINOMA OF THE ANUS

Epidemiology

This is a rare tumour. For example, in England and Wales, there are only 300 new cases and 200 deaths registered per annum. It comprises about 4 per cent of large bowel tumours with a peak incidence at 50–70 years and a slight female predominance overall. Anal margin tumours are more common in men, whilst anal canal tumours are more common in women.

Aetiology

Homosexual activity, in particular anoreceptive intercourse, is associated with anal cancer, and there is evidence that this is due to transmission of the human papilloma virus types 16 and 18,

50 per cent of cancer sufferers testing positive for these, which is analogous to carcinoma of the cervix. There is also evidence among attenders at sexually transmitted disease (STD) clinics that up to 60 per cent of homosexuals will have asymptomatic anal intraepithelial neoplasia (AIN), which is comparable to cervical intraepithelial neoplasia (CIN).

Pathology

The tumour can arise from skin at the anal margin or from the anal canal, appearing as a nodule, polyp or ulcer with everted edges; 90 per cent are squamous carcinomas, most of the remainder adenocarcinomas arising from mucous glands. Anal margin tumours are well differentiated as they are akin to squamous carcinomas of the skin, whereas 75 per cent of anal canal tumours are poorly differentiated. There may be in situ carcinoma in the surrounding epithelium.

Natural history

The tumour will spread circumferentially and longitudinally within the anus and can invade the lower rectum or perianal skin. Deeper infiltration leads to involvement of the sphincters, ischiorectal fossae, vagina and urethra. Lymphatic spread occurs in 10 per cent and is more common with anal canal tumours. The first station lymph nodes are the inguinal groups, from which there can be spread to the iliac nodes. Involvement of the distal rectum can lead to infiltration of the inferior mesenteric nodes. Haematogenous spread is very uncommon at presentation. Sites of distant metastases include the liver, lungs and skeleton.

Symptoms

Patients present with anal symptoms such as:

- discharge
- irritation/discomfort
- bleeding
- tenesmus.

Minor symptoms are frequently neglected by both patients and physicians alike as they resemble those from haemorrhoids, which are far more prevalent.

Signs

Tumours of the anal verge or most distal part of the anal canal should be easily seen on parting the buttocks (Fig. 9.11). The tumour should be palpable as an indurated ulcer or nodule on digital examination. Enlarged inguinal nodes should be sought, although a proportion of enlarged nodes will be secondary to infection.

Differential diagnosis

This includes:

- genital warts – these may be confused with a papilliform, well-differentiated carcinoma
- Crohn's disease of the anus
- syphilis
- basal cell carcinoma/melanoma.

Investigations

Proctoscopy

This is an essential investigation, allowing direct visualization and biopsy of the tumour, and complements the findings of a digital rectal examination.

Examination under anaesthetic (EUA)

This is the best staging investigation in an anxious or uncooperative patient. In a woman, a full bimanual examination is mandatory to assess the extent of local spread. An EUA will also allow the taking of a generous biopsy with minimal distress and discomfort.

Fine needle aspiration (FNA) of any enlarged inguinal lymph nodes

This will help to distinguish reactive lymph nodes from malignant ones, which is important in planning treatment.

Chest X-ray

This should be performed to exclude lung metastases.

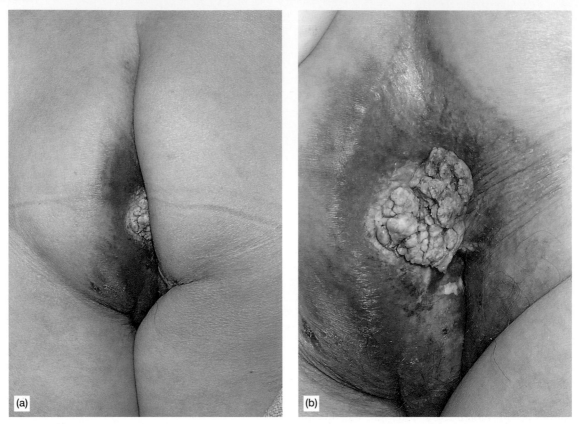

Figure 9.11 Anal margin carcinoma. Papilliform tumour arising from skin at anal verge. (a) Distant view. (b) Close view with buttocks parted.

Computed tomography (CT) of the pelvis

This allows an assessment of the degree of deep invasion of the tumour and is of value in excluding impalpable pelvic lymphadenopathy when the inguinal nodes are involved. It also surveys the liver.

Endo-anal ultrasound/magnetic resonance imaging

This can offer more precise information regarding the local extent of the tumour.

Staging

The TNM staging system is used:

- Tis – Carcinoma in situ
- T0 – No evidence of primary tumour

- TX – Primary tumour cannot be assessed
- T1 – Tumour 2 cm or less in greatest dimension
- T2 – Tumour more than 2 cm but not more than 5 cm in greatest dimension
- T3 – Tumour more than 5 cm in greatest dimension
- T4 – Tumour of any size that invades adjacent organ(s), e.g. vagina, urethra, bladder (involvement of the sphincter muscle(s) alone is not classified as T4)
- NX – Regional lymph nodes cannot be assessed
- N0 – No regional lymph node metastasis
- N1 – Metastasis in perirectal lymph node(s)
- N2 – Metastasis in unilateral internal iliac and/or inguinal lymph node(s)
- N3 – Metastasis in perirectal and inguinal

lymph nodes and/or bilateral internal iliac and/or inguinal lymph nodes

- MX – Distant metastasis cannot be assessed
- M0 – No distant metastasis
- M1 – Distant metastasis.

Treatment

Radical treatment

Surgery

Anal margin tumours can be treated by sphincter-sparing wide local excision alone, with more extensive surgery reserved for salvage of local relapse. In anal canal tumours, an abdominoperineal resection (APR) is necessary, which will result in the patient having a permanent colostomy. Preoperative counselling by a stomatherapist should be arranged in all patients in whom an APR is planned. Patients with cytologically positive inguinal nodes should undergo a block dissection of the groins.

Chemoradiotherapy (CRT)

Non-surgical treatment has the advantage of allowing sphincter preservation. Most local recurrences occur within 1 year of completing treatment and can still be salvaged by an APR. Radiotherapy alone is associated with a 60 per cent local recurrence rate, compared with 40 per cent for CRT. CRT has therefore become the standard of care for this disease. With CRT, 5FU is delivered continuously during the first and fifth weeks of radiotherapy with bolus mitomycin C on the first day of radiotherapy. Radiotherapy is delivered to the pelvis and inguinal nodes bilaterally, typically at a dose of 45 Gy in 25 fractions over 5 weeks. This is followed, after a short break, by a boost dose of 15–20 Gy to the anal tumour alone, either by external beam radiation over 1.5 weeks or by interstitial brachytherapy (Fig. 9.12). A poor objective response after the initial phase of CRT is an indication to proceed immediately to APR. CRT is associated with an increased severity of acute treatment reactions, particularly with respect to perineal skin reactions and diarrhoea. Five-year survival is approximately 60 per cent.

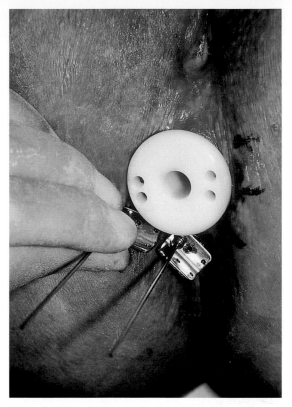

Figure 9.12 Brachytherapy. Implant of small bore tubes around the anal canal, which will be loaded with radioactive iridium wire.

Palliative treatment

Surgery

In the exceptional case of a very advanced inoperable tumour leading to anal occlusion, a defunctioning colostomy may be justified.

Radiotherapy

Pelvic/perineal radiotherapy can be used to palliate symptomatic local recurrence after radical surgery.

Tumour-related complications

An advanced tumour can lead to an aberrant connection between the anal canal and the perineum, vagina or urethra leading to faecal incontinence. The ischiorectal fossae are anatomically close to the anus and particularly prone to secondary infection and abscess formation.

Treatment-related complications

Radiotherapy

The perianal region does not tolerate radiotherapy well as the skin is constantly subjected to friction when sitting or walking, trauma when patients are having to defaecate frequently, moisture owing to sweating and perhaps discharge from the anus. During radiotherapy the patient can be expected to experience diarrhoea, tenesmus and perianal irritation/soreness. These symptoms will begin 1–2 weeks after starting radiotherapy and persist for 4–8 weeks after it has finished. In the longer term, chronic proctocolitis might manifest as diarrhoea, tenesmus, bleeding and mucus per rectum, which can be treated conservatively with topical steroids. Small bowel stricture, intestinal obstruction and bladder contracture occur in 10–20 per cent of cases. Infertility is inevitable for both males and females. High doses of radiation to the groins can lead to occlusion of the lymphatics, then leading to chronic lymphoedema best managed with pressure garments.

Surgery

The main morbidity in the short term is from dehiscence of the perineal wound and pelvic infection. Extensive pelvic surgery such as an abdominoperineal resection might damage autonomic nerves leading to urinary incontinence and impotence in men. The psychosexual trauma and effect on body image can be considerable.

Chemotherapy

Apart from the usual complications from these chemotherapy drugs, CRT leads to severe gastrointestinal toxicity causing anorexia, nausea, vomiting, diarrhoea and intense cutaneous inflammation.

Prognosis

The overall 5-year survival is 70 per cent. Adverse features include anal canal versus margin tumours, increasing TNM stage at presentation, and poorly differentiated tumours.

Screening/prevention

The high incidence of anal intraepithelial neoplasia in STD clinics can make screening a worthwhile exercise in this small group, particularly in male homosexuals. Health education could lead to earlier diagnosis. 'Safe sex' practices amongst homosexual males might also help prevent human papilloma virus transmission. A greater awareness of the disease could lead to earlier diagnosis rather than ad hoc prescription or purchase of proprietary haemorrhoid remedies.

TUMOURS OF THE PERITONEUM

The commonest presentation is with ascites where there is an abnormal accumulation of peritoneal fluid leading to abdominal discomfort and distension. As the peritoneum invests the gastrointestinal tract, abnormal areas of constriction of the bowel can lead to symptoms and signs of subacute or acute bowel obstruction.

The peritoneum is most frequently a site of transcoelomic spread from abdominal or pelvic malignancies. Occasionally, extra-abdominal

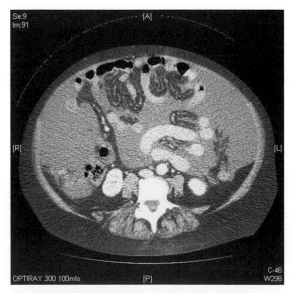

Figure 9.13 Pseudomyxoma peritonei. The CT image shows the abdomen is filled with mucoid material.

malignant tumours will spread to the peritoneum, e.g. lobular breast cancer or lung cancer.

Primary peritoneal mesothelioma is well described and has many features in common with pleural mesothelioma (see Chapter 7). Pseudomyxoma peritoneii is a rare, low-grade malignant condition, which may have a very protracted natural history (Fig. 9.13). It is characterized by the accumulation of large amounts of intra-abdominal mucin, often originating from a low-grade tumour of the appendix, ovary or pancreas. Both conditions are potentially treatable by cytoreductive radical peritonectomy (Sugarbaker procedure) and heated intraoperative intraperitoneal chemotherapy. The surgery is radical, involving:

- removal of the right hemicolon, spleen, gallbladder, greater omentum and lesser omentum
- stripping of peritoneum from pelvis and diaphragm
- hepatic capsulectomy
- hysterectomy and bilateral salpingo-oophorectomy in women
- removal of rectum in selected cases.

Not surprisingly, the procedure is associated with high morbidity and mortality. However, comparative studies suggest that it can increase median survival if performed well.

FURTHER READING

Carr B. *Hepatocellular Cancer – diagnosis and treatment.* Blackwell, Oxford, 2005

Jankowski J, Sampliner RE. *Gastrointestinal Oncology.* Blackwell, Oxford, 2008

Kelsen DP, Daly JM. *Principles and Practice of Gastrointestinal Oncology.* Lippincott Williams and Wilkins, London, 2007

Lowy AM, Leach SD. *Pancreatic Cancer.* Springer, New York, 2008

Meyerhardt J, Saunders M. *Colorectal Cancer.* Mosby Elsevier, Edinburgh, 2007

Scholefield JH. *Challenges in Colorectal Cancer.* Blackwell, Oxofrd, 2006

Williams CD. *Cancer of the Esophagus: a reference guide and bibliography.* Nova Science, Hauppauge, New York, 2006

SELF-ASSESSMENT QUESTIONS

1. Which three of the following statements are true about oesophageal cancer?
   a. Is rare in Africa
   b. A family history is common
   c. Tumours of the upper third are commoner in women
   d. May be caused by chronic acid reflux
   e. There is no association with smoking tobacco
   f. May be associated with asbestos exposure
   g. May be caused by excessive alcohol consumption

2. Which one of the following is not a presenting feature of oesophageal cancer?
   a. Dysphagia
   b. Acid reflux
   c. Regurgitation of food
   d. Weight loss
   e. Pulmonary aspiration

3. Which three of the following statements are true for oesophageal cancer?
   a. Radiotherapy alone cures >10 per cent of cases
   b. Surgery offers the best chance of cure
   c. Upper third cancers are best treated by radiotherapy
   d. Distant spread to the liver is rare
   e. Cisplatin is a useful drug
   f. Docetaxel is a drug of choice for metastatic disease
   g. Cetuximab is a useful treatment

4. Which three of the following statements are true for stomach cancer?
   a. It is commoner in lower socioeconomic groups
   b. It is three times commoner in males than females
   c. Often presents with abdominal pain
   d. Spread outside the stomach is common
   e. May be associated with non-malignant skin eruptions

f. Docetaxel is a drug of choice for metastatic disease
g. Cetuximab is a useful treatment

5. Which one of the following is not true about gastrointestinal stromal tumours?
   a. They are rare tumours
   b. Commoner in older age groups
   c. A specific cytogenetic abnormality is characteristic
   d. Chemotherapy is an effective treatment
   e. They are amenable to treatment with immunotherapy

6. Which three of the following statements are true about pancreatic cancer?
   a. Commonest in 40–60 age group
   b. A family history is common
   c. Mainly arises from the ducts of the gland
   d. Most cases are caused by gallstones
   e. Commonly presents with obstructive jaundice
   f. CA125 is a useful serum tumour marker protein
   g. CEA is a useful serum tumour marker protein

7. Which one of the following is true about the treatment of pancreatic cancer?
   a. Surgery offers the best chance of cure
   b. 10–20 per cent will be long-term survivors
   c. Chemotherapy has no role in the management of early pancreatic cancer
   d. 5FU is the most active chemotherapy agent
   e. Tamoxifen is a useful treatment

8. Which three of the following statements are true about hepatocellular carcinoma?
   a. It is common in Africa
   b. Has a viral aetiology in some cases
   c. Human chorionic gonadotrophin is a useful serum tumour marker

SELF-ASSESSMENT QUESTIONS

d. Diarrhoea is a common symptom
e. It is highly sensitive to chemotherapy
f. Can be successfully treated with bevacizumab
g. Has a very poor prognosis

9. Which one of the following is not true about cancer of the gallbladder and biliary tree?
a. Can be associated with gallstones
b. Can be associated with typhoid carriage
c. They are common tumours
d. They generally have a low probability of long-term cure
e. Adjuvant chemotherapy has no proven role in these diseases

10. Which three of the following statements are true about the epidemiology and aetiology of colorectal cancer?
a. It is commoner than breast cancer
b. It causes more deaths per annum than breast cancer
c. It is relatively common in Africa and Asia
d. There is a strong male predominance
e. Colon cancer is commoner than rectal cancer
f. It is commoner in more affluent socioeconomic groups
g. There is a strong association with HIV infection

11. Which three of the following statements are true about the presentation of colorectal cancer?
a. Bleeding is a common symptom
b. Vitamin B12 deficiency can occur
c. A normal digital rectal examination excludes rectal cancer
d. Abdominal obstruction is a sign of locally advanced disease

e. Abdominal distension is common
f. Many will have overt metastatic disease in the liver at diagnosis
g. Supraclavicular lymph nodes are uncommon

12. Which one of the following is true about the treatment of colorectal cancer?
a. Surgery alone is not curative
b. Those having a colostomy have a worse prognosis
c. Preoperative radiotherapy for rectal cancer substantially increases the risk of operative complications
d. Platinum compounds have no significant activity in this disease
e. Advanced stages of the disease responds to VEGF inhibitors

13. Which three of the following statements are not prognostic factors for colorectal cancer?
a. Duke staging
b. Presentation with rectal bleeding
c. Previous colonic polyps
d. Number of involved lymph nodes
e. Normal colonoscopy in preceding 3 years
f. Complete surgical excision of tumour
g. Vascular invasion

14. Which one of the following is not true about anal cancer?
a. It is associated with human papilloma virus
b. Associated with HIV infection
c. Nearly always treated by abdominoperineal resection
d. Relatively sensitive to radiotherapy
e. Has a high rate of local control

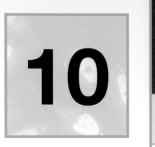

10 UROLOGICAL CANCER

■ Renal cell carcinoma   160
■ Prostate cancer   163
■ Bladder cancer   172
■ Cancer of the testis   177

■ Cancer of the penis   180
■ Further reading   182
■ Self-assessment questions   183

RENAL CELL CARCINOMA

Epidemiology

This accounts for 2 per cent of all malignancies with over 7000 cases each year in the UK and over 3000 deaths per year. It is more common in males than females. The incidence is high in Europe, particularly Denmark, and lowest in Japan and an overall increase in incidence has been reported worldwide, much of which is attributed to increased access to investigations such as abdominal CT scan, which can identify previously occult disease.

Aetiology

There are several possible aetiological factors:

■ smoking tobacco (increasing the risk of renal cell carcinoma)
■ cadmium exposure
■ a rare familial pattern associated with *HLA-BW44* and *HLA-DR8*
■ increased incidence in von Hippel–Lindau (VHL) disease, horseshoe kidneys and adult polycystic kidneys.

Pathology

Tumours can arise from any part of the renal tissue: a quarter involve the whole kidney, one-third the upper pole, and one-third the lower pole. Macroscopically, the tumour is usually solid, expanding the renal tissue with a central area of necrosis or cystic degeneration and other haemorrhagic areas. Occasionally a tumour arises within the wall of a cyst. Renal cell tumours are thought to arise from the lining cells of the proximal convoluted tubule.

Microscopically, they are adenocarcinomas composed of characteristic clear cells, although the degree of differentiation can vary from a well-differentiated tumour to a highly anaplastic appearance. The most commonly used grading system is the Fuhrman grading system based predominantly on nuclear size and shape.

The majority show aberrant expression of the VHL gene and upregulation of vascular endothelial growth factor (VEGF) with prominent neoangiogenesis.

Natural history

The tumour invades the surrounding kidney and can grow into the renal vein and thence into the inferior vena cava (IVC).

Lymph node spread involves the renal hilar nodes and progresses to the para-aortic chain. Blood-borne metastases characteristically go to the lung and bone, although many other sites including skin, central nervous system and liver are also recognized. Approximately 25 per cent of patients will present with metastatic disease and of the remainder a further 30–40 per cent will eventually express distant metastases.

Spontaneous regression of metastases, typically lung deposits monitored on chest X-ray, is often referred to in the context of renal cell cancer. While such events undoubtedly occur, the true incidence is extremely low, the verified incidence being around 7 per cent of patients with metastatic disease. Spontaneous regression of the primary tumour is virtually unknown.

Symptoms

Haematuria, typically painless, is the most common presenting symptom. Loin pain can occur acutely from haemorrhage within the tumour or chronically as the tumour enlarges.

Symptoms of metastases might be present, in particular bone pain or even pathological fracture (bone metastases) and cough with or without haemoptysis (lung metastases).

Symptoms of paraneoplastic conditions associated with renal cell cancer may be present: these include hypercalcaemia and polycythaemia. There might also be general symptoms of malignancy such as malaise, anorexia and weight loss.

Signs

The primary tumour can be felt as a mass in the loin, and in 10–20 per cent of patients there is associated fever.

Differential diagnosis

Other causes of haematuria should be considered, in particular benign renal adenomas, tumours of the renal pelvis, renal tract stones and bladder tumours.

Other causes of loin pain which should be taken into account include renal stones or hydronephrosis.

Investigations

Blood tests

A full blood count sometimes shows anaemia owing to chronic haematuria, or polycythaemia from tumour production of erythyropoietin-like substances. Serum calcium may be raised.

Radiography

Chest X-ray might show typical 'cannon-ball' metastases.

CT scan

The renal tumour will be imaged on either ultrasound or CT scan. The latter will also give information on renal vein/IVC invasion and involvement of surrounding structures. The role of intravenous urography (IVU) to demonstrate the primary tumour where CT is widely available is debatable. Figure 10.1 shows the appearances of a renal carcinoma on CT scan.

CT of the abdomen and thorax is also essential to screen for metastases in the lungs and liver.

Fine needle aspirate or biopsy

The radiological appearances of renal carcinoma are usually typical. Fine needle aspirate cytology or biopsy are usually avoided because of the risk of tumour seeding in the biopsy tract unless there is doubt on CT scan.

Isotope bone scan

Isotope bone scans are not routinely recommended but X-ray skeletal survey may be of value. The typical lytic bone lesions of renal cell carcinoma can give false negative bone scan images.

Staging

Important features of the TNM staging are the size of the primary tumour and involvement of

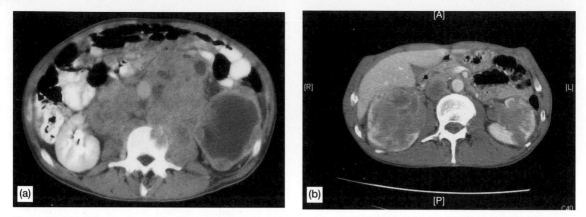

Figure 10.1 (a) CT scan demonstrating a large renal carcinoma rising from the right kidney. (b) CT scan demonstrating bilateral renal carcinomas more advanced on the right than the left.

surrounding structures including the renal vein, which will determine operability of the primary, and the presence of distant metastases.

TNM staging for renal carcinoma (revised 2002) is used:

- T1 – Tumour ≤7 cm limited to kidney
  - T1a – Tumour ≤4 cm
  - T1b – Tumour >4–7 cm
- T2 – Tumour >7 cm limited to kidney
- T3 – Tumour extends into major vessels, adrenal glands or surrounding tissues but not beyond Gerota's fascia
  - T3a – Invasion into adrenals or perinephric tissues
  - T3b – Extension into vena cava above diaphragm
- T4 – Tumour extends beyond Gerota's fascia
- N0 – No lymph node involvement
- N1 – 1 lymph node involved
- N2 – >1 lymph node involved.

Treatment

Surgery

Radical nephrectomy in which the perirenal fat, perirenal fascia, adrenal gland and regional nodes are removed en bloc is the operation of choice with superior local control rates to simple nephrectomy. Tumour invading the renal vein can be successfully removed and this is therefore not an absolute contraindication to radical treatment.

Small peripheral tumours can be considered for partial nephrectomy and there is increasing use of cryotherapy and high-frequency ultrasound ablation for such lesions.

Palliative treatment

Local irradiation of painful bone metastases may be required. Brain metastases can benefit from cranial irradiation, or if it is solitary without extensive disease elsewhere, surgical excision can be considered.

Lung metastases can also be amenable to surgical excision in the occasional patient who presents some years after treatment of the primary tumour with a solitary lung metastasis.

Systemic treatment

Renal cancer is responsive to biological therapies such as interferon and interleukin (IL-2). Response rates of around 15 per cent are seen with interferon and 20–30 per cent with IL-2. The antiangiogenic agents sumatinib, sorafinib and bevacizumab, which target VEGF, have been shown to be active in renal cancer with improvements in response rates over conventional management with interferon.

Treatment with biological agents is at best palliative in the setting of widespread metastatic disease. A trial comparing interferon with medroxyprogesterone reported a 1-year survival of 12 per cent and overall a 1-month advantage in progression-free survival for interferon. A more recent trial compared sunitinib with interferon and reported an increase in median survival from 5 months to 11 months with improved quality of life also in the sunitinib group.

Tumour-related complications

Complications of renal cell carcinoma include hypercalcaemia and polycythaemia. Renal function is usually unaffected provided the contralateral kidney is normal.

Prognosis

The prognosis for tumour localized to the kidney is good, with 5-year survival after radical nephrectomy of around 50 per cent.

Even in the presence of metastases, renal cell cancer often has a long and indolent course so that 5–10 per cent of patients with lung metastases will survive for 5 years or more.

Screening and future prospects

Simple urinalysis for microscopic haematuria and cytology are readily available. However, while sensitive, it is non-specific and results in unacceptably high false positive rates for routine application.

The recent success of drugs targeting VEGF has encouraged research into combination therapies using vascular targeting and antiangiogenic agents with conventional chemotherapy, biological agents and the new drugs such as tyrosine kinase inhibitors, with the hope of prolonging survival in advanced disease.

PROSTATE CANCER

Epidemiology

Each year in the UK there are 35 000 cases of prostate cancer, making it the commonest form of cancer in men, accounting for 12 per cent of all cancer cases and leading to a total of 10 000

deaths per annum. In the UK it is the second most common cause of death from cancer in men after lung cancer. The UK incidence of 52 in 100 000 compares with 274 in 100 000 in US black men, 171 in 100 000 in US white men and 6 in 100 000 men in Japan. The high rates in the US are again attributed at least in part to the widespread prostate-specific antigen (PSA) screening that occurs there.

The incidence of prostate cancer is rising. This may reflect an increasing proportion of the population over 70 years, a greater diagnostic rate and possibly a true increase in incidence in younger men. Despite this, mortality has been stable over recent years supporting the view that the increase in diagnosis is largely due to identification of early previously undetected disease mainly through PSA screening of healthy individuals.

Aetiology

- *Age*: It is rarely found in men under 45 years but increases with age, being almost universal at post mortem in men aged over 80 years.
- *Familial*: A family history of prostate cancer in a first-degree relative increases the risk in an individual by two to three times. When seen in young men under 45 years there can be a stronger genetic basis. Recently a seven-gene signature for prostate cancer has been identified. The most frequent alteration in prostate cancer is methylation of the promoter of *GSTP1*, a gene involved in carcinogen detoxification. An association with breast cancer in female relatives has also been described linked to the *BRCA2* gene which carries a 5-fold increased risk of prostate cancer and accounts for 2 per cent of all cases.
- *Other factors*: It is more common in city dwellers than rural communities, and is associated with a high fat and meat diet, and an occupational exposure to cadmium. It is more common in married men, related to the number of sexual partners, frequency of sexual activity and a history of sexually transmitted disease. The androgen receptor

signalling pathway is thought to play an important role in the early development of prostate cancer.

It is important to note that benign prostatic hypertrophy can co-exist with prostate cancer but is not causally related.

Pathology

Cancer of the prostate develops most commonly in the peripheral part of the gland, accounting for 70 per cent, while only 10 per cent arise centrally. The remainder arise in the transitional zone. Eighty-five per cent are diffuse multifocal tumours. In situ cancer (prostate intraepithelial neoplasia – PIN) is now a recognized precursor to invasive disease and may be seen in adjacent parts of a gland containing invasive cancer.

Microscopically, prostate cancer is typically an adenocarcinoma of varying differentiation. Various grading systems based on morphological appearances have been described, all of which correlate with outcome. The commonly used system is the Gleason score, which is based on the pattern of growth of the tumour and is recorded as the sum of a primary and secondary grade giving a summed score from 2 to 10. A Gleason score of 8 or above correlates with a relatively poor outcome. Another poor prognostic feature is perineural invasion.

Where there is doubt as to the primary origin of a tumour deposit, a prostatic primary will be characterized by staining for acid phosphatase and prostate-specific antigen. Androgen and progestogen receptors have been demonstrated on the surface of prostate cancer cells, although the value of this in routine clinical use remains uncertain.

Natural history

Local growth results in infiltration of the prostate gland and surrounding tissues, particularly into the seminal vesicles, bladder and rectum as shown in Figure 10.2. Predictive tables (the Partin tables) are available that correlate the risk of extracapsular extension and

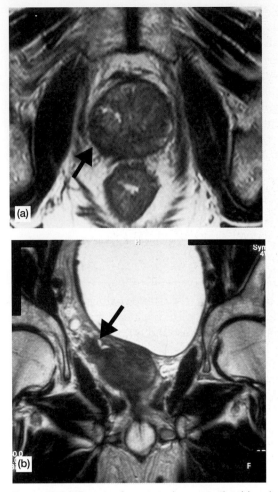

Figure 10.2 MR scan of prostate demonstrating (a) early extracapsular invasion and (b) seminal vesicle invasion.

seminal vesicle invasion with PSA, T stage and Gleason score. A patient with a PSA of 4.1–6.0 ng/ml, Gleason score 5–6 and stage T2a has a 19 per cent risk of capsular penetration and zero risk of seminal vesicle invasion. In contrast when the PSA is 6.1–10.0 ng/mL and Gleason score 7 (4+3) with the same stage, the risk of capsular penetration is 58 per cent and seminal vesicle invasion 11 per cent.

Lymph node metastases occur with initial involvement of pelvic nodes, which increases with clinical stage, presenting PSA and Gleason score. The probability of lymph node metastases can be calculated from the Roach score;

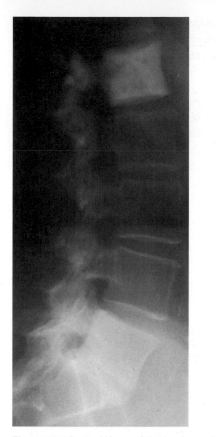

Figure 10.3 Lateral X-ray of the lumbar spine showing metastases in L1 causing extensive sclerotic changes compared with surrounding normal vertebrae.

the percentage risk is given by the formula (PSA/3) + 10 (Gleason Score –6).

Distant spread is usually blood-borne, typically by retrograde venous spread through the vertebral plexus of veins, so that bone metastases to the spine are common, although all parts of the skeleton may be affected (Fig. 10.3).

Soft tissue metastases, e.g. lung or liver, although well recognized are uncommon in prostatic cancer.

Symptoms

Prostate cancer is often asymptomatic and found either at post mortem or incidentally during the investigation of another condition. The following symptoms may be present:

- prostatic outflow obstructive symptoms, with frequency, hesitancy, poor stream, nocturia and terminal dribble
- haematospermia
- erectile dysfunction
- bone pain or, less often, spinal cord compression, owing to bone metastases
- hypercalcaemia
- general symptoms of malignancy, including malaise, anorexia and weight loss.

Signs

The tumour may be palpable per rectum as a hard nodule or diffusely infiltrating abnormality, which in more advanced cases might be invading surrounding pelvic tissues. Typically there is loss of the midline sulcus of the gland, which is present in the normal or hypertrophied prostate.

Bone metastases might be clinically apparent when complicated by pain, pathological fracture or neurological signs.

Differential diagnosis

Benign prostatic hypertrophy can produce the same symptoms of bladder outflow obstruction and indeed can co-exist with prostatic cancer.

The most common cause of a raised PSA is prostatitis.

Investigations

Routine blood tests

A full blood count might show a reduction of haemoglobin, white cells or platelets with widespread bone metastases. Hypercalcaemia and uraemia should be excluded on routine biochemistry.

Prostate-specific antigen

PSA is now the most common means of diagnosing prostate cancer; however, whilst very sensitive, it is relatively non-specific for prostate cancer distinct from benign prostate pathology. Up to two-thirds of men with a modestly raised PSA will not have prostate cancer and around

20 per cent of patients with prostate cancer can have a PSA in the normal range. As a sole screening test for prostate cancer it is therefore relatively poor and has to be supplemented by further investigations, in particular digital rectal examination and transrectal biopsy before a diagnosis can be confirmed. Exceptions to this are patients presenting with typical bone metastases and a PSA of >100 ng/ml.

PSA also has an important role in monitoring patients once a diagnosis has been confirmed. Prognosis is related to the rate of PSA change measured by the PSA doubling time.

Magnetic resonance scanning

MRI gives excellent views of the prostate gland and its relation to surrounding normal soft tissue structures such as bladder and rectum. Best definition is obtained using specific rectal coils. It is now the investigation of choice for staging prostate cancer; an example is shown in Figure 10.2.

MRI can also be used where there is uncertainty over the presence of bone metastases, particularly in the spine where, in an aging population, degenerative disease is common and might cause uptake on an isotope scan.

Ultrasound

Transrectal ultrasound is the most sensitive means of assessing the prostate gland and can be used to direct needle biopsy towards suspicious areas of the gland. Doppler flow studies can give even greater detail of the internal structure of the gland and highlight abnormal areas.

Intravenous urography

IVU will demonstrate the enlarged gland indenting the bladder and any associated hydronephrosis.

CT scan

This may give more detail of distal lymph node changes in the common iliac and para-aortic regions but will only be used for staging of prostate cancer where MRI is contraindicated, e.g. a patient with a pacemaker.

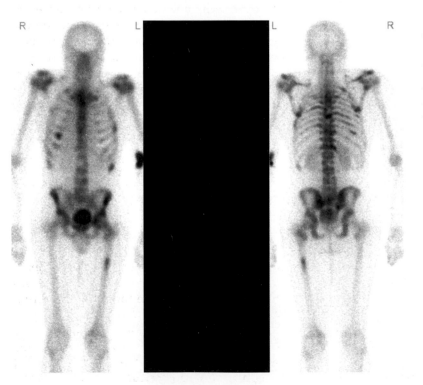

Figure 10.4 Isotope bone scan demonstrating multiple areas of increased uptake in spine, ribs and left femur due to bone metastases from carcinoma of the prostate. Anterior view is on the left and posterior view on the right.

Isotope bone scan

Isotope bone scan is the most useful screening test for bone metastases. A positive scan is shown in Figure 10.4.

Biopsy or resection

Histological confirmation is made either at transurethral resection of the prostate (TURP) or on transrectal ultrasound-guided needle biopsy per rectum. Wide sampling of the gland from all four quadrants should be undertaken with a minimum of 12 samples for a representative result. Previous fears that TURP could cause dissemination of cancer cells are unfounded but, in the absence of major bladder outflow symptoms, a needle biopsy is to be preferred.

Staging

Staging of cancer of the prostate is defined in the TNM system shown below. The important principles are to distinguish early localized carcinoma of the prostate from locally extensive disease from that which has already metastasized.

- T0 – No evidence of primary tumour
- TI – Asymptomatic or incidental finding
  - T1a – Incidental finding in ≤5 per cent resected tissue
  - T1b – Incidental finding in >5 per cent resected tissue
  - T1c – Diagnosis at needle biopsy because of asymptomatic raised PSA
- T2 – Tumour confined within capsule of gland
  - T2a – Tumour involves one half of a lobe or less
  - T2b – Tumour involves less than one half of a lobe but not both lobes
  - T2c – Tumour involves both lobes
- T3 – Tumour extension beyond capsule of gland
  - T3a – Tumour extends beyond capsule unilaterally
  - T3b – Tumour extends beyond capsule bilaterally
  - T3c – Tumour involves seminal vesicles

- T4 – Invasion of rectum or other pelvic structures
  - T4a – Tumour involves bladder neck, external sphincter or rectum
  - T4b – Tumour involves levator muscles or is fixed to pelvic side wall.
- NI, N2, N3 – Involvement of regional nodes
- M1 – Distant metastases.

Treatment

Radical treatment is indicated for prostatic cancer localized to the prostate gland with no evidence on the basis of MRI or isotope bone scan of distant metastases. A PSA level of under 20 ng/mL virtually excludes the possibility of bone metastases, whilst a level of >50 ng/mL carries a very high probability of distant spread even if the bone scan is 'normal', and such levels will usually exclude radical treatment approaches.

Active surveillance

It is clear that many men who are diagnosed with early low risk disease, having a PSA <10 ng/mL and a Gleason score <7 have indolent disease, which may never compromise their survival; this is evident in the large proportion of men dying from other causes who, as their age increases, have an increasing likelihood of harbouring asymptomatic undiagnosed prostate cancer. The ever-increasing use of PSA screening has amplified the problem of managing this group of patients in whom it is clearly important to identify those who have the potential to develop more aggressive prostate cancer and equally to enable those with indolent disease to avoid potentially morbid treatment. At present there is no reliable marker to separate out these two populations.

Many patients over 70 years with low PSA and Gleason scores at diagnosis will be offered active surveillance as a treatment option. This will require regular monitoring of the serum PSA, typically every 3 months, with repeat biopsies after 2 years to ensure there has been no change in the nature of the cancer. Treatment can be introduced if the PSA rises above 10 ng/mL or if the calculated PSA doubling time is >2 years, or if the patient indicates that he wishes to do so. Whilst this approach suits some patients, who are only too pleased to avoid major treatment intervention, many find the associated anxiety and uncertainty unacceptable.

Radical prostatectomy

This is indicated for disease that is localized to the gland, i.e. stages T1 and T2. The operation involves removal of the entire prostate and adjacent bladder neck, both seminal vesicles, the vasa deferentia and surrounding fascia. It requires considerable surgical expertise. Complications include erectile impotence and occasional urinary incontinence. 'Nerve sparing' techniques to preserve the neurovascular bundle responsible for penile erection are used but may not be possible where there is tumour infiltration close to these critical structures.

Postoperative radiotherapy may play a role where excision margins are close to or involved with tumour or when pelvic lymph nodes are involved. After prostatectomy the PSA should be undetectable; any presence of PSA even at very low levels suggests residual prostatic tissue and is an indication for postoperative radiotherapy. There is evidence that this is most effective when the PSA remains <0.6 ng/mL. The role of antiandrogen treatment in this setting remains under investigation.

Radical radiotherapy

This is indicated for all patients with disease localized to the pelvis. A small treatment volume encompassing known disease in the prostate and seminal vesicles is adequate, although there are advocates of prophylactic treatment of pelvic lymph nodes in patients with higher PSA levels and high Gleason scores (>7). CT scanning to enable three-dimensional conformal radiotherapy is now routine to deliver a standard dose of 74 Gy in 37 fractions; intensity-modulated radiotherapy (IMRT) is increasingly used to escalate the dose even further with doses of over 90 Gy, now technically feasible with these new techniques. There is also some evidence from the biological response of prostate cancer to radiation that larger single

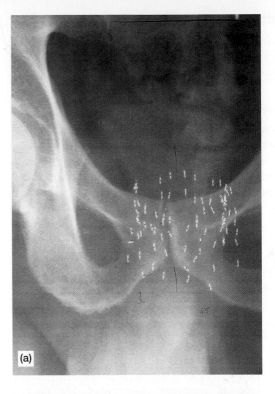

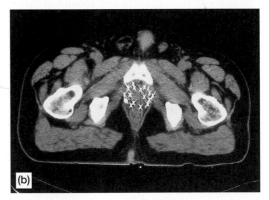

Figure 10.5 Plain X-ray showing iodine seeds after implantation into prostate gland and CT scan showing position taken 1 month after the implant procedure.

doses might be more effective and this approach is currently under investigation.

Brachytherapy techniques with permanent implants of radioactive iodine-125 or palladium-103 offer an alternative approach to external beam radiotherapy in patients with early localized disease. A permanent iodine seed implant is shown in Figure 10.5. Combined treatments using external beam with a brachytherapy boost, usually by a temporary implant using an iridium afterloading technique, are also advocated as a means of increasing radiation dose without additional side-effects.

Principle side-effects include bowel and bladder irritation but in the majority of patients potency is preserved. Brachytherapy is associated with very few bowel effects and a low level of impotence, although acute prostatitis and urethritis immediately following the procedure might be more pronounced than with external beam treatment.

Hormone therapy

Hormone therapy by androgen deprivation or blockade is effective when first introduced in most patients (see Chapter 6 and below). It may be used as:

- *primary treatment* in frail or medically compromised patients
- *metastatic disease treatment* at presentation
- *neoadjuvant or adjuvant treatment*. It has a role in primary treatment for locally advanced tumours prior to definitive radiotherapy by allowing initial reduction of tumour bulk and early control of local symptoms. When used as an adjuvant treatment for 3 years after definitive radiotherapy or surgery for stage T3 prostate cancer an improvement in survival has been demonstrated. Current evidence also shows an advantage in disease-free but not overall survival for at least 6 months adjuvant anti-androgen treatment in 'intermediate risk' disease defined by a PSA >10 ng/mL, Gleason score of 7 or above and stage T2
- *relapse* after definitive primary treatment.

Palliative treatment

For metastatic disease, hormone therapy will achieve a response in most patients, although eventually resistance to this approach will be seen. Hormone therapy can be given in a number of forms as shown in Table 10.1. All of these are equally effective and the choice will in general be based on patient acceptability and availability.

Anti-androgen drugs include cyproterone acetate, flutamide and bicalutamide. Gonadotrophin-releasing hormone (GnRH) analogue drugs include goserelin and leuprorelin.

First-line treatment for a patient presenting with metastatic prostate cancer will generally be either a GnRH analogue or an oral antiandrogen such as flutamide or bicalutamide. Over 80 per cent of patients will respond to this manoeuvre. When a GnRH analogue drug is started, the initial exposure should be covered by a period of 10–14 days oral antiandrogen administration to cover the initial flare seen with these agents. There is no evidence that continuing combination therapy, sometimes referred to as MAB (maximal androgen blockade) has major advantages over single-agent therapy. Permanent androgen deprivation by orchidectomy may be offered to responders with the alternative of continuing with medical treatment.

Patients will inevitably relapse despite an initial response, the median duration of response being around 18 months. Unfortunately response to a second hormone manoeuvre is usually disappointing; stilboestrol can be used when resistance is first seen with further short-lived responses in many patients.

Chemotherapy should be considered for selected patients with relapse after hormone treatment. Taxotere with prednisolone is now the schedule of choice having been shown to be

TABLE 10.1 Hormone therapy for prostate cancer: relative clinical merits

Bilateral orchidectomy	Anti-androgen drugs	GnRH analogue
Surgical procedure	Oral medication	Monthly injection
Permanent	Reversible	Reversible
Compliance guaranteed	Tablets may be missed	Compliance guaranteed
Patient acceptance variable	Readily accepted	Readily accepted

CASE HISTORY: PROSTATE CANCER

MJ, a 68-year-old man, had been noticing for some weeks a nagging pain in the back with some local tenderness over the lumbar spine. The pain was worse on standing and walking but never went away completely. He had done no recent heavy work to provoke it. For several years he had noted that he passed water more frequently and had started having to get up at night two or three times to pass water also. He consulted his GP who confirmed some local tenderness in the lumbar spine and in view of his urinary symptoms performed a rectal examination. This revealed an enlarged hard irregular prostate gland.

His GP arranged for X-rays of the spine and some blood tests including a serum PSA. This returned with an elevated level at 385 ng/mL and the X-rays showed scattered sclerotic changes compatible with metastatic disease. He was referred to a specialist oncology clinic where it was confirmed that the above findings were compatible with a diagnosis of metastatic prostate cancer. The raised PSA level was considered sufficient to confirm the diagnosis and no biopsy of the prostate gland was recommended. Treatment was started with cyproterone acetate tablets for 2 weeks and a goserelin subcutaneous implant was given. When reviewed 6 weeks later MJ reported a considerable improvement in his back pain but was complaining of intermittent hot flushes. It was explained that these were a common side-effect of the goserelin injections. A repeat PSA had fallen to 26 ng/mL and he was recommended to continue with the goserelin at 3-monthly intervals.

MJ remained well for the next 2 years, the hot flushes regressing and his pain remaining well controlled. He then noted over a period of a few days increasing difficulty in climbing stairs accompanied by a return of his backache. The following day he was unable to pass water and reported a loss of feeling in his legs. His GP referred him for an urgent assessment to his local casualty department. There he was found to be in urinary retention, with a Grade 3 to 4 weakness of the lower limbs and a reduction in pin prick and light touch sensation to the level of the umbilicus. A urinary catheter was inserted and an urgent MR scan was performed. This showed extensive spinal metastases with involvement of the spinal canal at T10. Urgent transfer to the local cancer centre was arranged. He was started on dexamethasone and immediate local radiotherapy to the lower thoracic spine was given over the next week. A repeat PSA level was found to be 376 ng/mL. Following completion of radiotherapy his pain settled once more. The power in his lower limbs improved and he was able to walk independently with the aid of a stick. He also regained control of his bladder function.

In view of his rising PSA despite taking goserelin he was recommended to add a peripheral antiandrogen and started bicalutamide tablets. When reviewed 2 months later his PSA had fallen to 230 ng/mL but he was complaining of discomfort and swelling in his breasts; it was explained that this was a recognized side-effect of the bicalutamide tablets.

He remained well for the next few months slowly becoming more active but 6 months later he started complaining of scattered pains in the spine, pelvis and ribs despite increasing his analgesia. His PSA had risen to 416 ng/mL. It was recommended in view of his relatively good general fitness that he consider a course of chemotherapy. He started docetaxel attending the hospital chemotherapy unit every 3 weeks. In addition he was given prednisolone tablets with the chemotherapy. After three courses of chemotherapy he noticed that his finger nails had developed brown discolouration and his skin was dry and flaky; he had also lost most of his hair. Otherwise he was feeling better, with no significant pain, an improved appetite and he had regained his previous levels of activity. He continued to receive a total of ten cycles of chemotherapy.

Three months later he returned to his GP complaining of a poor appetite, scattered aches and pains in his ribs and spine, and severe constipation. His wife who accompanied him reported also that he had become increasingly confused. His GP performed some further blood tests and his serum calcium was found to be elevated at 3.7 nmol/L. Urgent admission to his local hospital was arranged and he was treated with intravenous saline and an infusion of zolendronate. Over the next few days his symptoms improved and his calcium fell to 2.9 nmol/L. He was discharged home a week later and returned for further zolendronate infusions every 3 weeks. When he attended for his third infusion he mentioned that he was having more difficulty walking and felt his legs were getting weaker. An urgent MRI showed recur-

rence of his spinal canal compression. The risks of further radiotherapy to the spine were discussed and he felt that he was willing to take the chance of radiation damage to the spinal cord from further radiotherapy rather than allow the cancer to cause progressive spinal cord damage. Further irradiation was given but his general condition deteriorated and he became unable to mobilize himself without help. He required increasing levels of morphine to control his discomfort. He continued to deteriorate whilst remaining comfortable. A few weeks later he developed a productive cough and a chest X-ray showed patchy consolidation. His condition deteriorated further as he developed bronchopneumonia from which he died 3 days later.

superior to mitozantrone. It will achieve an improvement in quality of life scores and a median improvement in survival of 2 months has been demonstrated. Toxicity can counterbalance this, however, with many patients experiencing fatigue, neuromuscular symptoms, skin and nail changes and bone marrow depression.

Other palliative treatments that will be of value in these patients include the appropriate use of analgesics and co-analgesics, together with palliative radiotherapy using either external beam therapy or the radioisotope strontium-89 for bone pain. Palliative radiotherapy is also indicated for neurological complications.

Hypercalcaemia will require active management when symptomatic (see Chapter 22).

Tumour-related complications

These include:

- obstructive hydronephrosis
- hypercalcaemia
- spinal cord compression.

Treatment-related complications

Surgery

Surgery can lead to impotence and urinary incontinence.

Radiotherapy

Bowel and bladder damage can result from external beam radiotherapy.

Impotence also occurs but less often than after surgery; in both settings there is good response to drugs such as sildenafil.

Brachytherapy is associated only rarely with long-term bowel or bladder problems but can be followed by an immediate period of post-implant acute urethritis.

Hormone therapy

Androgen blockade is commonly associated with hot flushes, lethargy, gynaecomastia, reduced libido and varying degrees of impotence. Oral antiandrogens can cause nausea and, rarely, hepatic dysfunction.

Prognosis

While aggressive forms of prostatic cancer are recognized, particularly in young men, in the majority of cases the natural history of the disease will span several years. Because of this, it is difficult to judge the results of treatment on short-term survival figures.

Untreated, localized carcinoma of the prostate will still give a 5-year survival of 80 per cent, although many will have locally progressive disease. After radical treatment, surgical or radiotherapeutic, 10-year survivals in excess of 80 per cent are to be expected, falling to around 50 per cent for disease extending outside the capsule of the gland. In general the majority of men diagnosed with early localized disease having a low PSA and Gleason score will not die from their prostate cancer.

In contrast, patients presenting with metastatic disease have a median survival of 18–24 months.

Screening and future prospects

Digital rectal examination, serum prostate-specific antigen and transrectal ultrasound offer a high chance of detecting preclinical prostate cancer. A new urine test, PCA3 (Prostate Cancer Gene 3), may refine this further. Extensive studies are currently underway in Europe to evaluate the effect of screening healthy men and this is already common practice in the US, where 50 per cent of prostate cancers are detected while still localized to the gland, compared with smaller proportions where screening is not actively promoted such as in the UK. The impact of screening on overall survival remains unproven.

More specific antiandrogen drugs, eg abiraterone, are under evaluation to optimize the hormone responsiveness of prostate cancer.

Vaccine therapy for prostate cancer is currently under evaluation in combination with taxotere chemotherapy with encouraging improvements in response rates being seen.

Radium-223, an alpha particle-releasing isotope is being evaluated as a means of delivering fractionated targeted systemic radiation which, because of the short range of alpha particles even in patients with extensive bone metastases, does not cause significant bone marrow depression.

Denosumab is a monoclonal antibody to RANKL, a molecule pivotal in the osteoclast activation cascade when bone metastases develop. It is currently under evaluation both as a therapeutic and prophylactic agent in prostate cancer.

Rarer tumours

Transitional cell tumours of the prostate arising from the urethra usually present and are managed in the same way as other urothelial tumours.

BLADDER CANCER

Epidemiology

Each year in the UK there are 10 000 cases of bladder cancer, 7000 cases in men and 3000 cases in women, making it the fifth commonest form of cancer, accounting for 3.5 per cent of all cancer cases and leading to a total of 4800 deaths per annum. There is a male to female ratio of 5:2. It is unusual under the age of 50 years, being most common in people in their 70s and 80s. The UK incidence at 25.3 per 100 000 is below that of European average which is 34.4 per 100 000. In contrast to prostate cancer, it is twice as common in white US males with an incidence of 40.2 per 100 000 compared with black US males at 19.8 per 100 000. This may be accounted for by genetic differences.

Aetiology

- *Chemical carcinogens and smoking.* Bladder cancer is more common in industrialized societies than agricultural areas. Specific carcinogens include aniline dyes; rubber industry by-products such as β-naphthylamine and benzidine; and drugs, e.g.exposure to excessive amounts of phenacetin or cyclophosphamide. This may be associated with genetic changes in genes that code for enzymes important in the detoxification of chemicals. Glutathione S-transferase (GST) is involved in the detoxification of polycyclic aromatic hydrocarbons found in tobacco smoke. Individuals with absent or only single copies of the *GSTM1* gene have increased bladder cancer risk compared with those having two copies of the gene. The *N*-acetyl transferase 2 (NAT2) enzyme is important in the inactivation of aromatic amines; individuals who have a 'slow' variant, particularly those who smoke, are also at increased risk of bladder cancer. There is also evidence that genetic variation in the nucleotide excision repair pathway is associated with risk of bladder cancer.

- *Chronic irritation.* This is related to bladder diverticulae and infection with schistosomiasis is also important in those areas where this is common, being associated with squamous carcinomas in younger age groups.
- *Familial cases* are rare and usually seen in the hereditary non-polyposis colon cancer (HNPCC) syndrome.

Pathology

Macroscopically, bladder cancer can appear as papillary or solid lesions and may be solitary or more usually multiple. The usual area of the bladder affected is the lateral wall and involvement of the bladder base is also common.

Microscopically, the majority of cancers are transitional cell tumours (TCC) of varying differentiation graded from well to poorly differentiated using a numerical scale G1–G3. These account for 90 per cent of all bladder cancers. Of the remainder, 7 per cent are squamous carcinomas and 3 per cent are adenocarcinomas.

The majority of bladder TCCs are superficial indolent tumours that do not progress beyond this stage. However, around 25 per cent of superficial bladder cancer will progress to become muscle invasive; other than tumour grade there are no clear markers as to which tumours will undergo this change. In around 60 per cent of both superficial and invasive TCC deletions affecting chromosome 9 are seen and in over 70 per cent of superficial cancer mutations of fibroblast growth factor 3 gene (*FGFR3*) are seen. Numerous other genetic changes have been reported in invasive cancers including *cyclin D1*, *ERB-B2* and *TP53*, but no consistent picture has yet emerged to account for the change in behaviour between the superficial and invasive variants.

Natural history

Most bladder cancers probably arise as fairly indolent papillomas, which, left untreated, progress both in terms of dedifferentiation and local invasion. The primary tumour invades locally into the bladder muscle wall and thence into perivesical fat. More advanced disease can involve prostate, anterior vaginal wall or rectum.

Lymphatic spread involves pelvic lymph nodes and then para-aortic nodes. Blood-borne metastases particularly arise in lungs and bone.

In many, if not all, patients there is a generalized instability of the urothelium and a risk of further tumours developing not only elsewhere in the bladder but also throughout the ureters and renal pelves. Biopsies of adjacent sites frequently demonstrate dysplasia and a clinical picture of multiple recurrent transitional cell tumours throughout the tract is well recognized.

Symptoms

These may include:

- painless haematuria and other urinary symptoms such as frequency, urgency and dysuria
- cough, haemoptysis or bone pain caused by metastases – less frequent presentations of bladder cancer
- general symptoms of malaise, anorexia and weight loss.

Signs

In most patients there will be no clinical signs of bladder cancer. Bladder tumours are rarely palpable per rectum or per vaginam and only in advanced cases will a suprapubic mass be palpable.

Differential diagnosis

Other causes of haematuria should be considered, including urinary tract infection, stones and renal tumours.

Investigations

Blood tests

Routine blood investigations could reveal anaemia owing to chronic haematuria and renal impairment if there is obstructive hydronephrosis.

Radiography

Chest X-ray will demonstrate metastases if present.

Urine tests

Urine cytology can reveal malignant cells and is a useful screening test. Negative urinalysis, however, should not exclude further investigations.

Intravenous urography

IVU can demonstrate a filling defect in the bladder and renal tract obstruction if present. It is also important to exclude tumours in other parts of the urinary tract since a generalized instability of the urothelium is often present with multiple tumours developing between the renal pelvis and the urethra.

Cystoscopy

Cystoscopy is the definitive investigation at which mucosal abnormalities can be carefully documented and biopsies taken. Transurethral resection of bladder tumour (TURBT) can also be performed during the course of this.

Magnetic resonance imaging

MRI will demonstrate extravesical extension of tumour and lymph node enlargement if present. It is now the imaging modality of choice for staging bladder cancer. Typical appearances of a large bladder cancer are shown in Figure 10.6.

CT scan

This will be used to stage abdominal lymph nodes, liver and lungs for metastases. It also has a role in staging the primary tumour where MRI is contraindicated.

Isotope bone scan

Since bone metastases are relatively common in bladder cancer, this is an important part of the

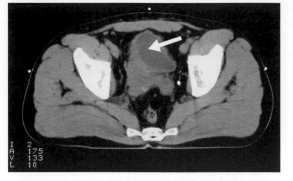

Figure 10.6 MR scan showing extensive bladder cancer filling the bladder cavity and with invasion through the bladder wall on the right side.

staging for a patient newly diagnosed with invasive high-grade bladder TCC.

Staging

The TNM staging system is commonly used:

- Tis – In situ carcinoma
- TI – Superficial invasive carcinoma confined to subepithelial connective tissue
- T2 – Invasion of bladder muscle
  – T2a – Invasion of superficial muscle
  – T2b – Invasion of deep muscle
- T3 – Invasion through muscle wall of bladder
- T4a – Invasion of surrounding pelvic structures
- T4b – Distant metastases.

The important features in deciding on appropriate therapy are the extent of local invasion into the bladder wall, tumour differentiation and distant spread.

Treatment

Local resection

Transurethral resection is performed for superficial (T1) bladder tumours followed by careful cystoscopic surveillance. Recurrence will occur in around 50 per cent and progression to a higher stage or worse grade will occur in around 15 per cent. This is particularly the case in large

CASE HISTORY

CASE HISTORY: BLADDER CANCER

A 56-year-old man has an episode of passing blood in his urine; he has no pain associated with this or other symptoms. He consults his GP who refers him to the Haematuria Clinic at his local hospital. There he undergoes an ultrasound examination of the kidney and bladder, an IVU and a flexible outpatient cystoscopy. When he returns for the results he is told that the ultrasound and IVU are clear but at cystoscopy an abnormal raised reddened area had been seen on the lateral wall of the bladder. He was advised to undergo a further cystoscopy with transurethral resection and biopsy of this area. The histology from the biopsies taken showed flat transitional cell carcinoma in situ (CIS). He was advised to have a course of BCG treatment. He attended the urology ward weekly for 6 weeks to have a urethral catheter passed and the BCG infusion into the bladder. He was allowed home the same day; he noted for the next 24 hours that he had burning when he passed urine and it was more frequent and urgent. On one occasion he had a further small amount of blood. He was reassured that this was a common side-effect after BCG.

Three months after completing the BCG he had a further cystoscopy; he was delighted to learn that no abnormality was seen. It was recommended that he receive a further maintenance course of 3-weekly BCG infusions before his next cystoscopy 6 months later.

He continued with regular cystoscopies for the next 2 years. He was then told after a routine check cystoscopy that a further reddened raised area had been seen in the bladder. He returned for a repeat cystoscopy and biopsy. This showed a return of the transitional cell CIS; one or two areas of poorly differentiated cells were noted where there was early invasion; the tumour was therefore staged T1G3 with associated CIS. After discussion with his urologist and oncologist he was advised that surgery could be curative but would involve a radical cystectomy; radiotherapy was not very effective in this setting and there was no role for further BCG or chemotherapy. He agreed to proceed with surgery. Radical cystectomy with construction of a neobladder from small bowel was performed. He made a good postoperative recovery, and was discharged after 7 days with an indwelling catheter. When this was first removed he had difficulty training his pelvic muscles to control his new bladder and was taught to pass a catheter himself at home twice a day to ensure it was empty. After a couple of months, however, he adjusted to controlling his new bladder and was able to pass water through the penis and remain continent. He had been told to expect difficulties with erectile function but was pleased to find that treatment with tadalafil enabled him to return to normal sexual activity.

He remained under review in the urology clinic with occasional X-rays of his remaining urinary tract to ensure any further tumours of the urothelium are detected at an early stage.

---

tumours, high-grade tumours and those with multiple areas of mucosal dysplasia or frank malignancy. In patients who fail initial resection, further local resection may be attempted. Where there are multiple recurrences and when there is progression to a high-grade tumour, then alternative therapies could be required.

Intravesical chemotherapy

This will improve local control of superficial bladder cancer. Various agents have been used, including Adriamycin, thiotepa and mitomycin C. Currently, BCG is used, which gives better results, although a higher incidence of local complications with acute cystitis can occur and, rarely, a generalized syndrome including joint pain and pulmonary infection has been reported. Typically an initial course of weekly instillations for 6 weeks is given; there is some evidence that maintenance treatment thereafter will reduce the incidence of relapse.

Radical radiotherapy

This is indicated for the treatment of T2 and T3 tumours. Paradoxically in non-invasive (stage Ta) and superficial (stage T1) tumours, radiotherapy has low response rates.

Three-dimensional CT planned conformal treatment will be standard delivering doses of up to 65 Gy; the role of chemoradiation, i.e. adding chemotherapy as a radiation sensitizer, is still under evaluation in bladder cancer.

Cystectomy

This may be considered for progressive superficial bladder cancer and locally advanced muscle-invading tumours. It is also used to salvage recurrence after radical radiotherapy and involves removal of the bladder and perivesical tissues together with pelvic lymphadenectomy. For multifocal lesions, urethrectomy is also recommended. Urine is diverted via an ileal conduit to the abdominal wall or into a neobladder fashioned from bowel, which can be retrained to void or be drained by intermittent self-catheterization.

Partial cystectomy is occasionally used for a localized superficial tumour or where there is only minimal muscle invasion.

Chemotherapy

Whilst chemotherapy is not effective alone as a primary treatment, there is now good evidence that the use of neoadjuvant chemotherapy, i.e. preceding definitive surgery or radiotherapy, will result in improved results, both local control and survival. The absolute benefit, however, is relatively modest with an overall survival advantage of 5 per cent in favour of adding chemotherapy. It is now usual to include three cycles of chemotherapy prior to cystectomy or radical radiotherapy for locally advanced bladder cancer. The standard combinations are gemcitabine with cisplatin (GC) or methotrexate, vinblastine and cisplatin (MVC) to which may also be added Adriamycin (MVAC).

Choice of radical treatment

There are two prevailing philosophies in the treatment of invasive bladder cancer. Some centres offer all patients radical radiotherapy and reserve surgery for salvage. This approach results in initial bladder preservation and complete regression of the bladder tumour in around 60 per cent, but local recurrence requiring salvage surgery may occur in over half of these. The alternative approach is to offer selected patients, particularly those under 65 years, preoperative chemotherapy and elective cystectomy with which 5-year survivals of around 35 per cent are to be expected, although without bladder preservation. No survival advantage between these two approaches has become apparent.

Palliative treatment

Palliative local treatment might be required for advanced tumours or in the frail and elderly who cannot tolerate radical treatment. Local radiotherapy will help haematuria and local pain, given in short, low-dose schedules over 1 or 2 weeks.

Bladder cancer is sensitive to chemotherapy using the GC, MVC or MVAC combinations defined above. Response rates of 50–60 per cent can be achieved, some of which are complete responses resulting in useful palliation in selected patients with symptoms related to uncontrolled local tumour or soft tissue metastases.

Palliative radiotherapy for bone metastases, a relatively common feature of advanced bladder cancer, should also be available.

Tumour-related complications

Haematuria leading to clot retention and clot colic may occur as well as ureteric obstruction leading to hydronephrosis and renal failure.

Treatment-related complications

Surgery

Cystectomy has an operative mortality particularly in the elderly. Stoma problems (e.g. prolapse, bleeding or stricture) can arise and impotence occurs.

Radiotherapy

This can result in both bowel and bladder damage.

Prognosis

Ten-year cause-specific survival ranges from around 70 per cent for T1 bladder cancer to 40 per cent for T3 and <5 per cent for T4 tumours.

Screening and future developments

Urine cytology is currently in use for patients at high risk by virtue of industrial exposure to known bladder carcinogens.

Chemoradiation and other radiosensitizing combinations are under investigation to improve the results of local treatment; surgical developments in reconstructive surgery enable increasing numbers of patients to consider bladder reconstruction after cystectomy.

Rarer tumours

The squamous and adenocarcinomas of the bladder are treated in the same way as the transitional cell tumours. Generally their prognosis is worse and they respond less well to non-surgical treatments.

CANCER OF THE TESTIS

Epidemiology

Each year in the UK there are 2000 cases of testicular cancer, accounting for 0.7 per cent of all cancer cases and leading to a total of 80 deaths per annum. Testicular tumours occur most commonly in men aged between 20 and 40. The UK incidence of 57 per million is five times the incidence in Japan. In the US it is more common in white people than in black people. A slow but steady increase in incidence has been observed over recent years. The success of treatment, however, is reflected in the very low mortality rates with around 70 deaths per year in the UK.

Aetiology

Many testicular tumours are thought to arise as a developmental abnormality in those with mal-descent, which increases the likelihood of a testicular tumour by up to 40-fold. Other factors are a contralateral testicular tumour (the incidence of second malignancy in the other testis being around 3 per cent) and possibly previous orchitis, although this remains speculative.

Men with a first-degree relative having testicular cancer have an increased risk with a relative risk of 8–10 amongst siblings and 4–6 between father and son. Genetic changes in the region of the short arm of chromosome 12 are thought to be relevant to the development of testicular cancer.

Pathology

There are two main types of testicular tumour: seminoma and teratoma. Around 40 per cent are seminomas and 32 per cent teratomas, with a further 14 per cent containing components of both seminoma and teratoma.

Macroscopically, seminomas are solid tumours, well-circumscribed, often lobulated and pale in appearance. In contrast teratomas are often haemorrhagic and contain cystic areas.

Microscopically, seminoma is composed of sheets of uniform rounded cells and may contain granulomata. Particularly well-differentiated variants are recognized (spermatocytic seminoma) as are more aggressive types (anaplastic seminoma). In contrast, teratoma can contain a range of cell types with varying differentiation. Undifferentiated teratoma contains no recognizable mature elements. Trophoblastic elements may predominate and there might be recognizable yolk sac elements.

Natural history

Testicular tumours invade locally into the tunica vaginalis and along the spermatic cord. Lymph node spread occurs relatively early to para-aortic nodes and thence to mediastinal nodes. Blood-borne spread is most commonly to the lungs and liver.

Symptoms

These include:

- testicular swelling or discomfort, particularly with a past history of maldescent
- gynaecomastia owing to excess HCG secretion from the tumour
- backache from enlarged para-aortic nodes
- cough, haemoptysis or dyspnoea from lung metastases.

Signs

These may include:

- testicular swelling which may have an associated hydrocele
- central abdominal mass owing to palpable para-aortic nodes
- pleural effusion
- gynaecomastia owing to stimulation by high levels of HCG.

Differential diagnosis

The following conditions will need to be ruled out:

- benign hydrocele
- testicular torsion
- other causes of backache such as degenerative spinal disease
- other causes of lymphadenopathy, e.g. lymphoma.

Investigations

Routine investigations may demonstrate renal impairment owing to ureteric obstruction by enlarged para-aortic nodes. Abnormal liver function tests could reflect liver metastases. Chest X-ray can also demonstrate metastases as either lung deposits or pleural effusion.

Ultrasound

Testicular ultrasound will demonstrate a solid mass, sometimes with cystic elements in the testis.

Serum markers

There are specific serum markers for germ cell tumours. These are serum α-fetoprotein (AFP) and β-human chorionic gonadotrophin (HCG)

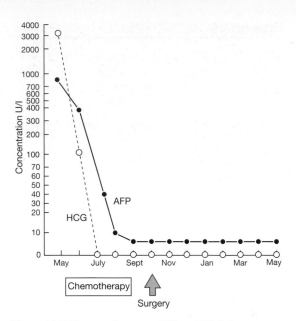

Figure 10.7 Changes in serum AFP and HCG from diagnosis through treatment with chemotherapy and later surgical removal of a residual tumour mass in a patient presenting with advanced testicular germ cell tumour.

and should be measured both prior to any surgical intervention and serially thereafter. Their value in monitoring response to treatment is shown in Figure 10.7. Placental alkaline phosphatase is of value for seminoma but is also affected by cigarette smoking and may therefore be misleading in smokers; lactate dehydrogenase (LDH) is a further marker of use in seminoma.

Around 90 per cent of patients with teratoma will have either AFP or HCG elevated and 40–50 per cent will have both markers raised. The absolute level and rate of fall after treatment are useful prognostic features.

CT scan

CT scan of the pelvis and abdomen is essential to evaluate pelvic nodes and liver, and CT scan of the lungs will give accurate assessment of lung metastases. Figure 10.8 demonstrates the appearances of para-aortic lymph involvement and lung metastases on CT scan.

Staging

The TNM staging system is sometimes used to describe the extent of the primary tumour but

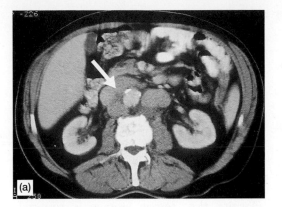
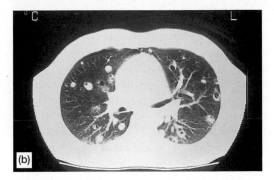

Figure 10.8 CT scans demonstrating (a) enlarged para-aortic lymph nodes and (b) lung metastases from testicular teratoma.

for the overall disease the Royal Marsden Hospital staging system is more widely applied. These are shown below.

TNM stage

- Tl – Limited to testis
- T2 – Involving tunica albuginea or epididymis
- T3 – Invading spermatic cord
- T4 – Invading scrotum
- NI – Single node <2 cm max diameter
- N2 – Single node 2–5 cm max diameter or multiple nodes <5 cm max diameter
- N3 – Any node >5 cm max diameter
- M1 – Distant metastases

Royal Marsden stage

- I – Limited to testis
- II – Involving nodes below diaphragm
- III – Involving nodes both sides of diaphragm
- IV – Distant metastases
  - IVL – Lungs
  - IVH – Liver.

Treatment

All patients will proceed to inguinal orchidectomy with removal of the affected testis. Scrotal interference should be avoided at all costs because of the risk of tumour implantation in the scrotal wound and subsequent relapse.

Stage 1 tumours

If there is no evidence of residual tumour after surgery, then the prognosis is extremely good and around 85 per cent of patients will be cured with no further treatment.

Patients with seminomas can be offered surveillance, radiotherapy to the para-aortic nodes or a single dose of carboplatin. Surveillance is less popular in seminoma than teratoma as the absence of detectable serum markers means that there is greater dependence on radiology. Current evidence suggests that both low-dose para-aortic node radiotherapy delivering only 20 Gy and a single dose of carboplatin are equivalent in preventing subsequent relapse.

Patients with teratomas are entered into a programme of intensive surveillance with monthly measurement of serum markers and regular abdominal and chest CT scans. Those with adverse features such as anaplastic tumour and vascular invasion will receive a short course of chemotherapy.

Stage 2, 3 or 4 tumours

Patients with seminomas will proceed to chemotherapy except those with very small para-aortic nodes. The drugs used are usually cisplatin or carboplatin with the possible addition of etoposide. Small volume disease can be treated by radiotherapy alone to the para-aortic and pelvic nodes, and radiotherapy can be given following chemotherapy in other patients if there is concern regarding residual disease.

Patients with teratomas will proceed to chemotherapy. For good prognosis tumours, standard chemotherapy will be 3-weekly cycles of BEP (bleomycin, etoposide and cisplatin). High-risk patients with extensive disease or very high markers (AFP >1000, HCG >10 000) will receive more intensive regimens with weekly administration of alternating drug schedules containing bleomycin, vincristine, cisplatin, methotrexate and etoposide (BOPP or POMBACE).

In recurrent or resistant cases high-dose chemotherapy is increasingly used with peripheral blood progenitor cell or autologous bone marrow support.

Pelvic surgery

Pelvic lymphadenectomy is advocated as part of the primary treatment of germ cell tumours in some centres, particularly in the United States. In the UK and Europe it is more usual to give initial treatment with chemotherapy and use surgery electively for those patients with primary teratomas who have residual tumour masses after full chemotherapy. This occurs in around 20 per cent of patients and excision of these masses is important to remove not only residual malignant teratoma but also benign differentiated teratoma since this retains the potential to develop into a malignant form at a later date. At surgery approximately 20 per cent are malignant teratoma, 50 per cent differentiated teratoma and the remainder are necrotic with no viable tumour.

Tumour-related complications

Gynaecomastia owing to high levels of HCG sometimes occurs.

Treatment-related complications

- Unilateral orchidectomy has no physiological effect on potency but this may be affected after pelvic lymphadenectomy.
- Abdominal radiotherapy can be related to subsequent peptic ulceration and an increased rate of second malignancies in later life.
- Chemotherapy causes alopecia which is reversible.

- Cisplatin can result in peripheral neuropathy and ototoxicity. Renal impairment which is usually reversible also occurs and an increased incidence of hypertension in later life has been reported.
- Bleomycin can cause skin changes and pneumonitis in high dose.
- Fertility is impaired after chemotherapy but recovery usually occurs after standard BEP chemotherapy, and there are increasing reports of success in fathering children after treatment for testicular cancer. Despite this, semen storage is routinely advised for patients undergoing this type of chemotherapy. Potency is not affected.

Prognosis

Few patients die from testicular cancer today. Cure is virtually guaranteed for stage 1 tumours and is expected in around 85 per cent of those with more advanced stages. However, relapse after primary chemotherapy heralds a poor outlook with only 20–30 per cent of patients surviving long term with salvage treatment.

Screening

Health education programmes aimed at self-examination are the main form of population screening.

Rarer tumours

The remaining tumours that occur in the testis are lymphomas (7 per cent) and the rare pure yolk sac tumours, Sertoli cell tumours and interstitial cell tumours. Mesotheliomas arising from the tunica vaginalis have also been described. Lymphomas are managed as for any extranodal lymphoma while other rare tumours are managed by surgical excision.

CANCER OF THE PENIS

Epidemiology

Each year in the UK there are 400 cases of penis cancer, accounting for 0.3 per cent of all cancer cases and leading to a total of 100 deaths per annum. It accounts for less than 1 per cent of deaths from cancer in men. It is more common in other parts of the world, in particular Africa and China where it accounts for around 15 per cent of male cancers.

Aetiology

It is virtually unknown in populations who practise circumcision. A relationship with papilloma virus has been proposed.

Pathology

Macroscopically, the tumour may be a papilliferous or solid growth on the shaft or glans of the penis. Ulceration can occur. It may develop insidiously beneath the foreskin.

Microscopically, penile cancer is a squamous carcinoma often well or moderately differentiated.

Natural history

The tumour will invade the shaft of the penis as shown in Figure 10.9 and spread to inguinal lymph nodes (Fig. 10.10). Blood-borne spread occurs relatively late to lungs and liver.

Symptoms

Tumours are usually asymptomatic but there might be local discharge and odour.

Signs

The primary tumour is usually obvious on clinical examination. Palpable inguinal nodes are present in up to half of patients.

Differential diagnosis

Other penile skin lesions should be considered, including lymphogranuloma venereum, condylomata acuminata, chancroid, traumatic ulceration, leukoplakia, Bowen's disease, erythroplasia of Queyrat and giant penile condylomata (Buschke–Lowenstein tumour).

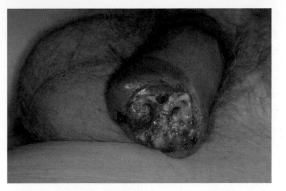

Figure 10.9 Locally advanced primary squamous carcinoma of the penis with destruction of the glans.

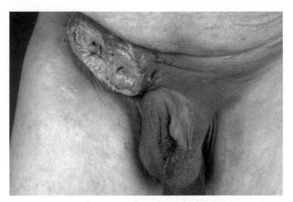

Figure 10.10 Advanced right inguinal nodes disease owing to metastases from a carcinoma of the penis. The primary tumour was treated some months earlier when no metastases were apparent by amputation.

Other causes of inguinal lymphadenopathy need to be taken into account, in particular chronic infection, which accounts for around 50 per cent of the associated lymphadenopathy.

Investigations

Routine investigations are rarely helpful although a chest X-ray will be necessary to exclude lung metastases.

Biopsy

A biopsy or cytological scrapings will confirm the diagnosis.

Fine needle aspiration

FNA of enlarged nodes should be used to distinguish metastatic nodes from infected and inflammatory nodes.

CT scan

Where inguinal nodes are involved, a pelvic CT scan is of value to assess further lymphatic spread.

Staging

The commonly used staging system is the Jackson staging, which is shown below as well as the formal TNM staging.

T stage
- T1 – Superficial subepithelial
- T2 – Invading corpus cavernosa
- T3 – Invading urethra or prostate
- T4 – Invading adjacent structures

Jackson stage
- I – Limited to glans or prepuce
- II – Invading shaft; no nodes
- III – Invading shaft; node positive
- IV – Fixed inoperable nodes or distant metastases.

Treatment

Surgery

This will usually involve partial or complete amputation as shown in Figure 10.10, unless the tumour is small and confined to the prepuce when local excision by circumcision may be adequate. Penile reconstruction can be offered after surgery.

Radiotherapy

This can be delivered by either external beam or by the use of brachytherapy with an interstitial implant or penile mould. The penis is preserved, with surgery reserved for salvage.

Treatment of involved nodes should be by block dissection of the groin. In the case of fixed inoperable nodes local irradiation can be performed. Advanced fixed fungating nodes are shown in Figure 10.10.

Palliative treatment

This might be indicated for locally advanced disease or where there are distant metastases. Usually a short palliative course of radiotherapy to the primary site, nodes or local recurrence will help prevent local pain and fungation.

There is no recognized chemotherapy for penile cancer although responses are seen in advanced disease using schedules containing drugs such as cisplatin, methotrexate, 5FU and mitomycin C.

Tumour-related complications

Interference with micturition and potency is seen.

Treatment-related complications

Radiotherapy can result in urethral stricture in about 10 per cent of cases.

Prognosis

Survival with stage 1 disease is over 85 per cent at 5 years falling to 35 per cent for stage 3 tumours. Long-term survival with stage 4 disease is unusual.

FURTHER READING

Cohen HT, McGovern FJ. Renal cell cancer. *New England Journal of Medicine* 2005;**353**:2477–90

Damber J-E, Aus G. Prostate cancer. *Lancet* 2008;**371**:1710–21

Lerner SP, Schoenberg NP, Sternberg CN. *Textbook of Bladder Cancer*. Informa Healthcare, New York, 2005

Horwich A, Shipley J, Huddart R. Testicular germ cell cancer. *Lancet* 2006;**367**:754–65

SELF-ASSESSMENT QUESTIONS

1. Which of the following applies to renal cell cancer?
   a. There are approximately 12 000 cases per year in the UK
   b. It occurs equally in males and females
   c. It is related to smoking
   d. It is common in Japan
   e. The mortality is similar to the incidence

2. Which of the following is correct in renal cell cancer?
   a. It arises from cells in the glomerulus
   b. Characteristically the cells are adenocarcinoma clear cells
   c. There is often detection of the retinoblastoma gene
   d. Lymph node spread is rare
   e. Most patients have metastases at presentation

3. Which three of the following are common presenting features of renal cell cancer?
   a. Dysuria
   b. Haematuria
   c. Urinary retention
   d. Loin pain
   e. Paraneoplastic neuropathy
   f. Renal failure
   g. Weight loss

4. Which of the following is true of prostate cancer?
   a. It is rare under 60 years
   b. Most cases have a family history
   c. It is related to smoking
   d. It is the most commonly diagnosed cancer in males in the UK
   e. It is more common where there is benign prostatic enlargement

5. Which three of the following are important in determining the prognosis from prostate cancer?
   a. PSA level
   b. Haemoglobin
   c. Urinary function
   d. Gleason grade
   e. Seminal vesicle involvement
   f. Bilateral tumour
   g. Urethral involvement

6. Which three of the following are recognized presenting features of prostate cancer?
   a. Weight loss
   b. Dysuria
   c. Erectile impotence
   d. Leg oedema
   e. Constipation
   f. Haematospermia
   g. Urinary retention

7. In the treatment of prostate cancer which of the following is true?
   a. Surgery with transurethral resection is adequate for localized tumour
   b. Radiotherapy is rarely used for localized disease
   c. Hormone manipulation is aimed at reducing levels of oestrogen
   d. Urinary incontinence is common after radiotherapy
   e. Goserelin works through the pituitary gland

8. Which of the following applies to bladder cancer?
   a. In men it is more common than prostate cancer
   b. The most common form is not life threatening
   c. It is related to alcohol consumption
   d. It is related to diet
   e. It is most common in the 50–60-year-old group

9. Which of the following is true in relation to bladder cancer?
   a. The common form is muscle-invasive squamous carcinoma

SELF-ASSESSMENT QUESTIONS

b. Exposure to schistosomiasis results in squamous carcinoma
c. Primary stage is related to extent of bladder surface involved
d. Carcinoma in situ is more dangerous than superficial tumour
e. Adenocarcinoma might be due to aniline dye exposure

10. In the treatment of bladder cancer which of the following is true?
   a. Intravesical therapy can be used for muscle-invasive tumour
   b. Chemotherapy has no role in primary treatment
   c. Metastases may respond to hormone therapy
   d. Radical radiotherapy may be used for superficial invasive cancer
   e. Cystectomy can be successful after radiotherapy

11. Which of the following is true of testicular tumours?
   a. They increase in frequency with age
   b. They typically have a rapidly fatal course
   c. They are related to previous measles infection
   d. There is an increased risk of a contralateral second testicular tumour
   e. They are most common in Asia

12. Which three of the following are characteristic of testicular tumours?
   a. Gynaecomastia
   b. Haematuria
   c. Impotence
   d. A family history of testicular tumour
   e. Raised blood levels of CEA
   f. Haematospermia
   g. A positive pregnancy test

13. Which is true of the treatment of testicular cancer?
   a. Biopsy of the testicular mass confirms the diagnosis
   b. Early cases may need no treatment after removal of the testis
   c. Seminoma will require more intensive treatment than teratoma
   d. Most patients will be impotent after treatment
   e. Maintenance chemotherapy will improve long-term prognosis

14. Which of the following applies to cancer of the penis?
   a. Circumcision protects against its development
   b. The common type is an adenocarcinoma
   c. It is most common in South America
   d. Early spread to the prostate and bladder occurs
   e. Local excision is usually adequate treatment for localized tumour

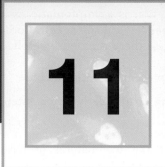

11 GYNAECOLOGICAL CANCER

■ Cervical cancer 185
■ Endometrial cancer 191
■ Ovarian cancer 194
■ Cancer of the vagina 198
■ Cancer of the vulva 200
■ Choriocarcinoma 202
■ Further reading 204
■ Self-assessment questions 205

CERVICAL CANCER

Epidemiology

Each year in the UK there are 2700 cases of cervical cancer, accounting for 1 per cent of all cancer cases and leading to a total of 900 deaths per annum. It has an annual incidence of 8 per 100 000. In contrast, largely as a result of effective screening, there are 24 000 cases of carcinoma in situ (CIN III) each year. Invasive cervical cancer is predominantly a disease of women in their 40s and 50s but is showing an increase in younger age groups. It is common in lower socioeconomic groups and there is a wide geographical variation, highest levels of the disease being in South America with incidence figures of up to 80 in 100 000.

Aetiology

Persistent human papilloma virus (HPV) is now thought to be a feature of all cervical cancers, although only a small proportion of women acquiring HPV infection will develop cervical intraepithelial neoplasia (CIN). Prevalence rates of HPV in the population are up to 48 per cent.

It is the subtypes HPV 16 and 18 that are most clearly linked to CIN.

It is associated with sexual activity, being increased in women starting intercourse at an early age and having multiple partners. It is more common in women who are or who have been married than in single women. There is some evidence that the male partner is implicated, being associated with partners of lower socioeconomic groups and those high-risk males who have more than one partner who develops cervical cancer. Other recognized aetiological factors include smoking, miscarriage, use of oral contraceptives, parity and co-infection with sexually transmitted diseases. It is a recognized HIV related malignancy.

Pathology

Macroscopically, there are two common presentations:

■ proliferative growth at the cervix with surface ulceration
■ diffusely infiltrating tumour with the mucosa intact owing to tumour arising in the endocervical canal. The latter is sometimes described as a 'barrel-cervix'.

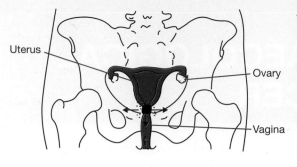

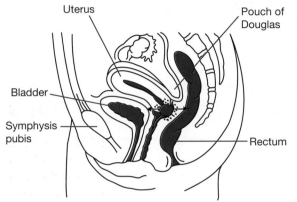

Figure 11.1 Patterns of local spread from cervical carcinoma. (a) Lateral and (b) anteroposterior spread.

Microscopically, 90 per cent of cervical cancers are squamous carcinomas of varying differentiation. The remaining 10 per cent are adenocarcinomas arising from the external os or endocervix. The relative proportion of adenocarcinomas has increased over the last decade, particularly in younger women.

Natural history

Local spread in all directions occurs predominantly laterally and anteroposteriorly as shown in Figure 11.1. Lymph node spread occurs relatively early, being identified in around 15 per cent of stage 1 tumours.

From paracervical nodes there is spread to internal and external iliac nodes, presacral and obturator nodes. Subsequent spread is then up the para-aortic node chain.

Blood-borne metastases occur, affecting in particular the lungs, liver and bone.

Symptoms

Frequently, presentation is asymptomatic as a result of an abnormal cervical smear test. Local pain is unusual unless there is extensive pelvic infiltration.

If symptoms are present they may include:

- vaginal bleeding, particularly after intercourse
- vaginal discharge
- renal failure owing to bilateral ureteric obstruction
- haematuria or rectal bleeding owing to local spread
- low back and sacral pain owing to pelvic and para-aortic lymphadenopathy
- general symptoms of malignancy, including anorexia, malaise and weight loss.

Signs

Pelvic examination is mandatory; the tumour will usually be apparent at the cervix as a proliferative or ulcerative growth or a diffuse infiltration. It is important to note extension onto the vaginal mucosa and, on rectal examination, any evidence of spread into the parametrium or rectal mucosa.

Differential diagnosis

Other cervical lesions should be considered, such as a cervical erosion.

Where bladder or rectal involvement is diagnosed it may be difficult to distinguish clinically between primary tumours of these sites invading the cervix, although this is usually apparent on histology.

Investigations

Routine investigations can reveal anaemia owing to bleeding and a raised white cell count where there has been chronic infection. Renal failure will be apparent on routine biochemical tests and a chest X-ray will be needed to exclude metastases.

Cervical cytology

This is performed to diagnose malignancy and vaginal swabs taken at the same time can demonstrate the nature of an infective discharge.

Biopsy

A full examination under anaesthetic including a cystoscopy should be performed in all cases, at which time biopsies can also be taken.

CT scan

A CT scan of the abdomen and pelvis will help assess local extension and enlargement of pelvic and para-aortic lymph nodes.

Intravenous urography

An IVU will assess ureteric obstruction, although this can now usually be seen clearly on CT.

Magnetic resonance imaging

For definition of soft tissue changes around the cervix and assessment of the primary tumour MRI is superior to CT, as shown in Figure 11.2.

Staging

The FIGO staging system is generally accepted in clinical assessment of cervical cancer:

- Stage 1
  - 1A – Microinvasive disease limited to the cervix
  - 1B – Confined to the cervix with invasion >5 mm depth from surface or >7 mm spread in a horizontal direction.
- Stage 2
  - 2A – Extension to vaginal mucosa but not into lower third of vagina
  - 2B – Extension to parametrium but not reaching pelvic side wall
- Stage 3
  - 3A – Extension to lower third of vagina
  - 3B – Extension to pelvic side wall
- Stage 4
  - 4A – Involvement of bladder and rectal mucosa
  - 4B – Distant metastases.

Treatment

Radical treatment will be considered for all patients except those with widespread metastatic disease or bladder or rectal involvement. Presentation with renal failure is not an absolute contraindication to radical treatment and in selected cases percutaneous nephrostomies to re-establish renal drainage should be performed prior to treatment as shown in Figure 11.3.

Localized to the cervix (stage 1)

Surgery

Radical surgery is the treatment of choice in the form of a radical hysterectomy (Wertheim's hysterectomy) during which, in addition to the removal of the uterus, tubes and ovaries, the upper vagina, parametrium and pelvic lymph nodes are also included in the resection.

Chemoradiotherapy

Radical chemoradiation can be given for early stage cancer of the cervix and the results in terms of survival are no worse than those after radical surgery, although there might be a greater incidence of long-term morbidity. It is usually therefore reserved for elderly patients and those medically unfit for surgery, but is an acceptable option for younger women who refuse surgery.

Postoperative radiotherapy can be given following Wertheim's hysterectomy where the

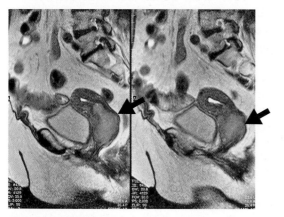

Figure 11.2 MR scan demonstrating locally advanced carcinoma of the cervix.

CASE HISTORY: CERVICAL CANCER

A 38-year-old woman presents with a 3-month history of postcoital bleeding. One year previously she had a normal cervical smear report when she saw her GP for family planning advice. The GP has referred her to a Consultant Gynaecologist having performed a pelvic examination at which he found a hard irregular cervix and considered the likely cause of bleeding to be a cervical carcinoma. The gynaecologist confirmed the clinical history and on examination found a hard ulcerating tumour at the cervix with no obvious extension beyond this site. He subsequently performed examination under anaesthetic confirming a stage Ib carcinoma of the cervix with no parametrial or vaginal extension. A biopsy showed moderately differentiated squamous carcinoma. A cystoscopy was normal.

Further investigations included a normal full blood count and chest X-ray; an MR scan confirmed a 3 cm mass at the cervix but no extension beyond that and a CT scan showed no hydronephrosis and no signs of metastatic disease in lymph nodes, liver or lungs. Treatment was recommended with radical hysterectomy at which the uterus and cervix with an upper cuff of vagina and parametrial tissue was removed together with a pelvic lymph node dissection. Histological examination of the specimen confirmed a moderately differentiated carcinoma of the cervix but three out of five left pelvic lymph nodes were positive and two out of eight right-sided pelvic lymph nodes were positive. As a result of this finding postoperative radiotherapy was recommended. The patient received a standard 5-week course of postoperative radiotherapy to the pelvis. During this time she experienced some diarrhoea and urinary frequency.

Three months later she was well but complaining of some bowel frequency attributed to the radiotherapy. When seen 6 months later she complained of some persistent low back pain. Clinical examination was normal but a CT scan showed large lymph nodes in the para-aortic region. The chest X-ray showed three small volume metastasis in the left lung field and five metastasis in the right lung.

Chemotherapy was recommended. The patient received a course of cisplatin and topotecan. During treatment she suffered nausea and vomiting and for the following week had some nausea but otherwise tolerated the treatment well. She returned 3 weeks later for a second course of treatment which was given with similar side-effects. Two weeks later she returned to the hospital earlier than planned with persistent nausea and vomiting. She was drowsy and slightly confused. Urgent investigations revealed a serum creatinine of 800. Abdominal ultrasound showed bilateral hydronephrosis and a CT scan identified enlarged common iliac and para-aortic lymph nodes obstructing both ureters. Bilateral nephrostomies were inserted; over the subsequent 3 days as urine drainage was re-established her creatinine fell to 260. At this point she developed a high fever and her full blood count had fallen with a profound neutropenia, total neutrophil count 0.3. She was treated with intravenous antibiotics using ceftazidime but continued to have a high fever. The culture from her urine draining through the nephrostomy showed a staphylococcal infection. Flucloxacillin was added to an antibiotic regimen and her fever settled. Two days later she complained of acute chest pain and shortness of breath. She became acutely hypotensive and despite active resuscitation died from a presumed pulmonary embolus.

excision margins are not clear of tumour and where there is involvement of the removed pelvic lymph nodes in the resection.

Preoperative radiotherapy has been advocated in the past but it has no proven value and, with the use of the above criteria, only 20 per

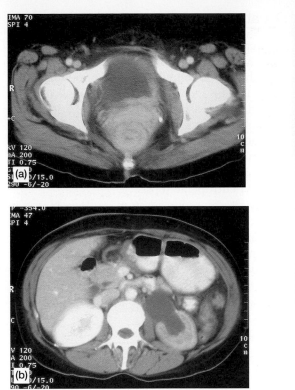

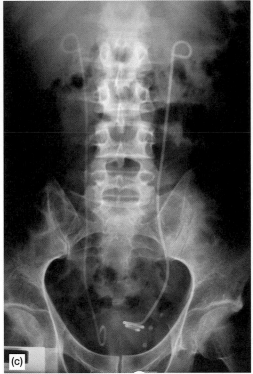

Figure 11.3 CT scan demonstrating (a) extensive local infiltration from cervical cancer into the bladder base with (b) associated hydronephrosis. Insertion of ureteric stents is necessary in this situation if renal function is to be preserved as shown in the plain X-ray (c).

cent of women will require irradiation in addition to surgery.

Tumour beyond cervix (stages 2 and 3)

Chemoradiotherapy

Radical chemoradiation will be the treatment of choice. This will involve a course of external beam treatment to the whole pelvis covering the major node chains up to the bifurcation of the aorta, delivering a dose of 40–50 Gy over 4–5 weeks with weekly cisplatin. Intracavitary brachytherapy treatment to the cervix will follow this by intrauterine tube and vaginal source to give a further 25–30 Gy to the cervix and surrounding tissues. A typical arrangement of intracavitary applicators is shown in Figure 11.4.

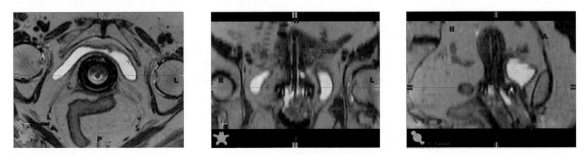

Figure 11.4 MR scan demonstrating intrauterine tube and vaginal ring source in position for treatment of carcinoma of the cervix using brachytherapy.

Chemotherapy

The results of radical radiotherapy for cervical cancer are improved if chemotherapy is given during radiotherapy and the usual schedule includes weekly cisplatin during external beam radiotherapy.

In contrast, the use of adjuvant chemotherapy usually given prior to radiotherapy in locally advanced disease has been disappointing and to date no proven advantage has emerged in clinical trials.

Palliative treatment

Where there are distant metastases or locally advanced pelvic disease, then radical local treatment is inappropriate. Chemotherapy for advanced and recurrent disease has only limited activity and complete response is extremely rare. The most effective drug schedule is cisplatin either alone or with topotecan. Other schedules include methotrexate and ifosfamide or taxotere. These can be associated with considerable toxicity.

Palliative radiotherapy for advanced local disease could be worthwhile and is particularly indicated for the control of local bleeding and pelvic pain. Other procedures such as a palliative colostomy might be required where there is rectal involvement, or fistulae develop.

Hormone replacement

Cervical cancer is not hormone dependent. This means that hormone manipulation is not a useful approach to treatment but also that, following radical treatment, in young women particularly, hormone replacement therapy should be offered.

Tumour-related complications

These include:

- renal failure owing to bilateral ureteric obstruction
- acute haemorrhage from the tumour occasionally resulting in hypovolaemic shock
- fistulae between bladder or rectum and vagina
- pyometra owing to obstruction of the cervical canal by tumour.

Treatment-related complications

Radical surgery can result in urinary urgency and urge or stress incontinence. Lower limb lymphoedema following pelvic node dissection may also be seen. It can also result acutely in bowel and bladder toxicity with radiation cystitis and diarrhoea.

Chemoradiation schedules sometimes enhance the above toxicities of radiotherapy and in addition cause pancytopenia with the risk of neutropenic sepsis.

Long-term sequelae from radiotherapy can include reduced bladder volume, telangiectasia causing haematuria or rectal bleeding, chronic diarrhoea and vaginal stenosis. Rarely bowel or bladder fistulae occur, although subsequent investigations often reveal recurrent disease in this setting.

Prognosis

Outcome is closely related to stage at presentation with a 5-year survival of around 80 per cent for stage 1 and 2A tumours, falling to only 20–30 per cent for stage 3 and less than 5 per cent for stage 4. Within stage 1 tumours, prognosis is related to tumour bulk and differentiation.

For microinvasive and in situ carcinoma of the cervix, surgery is almost always curative, emphasizing the importance of early diagnosis in this condition where curative treatment is readily available for early stage disease.

Screening

Screening for cervical neoplasia by cervical smear testing is widespread and there is good evidence that in the US and Scandinavia the rate of decline in cervical cancer can be related to intensity of screening.

Currently around 3 million cervical smears are performed in the UK each year and it has been estimated that this has reduced the incidence of invasive cancers by around 30 per cent. This accounts for around 80 per cent of all eligible women. Current recommendations are for all sexually active women below the age of 50 years to have cervical smears at 3–5 yearly intervals. A major problem with this, as with any screening programme, is to achieve good rates of compliance, particularly in those groups at high risk. It is also important to recognize the limitation of smear screening since a number of women will still be diagnosed having a normal smear. Overall, the accuracy of cervical smear cytology is only around 80 per cent despite technically good smears and accurate interpretation.

Future prospects

The greatest impact is likely to be made by extending the current screening programmes to reach all those women at risk with high rates of compliance in order to detect early curable disease.

Vaccines are now available against HPV 16 and 18; their use at present is sporadic but it is envisaged that in the future all girls will receive vaccination before becoming sexually active.

Rarer tumours

Five per cent of cervical cancers are adenocarcinomas. These are generally treated in the same way as the more common squamous cancers and, stage for stage, they have a similar prognosis.

ENDOMETRIAL CANCER

Epidemiology

Each year in the UK there are 6400 cases of endometrial cancer, accounting for 2.3 per cent of all cancer cases and leading to a total of 1700 deaths per annum. Compared with cancer of the cervix, cancer of the endometrium affects the older, predominantly postmenopausal age group, the median age at presentation being 61 years. The incidence in the UK is 16 per 100 000. There is far less geographical variation than with cervical cancer, although it is relatively rare in Japan where the incidence is about one-tenth of that in Europe and the US.

Aetiology

Endometrial carcinoma occurs typically in obese nulliparous women who have a tendency to diabetes and cardiovascular disease. Early menarche and late menopause increase the risk.

High levels of circulating oestrogens are a known cause and it is a recognized complication of an oestrogen-secreting granulosa cell tumour of the ovary. There is no proven association with therapeutic use of oestrogens in hormone replacement therapy but there is increasing evidence linking endometrial cancer with prolonged tamoxifen use for breast cancer.

Endometrial cancer can occur as part of the hereditary non-polyposis colorectal cancer (HNPCC) syndrome and daughters of women with endometrial cancer have approximately double the risk of developing endometrial cancer themselves.

Pathology

Macroscopically, the tumour arises within the uterine cavity and can be polypoid or a more diffuse even multifocal growth arising from the endometrium.

Microscopically, the tumour is an adenocarcinoma, which may be of varying grade, usually designated from G1 (well differentiated) to G3 (poorly differentiated).

Mutations in the *PTEN* tumour-suppressor gene are relatively common.

Natural history

There is local invasion into the myometrium and cervix. The tubes and ovaries are sometimes also involved and the tumour occasionally extends into parametrial tissues or involves the bladder or rectum. This is far less common than in cancer of the cervix.

Lymph node spread can occur, involving pelvic lymph nodes, and submucosal lymphatic permeation along the vaginal walls is well recognized.

Distant metastases by blood-borne spread most frequently involve lungs and bone.

Symptoms

The classic presentation of endometrial cancer is with postmenopausal bleeding. In the premenopausal woman heavy and/or irregular periods may be the only symptom. There might be an associated vaginal discharge.

General symptoms of malaise, anorexia and weight loss are usually mild and symptoms from metastatic disease are unusual at presentation.

Signs

On pelvic examination the uterus may feel bulky and a vaginal discharge or bleeding from the os may be apparent. Often no physical signs can be detected.

Differential diagnosis

Other causes of postmenopausal bleeding should be considered such as atrophic vaginitis and in premenopausal women other causes of irregular menstrual bleeding such as fibroids.

Investigations

Routine investigations can reveal anaemia owing to chronic blood loss. Other abnormalities are unusual.

Biopsy

Whilst positive cytology can be obtained from cervical smears or sampling of the endometrial cavity, this cannot be relied upon and the diagnosis is confirmed by examination of endometrial biopsies. These may be obtained by examination under anaesthetic at which time the cervical canal and uterine cavity are dilated in turn and fractional curettage performed to obtain endometrial samples, but increasingly this is being replaced by outpatient sampling using a pipelle and hysteroscopy and endometrial biopsy under direct vision.

Radiology

MRI scanning is now used routinely preoperatively and accurate estimates of the extent of myometrial invasion can be obtained together with information on spread beyond the body of the uterus. An example is shown in Figure 11.5.

For more advanced cases (stage 2, 3 or 4) a CT scan will be used to assess abdominal lymph node status and lungs.

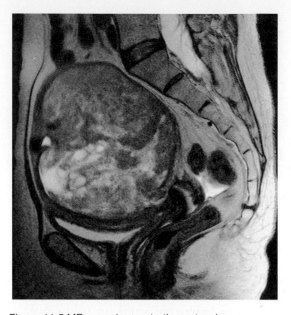

Figure 11.5 MR scan demonstrating extensive endometrial carcinoma expanding the uterine cavity and invading the muscle wall of the uterus; note bladder is flattened anteriorly from massive uterine enlargement with tumour. (Courtesy of Dr A Padhani)

Staging

Carcinoma of the endometrium is staged using the FIGO system:

- Stage 1
  - 1A – Confined to the endometrium; no myometrial invasion
  - 1B – Confined to the endometrium, invasion <50 per cent of myometrium
  - 1C – Confined to the endometrium; invasion >50 per cent of myometrium
- Stage 2 – Invasion of cervix
- Stage 3 – Spread to pelvic tissues
- Stage 4
  - 4A – Spread to bladder or rectum
  - 4B – Distant metastases.

Treatment

A major feature of endometrial cancer is the predominance of stage 1 tumours at presentation, accounting for 70–80 per cent of patients.

Surgery

Total abdominal hysterectomy and bilateral salpingo-oophorectomy is the treatment of choice for disease localized to the endometrium.

A Wertheim's hysterectomy (see above) is indicated when there is cervical involvement (stage 2).

Radiotherapy

Postoperative radiotherapy is considered for patients following hysterectomy for stage 1 disease who have poor risk features, in particular high-grade tumours and deep myometrial invasion (stage 1C).

Radical radiotherapy can on occasions be given for elderly unfit patients with stage 1 disease and is the treatment of choice for those with bulky stage 2 and stage 3 tumours. This will take the form of external beam treatment to the pelvis followed by intracavitary treatment to the uterine cavity and upper vagina.

Chemotherapy

The role of adjuvant chemotherapy for high-risk endometrial cancer is currently under evaluation using combinations of cisplatin, or carboplatin with taxotere.

Palliative treatment

Palliative radiotherapy can be given for locally advanced tumours and for painful bone metastases.

Endometrial cancer is a hormone-dependent tumour and metastatic disease will respond to progestogens such as medroxyprogesterone acetate or megestrol. Response rates are between 20 and 30 per cent and useful palliation of symptomatic metastases can be achieved. Responses to gonadotrophin-releasing hormone analogues such as leuprorelin are also recognized. There is no good evidence to support the use of these agents as adjuvant treatment.

Occasionally chemotherapy using cisplatin and Adriamycin or taxotere can be offered to younger fit patients with advanced disease; objective tumour responses are seen in 20–30 per cent of patients.

Tumour-related complications

Pyometra or haematometra can occur owing to obstruction of the uterine cavity.

Treatment-related complications

Hysterectomy can result in urinary urgency and urge or stress incontinence. Pelvic radiotherapy is sometimes associated with late bowel and bladder toxicity, causing frequency, haematuria, rectal bleeding and rectal or vaginal stenosis.

Prognosis

The prognosis for endometrial carcinoma is good since the majority of patients present with stage 1 disease for which there are cure rates in excess of 85 per cent. Prognosis for more advanced stages falls, as would be anticipated, with 5-year survival rates of around 65 per cent for stage 2, and 35 per cent for stage 3. Survival stage for stage is worse for women over 60 years than for younger women and also for those with the papillary serous type of cancer.

Prevention

The early diagnosis of endometrial cancer is helped by its early presentation with post-menopausal bleeding. It is therefore vital that all women with this symptom are investigated appropriately to exclude endometrial cancer.

Rarer tumours

Sarcomas of the endometrium can arise, presenting in the same way as endometrial cancer. They may be pure sarcomas such as a leiomyosarcoma arising from a fibroid or mixed tumours, such as the mixed mesodermal tumour, which contains both epithelial and stromal components, the latter in the form of malignant sarcomatous cells.

The prognosis for endometrial sarcomas is poor. Treatment is surgical removal at hysterectomy. There is no proven role for radiotherapy or chemotherapy, although regional and distant metastases are a common problem with these tumours.

OVARIAN CANCER

Epidemiology

Each year in the UK there are 6600 cases of ovarian cancer, accounting for 2.3 per cent of all cancer cases and leading to a total of 4400 deaths per annum. There is a similar incidence in the USA but a low incidence in Japan, which approaches that of American women in Japanese immigrants to the USA.

Aetiology

Ovarian cancer tends to occur in women over the age of 40 years who are nulliparous and of higher socioeconomic groups. Compared with women who have had more than four pregnancies, the relative risk for nulliparous women is 2.4. Paradoxically there appears to be a protective effect from oral contraceptive use, particularly for those using it for over 5 years, while a modest increase in risk is seen in women taking hormone replacement therapy for more than 10 years.

Genetic factors are important in the development of around 10 per cent of ovarian cancers. A link with the breast cancer-associated genes *BRCA1* and *BRCA2*, as well as with HNPCC, is recognized. The lifetime risk in a carrier of *BRCA1* is 50 per cent and in HNPCC 12 per cent.

No specific environmental agents have been identified as directly contributing to the development of ovarian cancer.

Pathology

The common appearance of ovarian cancer is that of a cystic enlargement of the ovary. Two common types are recognized macroscopically:

- the pseudomucinous cyst, characteristically a large, multiloculated tumour mass containing mucinous material
- the serous cyst, containing clear fluid within a thin-walled cyst containing papillary structures.

Other tumours may form solid masses (typical of a Brenner tumour) or characteristic teratomas.

The microscopic appearances of ovarian cancer are variable and the classification often complex.

Epithelial adenocarcinomas are the common ovarian cancers with several variants recognized, such as clear cell carcinomas and endometrioid carcinomas.

Germ cell tumours are the other major group of tumours of the ovary but, in contrast to the testis, the majority are benign teratomas.

Rarer tumours include those derived from gonadal stroma such as the *granulosa cell* and *Sertoli cell tumours*, which are oestrogen- and androgen-secreting, respectively, *mixed mesodermal tumours* analogous to those that grow in the uterus, and lymphomas.

Metastases may also present in the ovary, typically from carcinoma of the breast or stomach (Krukenberg tumours).

Natural history

Local growth occurs within the ovary, spreading through the cyst wall onto the surface. Transcoelomic spread across the peritoneal cavity results in the classic appearance of multiple seedlings visible throughout the pelvic and abdominal cavities studding the peritoneal surfaces. Involvement of the omentum is also common and ascites is frequently found at operation.

Lymph node spread occurs to para-aortic nodes in the first instance.

Blood-borne metastases to liver and lungs are seen in more advanced disease. Meig's syndrome is the presence of a pleural effusion accompanying an ovarian tumour and has the features of a transudate, cytologically negative for carcinoma cells.

Symptoms

Ovarian cancer can remain asymptomatic for some time and often presents with vague symptoms of abdominal discomfort and pelvic pain. In more advanced cases this may be associated with abdominal swelling owing to either tumour or ascites, and urinary and bowel disturbance owing to local pressure.

General symptoms of malignancy including malaise, anorexia and weight loss may also be present, and metastases can cause dyspnoea or bone pain.

Signs

Abdominal swelling and distension with a palpable mass or clinical signs of free fluid (shifting dullness to percussion and a fluid thrill) might be present. An ovarian mass may be palpable per vaginam or per rectum and a pleural effusion detectable clinically by dullness to percussion and absent breath sounds. A left supraclavicular node may be palpable in advanced cases.

Differential diagnosis

Other causes of abdominal swelling should be considered, including ascites from other causes, hepatomegaly or splenomegaly, benign ovarian masses and intestinal obstruction.

Investigations

Routine investigations will often be unremarkable, although in advanced cases there might be electrolyte disturbance from intestinal obstruction or ureteric obstruction causing renal failure.

Radiography

Chest X-ray may demonstrate metastases or a pleural effusion.

Ultrasound

This will image the ovaries and give information regarding the nature of ovarian cysts. Liver ultrasound will evaluate the presence or absence of liver metastases.

CT scan

CT scan of the abdomen and pelvis will demonstrate the primary tumour and also pelvic and para-aortic lymph node enlargement together with liver metastases if present. An example of a massive intra-abdominal tumour mass from carcinoma of the ovary is shown in Figure 11.6.

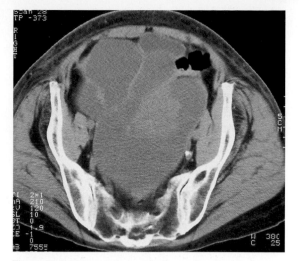

Figure 11.6 CT scan demonstrating extensive intra-abdominal tumour from carcinoma of the ovary.

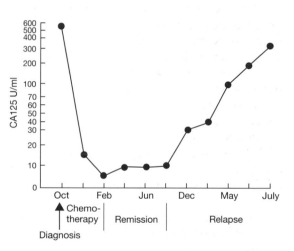

Figure 11.7 Changes in serum CA125 from high levels at diagnosis, falling through chemotherapy and later rising at relapse.

Serum markers

Serum CA125 is a valuable blood marker for ovarian cancer and is a useful monitor of response to treatment as demonstrated in Figure 11.7.

Creatinine or ethylene diamine tetra-acetic acid (EDTA) clearance

Creatinine clearance or EDTA clearance might be necessary to measure renal function for those patients requiring chemotherapy.

A 'Risk of Malignancy' index (RMI) has been described based on the findings on transvaginal ultrasound, serum CA125 and menopausal status.

Staging

The FIGO staging system for ovarian cancer is in common use:

- Stage 1 – Confined to the ovary
  - 1a One ovary involved
  - 1b Both ovaries involved
- Stage 2 – Spread to the pelvis
- Stage 3 – Spread to the abdominal cavity
- Stage 4 – Blood-borne metastases.

Treatment

Surgery

All patients with operable disease will proceed to laparotomy at which total abdominal hysterectomy, bilateral salpingo-oophorectomy and omentectomy are performed, together with careful examination of the para-aortic nodes, liver and peritoneal surfaces, including the sub-diaphragmatic regions and biopsy of any suspicious areas. Prognosis is directly related to the residual bulk of tumour and so maximum tumour debulking should be attempted in all patients, even where complete clearance is not possible.

For patients with stage 1a or 1b tumours that are well or moderately differentiated and with normal postoperative CA125 levels, no further treatment is indicated and close observation with serial pelvic ultrasounds and serum CA125 levels will be undertaken.

Surgery can have a role to remove persisting disease after chemotherapy, the 'second look laparatomy', at which residual tumour is removed to achieve macroscopic complete remission.

Chemotherapy

Primary chemotherapy can be chosen where patients present with inoperable disease which, in those who achieve a good response, will be followed by surgical removal of residual tumour.

Postoperatively, for high-grade stage 1 tumours, stage 1c tumours and more advanced disease localized to the abdominopelvic cavity, i.e. stages 2 and 3, chemotherapy is indicated. The drugs of choice are currently cisplatin or its analogue carboplatin, given for six cycles at monthly intervals together with paclitaxel.

For stage 4 disease with soft tissue metastases the outlook is poor and treatment might not influence the outcome. In patients with good general status, chemotherapy could be considered as for earlier stage disease.

Palliative treatment

Chemotherapy is of value where relapse occurs after a long period of remission (>1 year) with many patients responding to re-exposure to cisplatin-based schedules. Relapse within the first year responds less well to further chemotherapy and heralds a particularly poor prognosis. Alternative drugs to be considered include liposomal daunorubicin, etoposide containing schedules or topotecan.

Radiotherapy might be of value for symptomatic pelvic masses, vaginal bleeding from disease invading the vagina and bone metastases.

Tumour-related complications

Ascites and pleural effusions can occur. Intestinal obstruction is common in the advanced phases of the disease.

Treatment-related complications

Cisplatin can cause neurotoxicity with peripheral neuropathy or less frequently spinal cord damage. Ototoxicity can result in tinnitus and high tone deafness. Reduced renal function is common but overt renal failure need not occur provided the patient is well hydrated and renal function is properly monitored.

Both paclitaxel and carboplatin can cause significant bone marrow depression. Paclitaxel will in addition cause alopecia and it is associated with peripheral neuropathy.

Prognosis

The outlook for stage 1 ovarian cancer is good, with 10-year survival figures of over 80 per

CASE HISTORY: OVARIAN CANCER

A 48-year-old woman presents with a 1-year history of intermittent abdominal discomfort and a 1-month history of progressive abdominal distension. An abdominal ultrasound has shown a complex mass in the left ovary. Her CA125 is measured at 3562. Other investigations including a full blood count, renal function and chest X-ray are normal. She proceeds to laparotomy at which a large clinically malignant tumour is seen in the right ovary with multiple seedlings found throughout the abdominal cavity. Five litres of ascites are drained from the abdominal cavity. A total abdominal hysterectomy, bilateral salpingo-oophorectomy is performed leaving behind multiple small nodules on the peritoneum. Postoperatively a course of chemotherapy is recommended. She proceeds to receive five courses of carboplatin and paclitaxel. During treatment she suffers alopecia and is complaining at the end of her course of tingling in the fingers particularly when attempting to use them for fine movements. Her CA125 at completion of chemotherapy has fallen to 23.

Following chemotherapy she makes a good recovery and returns to a normal lifestyle.

Two years later she presents to her Casualty Department with a 3-day history of nausea, vomiting and constipation. On clinical examination intestinal obstruction is found. An emergency laparotomy is performed which reveals widespread multiple areas of obstruction of the small bowel secondary to scattered nodules of tumour. Biopsy confirms recurrence of her ovarian cancer. No attempt at resection is made and postoperatively she makes a slow but steady recovery with gradual resolution of her obstructive symptoms. Second-line chemotherapy is offered but she declines. Within 2 weeks she has a further episode of abdominal obstruction, which is managed conservatively with intravenous fluids and subcutaneous diamorphine and cyclizine. The symptoms are well controlled but her general condition deteriorates and she dies peacefully 10 days later.

cent. For more advanced disease the results of current chemotherapy give 5-year survival figures of 35–50 per cent. The survival of patients with stage 4 disease is usually only a few months.

Screening

Screening programmes for ovarian cancer have been proposed using serum CA125 measurements and abdominal ultrasound. Currently they are recommended for those with a strong positive family history but routine population screening is not justified.

Rare tumours

Brenner tumours

These are fibromas of the ovary and are usually benign in nature. Treatment is surgical removal.

Teratomas

Arising in the ovary, these are usually benign dermoid cysts. Malignant teratomas analogous to those arising in the testis are seen and, following surgical removal, adjuvant chemotherapy is recommended using drug combinations such as BEP (bleomycin, etoposide and cisplatin).

Dysgerminomas

These are germ cell tumours arising in the ovary analogous to seminomas arising in the testis. For stage 1 tumours surgery is often curative. Chemotherapy using drugs such as VAC (vincristine, actinomycin D and cyclophosphamide) can be used for more widespread disease and these tumours are usually very radiosensitive; pelvic radiotherapy could have a role in persisting and recurrent disease.

Granulosa cell tumours

These are usually low grade and generally cured by surgery, although local recurrence some years later is recognized. Characteristically they secrete oestrogens and can be associated with the synchronous development of an endometrial cancer.

Sertoli–Leydig cell tumours

These are usually of low malignant potential and cured by oophorectomy.

Sarcomas

These are rare and typically mixed mesodermal tumours having both sarcomatous and epithelial elements. Their prognosis is poor unless localized within the ovary at the time of surgery.

Lymphomas

These can arise within the ovary and are typically high-grade non-Hodgkin's lymphomas treated as extranodal lymphomas at any other site with adjuvant chemotherapy with or without pelvic radiotherapy.

Metastases

These can present in the ovary, usually from stomach or breast cancer. The classic bilateral ovarian metastases from carcinoma of the stomach are sometimes referred to as Krukenberg tumours.

CANCER OF THE VAGINA

Epidemiology

Carcinoma of the vagina is rare accounting for only 1 per cent of all gynaecological cancers. It is a disease predominantly of elderly women. In the past it was seen in young women associated with maternal use of stilboestrol.

Each year in the UK there are 250 cases of vaginal cancer, accounting for 0.1 per cent of all cancer cases and leading to a total of 100 deaths per annum.

Aetiology

Cancer of the vagina is closely related to HPV infection and other sexually transmitted infection including herpes simplex. There is therefore also an association with cervical neoplasia and women with a past history of CIN or invasive cervical cancer have a 20-fold risk of vaginal cancer also.

Unlike in cervical cancer, an association with genital warts, typically associated with HPV 6 and 11, is seen.

Chronic irritation of the vaginal mucosa following long-term use of a vaginal ring pessary for vaginal prolapse is also a risk factor.

Maternal use of stilboestrol during pregnancy was associated with the development of clear cell adenocarcinoma of the vagina during adolescence, fortunately no longer seen.

Pathology

Vaginal intraepithelial neoplasia (VAIN) is a recognized epithelial change analogous to CIN at the cervix and can progress to frank carcinoma.

Macroscopically, the tumour presents either as an ulcer, papilliferous growth or diffuse infiltration of the vaginal mucosa.

Microscopically, the usual histology is a squamous carcinoma. Rarely, adenocarcinomas arise and the clear cell variant related to stilboestrol can also be seen without this aetiology.

Natural history

Direct extension results in invasion of the parametrium, bladder or rectum. Lymph node spread is to internal iliac and pelvic nodes (from the upper two-thirds of the vagina) and to inguinal and femoral nodes (from the lower third).

Blood-borne spread to liver and lungs also occurs in advanced disease.

Symptoms

These include vaginal discharge and bleeding; local pain is unusual unless there has been extensive pelvic infiltration.

Signs

Tumour will usually be visible and palpable on speculum and digital vaginal examination.

Inguinal nodes might be palpable with tumours of the lower vagina.

Differential diagnosis

This includes: atrophic vaginitis; metastases from the cervix or endometrium; and a tumour of the urethra or Bartholin's gland.

Investigations

The diagnosis will be confirmed at examination under anaesthetic when biopsies can be taken. Routine investigations can show chronic anaemia from blood loss and, rarely, renal failure owing to ureteric obstruction from pelvic infiltration or lung metastases on chest X-ray.

Fine needle aspiration

Palpable inguinal nodes should be investigated further by FNA to distinguish inflammatory nodes from metastases.

CT scan

Staging should include CT scan of the pelvis to assess pelvic lymph nodes.

Magnetic resonance imaging

MRI will give most accurate details of the soft tissue anatomy of the pelvis and identify local extension of the tumour.

Staging

Vaginal carcinoma is staged using the FIGO classification:

- Stage 1 – Limited to the vaginal mucosa
- Stage 2 – Extension to submucosa and parametrium but not to pelvic side walls
- Stage 3 – Extension to pelvic side wall
- Stage 4 – Bladder, rectum or distant metastases.

Treatment

Surgery

Early disease can be treated by radical hysterectomy and total vaginectomy with pelvic lym-

phadenectomy. Inguinal node dissection is also undertaken for tumours in the lower third of the vagina. Vaginal reconstruction should be offered to women undergoing this procedure.

Radiotherapy

Radiotherapy is indicated for stage 2 and stage 3 disease. It could also be considered for those with early tumours who are unwilling to accept vaginectomy, reserving surgery to salvage patients whose disease recurs and for those unfit for surgery. External beam irradiation to the pelvis including the inguinal nodes for lower third tumours should be followed by intracavitary or interstitial treatment to give a high dose of radiation directly to the vaginal mucosa and surrounding local tumour extension. Chemoradiation using weekly cisplatin with radiotherapy is considered for younger patients.

Palliative treatment

Radiotherapy is helpful for locally advanced or recurrent disease. This takes the form of external beam treatment where there is a major pelvic component or intracavitary treatment for bleeding or ulcerated disease locally in the vagina.

There is no recognized effective chemotherapy for vaginal carcinoma.

Tumour-related complications

These may include vaginal haemorrhage and sepsis and renal failure owing to urethral obstruction.

Treatment-related complications

Recognized acute complications of pelvic radiotherapy include radiation cystitis and diarrhoea.

Late complications include vaginal stenosis and fistulae into bladder or rectum, particularly where there has been local infiltration by tumour.

Prognosis

Over 80 per cent of stage 1 patients can expect cure; 50 per cent of patients with stage 2 and 30 per cent of those with stage 3 tumours will survive 5 years.

Screening

Female offspring of mothers who received stilboestrol during pregnancy are at recognized high risk and will benefit from regular screening by clinical examination and vaginal smears.

VAIN seems to be related to earlier cervical malignancy and therefore these patients should also receive regular vaginal smears following treatment of a cervical cancer.

Rarer tumours

Adenocarcinoma and clear cell carcinoma are usually treated surgically, with radiotherapy reserved for palliation of advanced tumours.

CANCER OF THE VULVA

Epidemiology

Each year in the UK there are 1000 cases of vulval cancer, accounting for 0.4 per cent of all cancer cases and 5 per cent of all gynaecological cancers with 380 deaths each year. It is usually seen in older, postmenopausal women.

Aetiology

There is an association with HPV infection, both subtypes 16 and 18 related to cervical cancer, and genital wart viruses, subtypes 6 and 11. The risk in women having previous CIN or invasive cervical cancer is 10 times that of those without. There is an association with other sexually transmitted diseases including herpes simplex and HIV. Other immunosuppressed groups are also at increased risk with a 100-fold excess risk in patients after renal transplantation.

Vulval cancer is increased in smokers and chemical carcinogenesis was seen historically in the 'mulespinners' exposed to mineral oils.

Pathology

Vulval cancer may be preceded by or co-exist with dystrophic conditions of the vulval skin including leukoplakia, lichen sclerosus et atrophicus and Paget's disease of the vulva. True carcinoma in situ is also seen in the vulval skin.

Macroscopically, the invasive tumour is typically a papilliferous growth or an ulcer arising from the medial side of the labium majorum (Fig. 11.8). Bilateral tumours are also seen – the so-called 'kissing cancer'.

Microscopically, vulval carcinomas are squamous carcinomas. Other rare tumours that can arise in the vulva include basal cell carcinomas, melanomas, sarcomas and tumours of the female urethra and Bartholin's gland.

Natural history

Local invasion of surrounding soft tissue occurs early and in advanced cases pubic bone can also

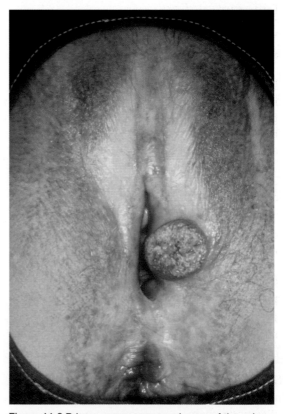

Figure 11.8 Primary squamous carcinoma of the vulva.

become involved. Lymphatic spread is to the inguinal nodes before progressing along the pelvic node chain. Blood-borne spread to lungs can occur but is a late event.

Symptoms

- There may be long-standing symptoms of skin dystrophy with local irritation.
- A lump may be obvious to the patient.
- Pain is usually a late symptom owing to bone invasion.
- Swelling of the legs can occur from inguinal nodes or femoral vein involvement.

Signs

- The local tumour will be apparent as an ulcer or papilliferous growth.
- Inguinal nodes can be palpable with associated leg oedema.

Differential diagnosis

Vulval dystrophies can be a forerunner of invasive cancer, as discussed above.

Infective conditions, such as condylomata, lymphogranuloma inguinale or lymphogranuloma venereum, should be considered. In the past tuberculous or syphilitic lesions have also been described in the differential diagnosis but are rarely seen today.

Investigations

The tumour is usually apparent clinically and diagnosis is confirmed by a full examination under anaesthetic and biopsy.

Fine needle aspiration

Palpable nodes should be investigated with FNA for cytological confirmation of malignancy as many will be only inflammatory.

CT scan

In the presence of palpable nodes CT scan of the pelvis will assess proximal spread into the iliac node chain.

Radiography

Chest X-ray will exclude the presence of lung metastases.

Staging

Staging uses the TNM classification:

- T1 – Confined to the vulva, 2 cm or less in diameter
- T2 – Confined to the vulva, >2 cm in diameter
- T3 – Involving the urethra, vagina, perineum or anus
- T4 – Invading the rectal or bladder mucosa, urethral mucosa or underlying bone
- N0 – No nodes palpable
- NI – Mobile nodes in either groin, not clinically suspicious of malignancy
- N2 – Mobile nodes in either groin, clinically suspicious of malignancy
- N3 – Fixed or ulcerated nodes.

Treatment

Surgery

Wide excision of the vulva (simple or radical vulvectomy) with bilateral femoral and inguinal node dissection is usually recommended.

Radiotherapy

For inoperable disease, radical radiotherapy can be given using both external beam treatment, often given as chemoradiation with weekly cisplatin and interstitial implantation of the tumour. A radical dose could be given but acute reactions in this area can be severe and are often dose limiting; they are particularly severe in patients receiving combined chemoradiotherapy.

Palliative treatment

Local toilet surgery might be required or, where there is extensive posterior infiltration, a defunctioning colostomy. Radiotherapy is of value for local pain, discharge and bleeding.

There is no recognized chemotherapy for vulval carcinoma although responses are described following combinations effective against squamous carcinomas, such as mitomycin C and 5FU or methotrexate and 5FU.

Tumour-related complications

These can include:

- local haemorrhage and discharge
- oedema of either or both legs from venous or lymphatic obstruction
- urethral invasion causing difficulty with micturition
- anal invasion possibly resulting in faecal incontinence.

Treatment-related complications

Radical surgery can be complicated by delayed wound healing. Leg oedema is sometimes seen where there has been extensive dissection of the groins.

Prognosis

Survival is related to the extent of disease at presentation and general condition, which in the frail and elderly might preclude radical surgery.

Following radical surgery for localized disease, over 80 per cent of patients will survive 5 years. The involvement of lymph nodes is a poor prognostic sign, reducing 5-year survival to around 40 per cent.

Rare tumours

Basal cell carcinomas

These are usually cured by local surgery unless they have invaded deeper structures. They can also be treated by radiotherapy.

Melanomas

These are best treated with wide surgical excision. For more advanced local lesions or patients with distant metastases, palliative radiotherapy could be of value in obtaining local control.

Sarcomas

These are also best treated by wide surgical excision.

CHORIOCARCINOMA

Epidemiology

Choriocarcinoma is a malignant tumour arising from the placental tissues. It is a rare tumour that may arise occasionally in association with a normal pregnancy, but is far more common as a complication of a hydatidiform mole.

The incidence of hydatidiform mole is around 1 in 1000 pregnancies in the UK of which 3 per cent will develop into choriocarcinoma. The incidence of choriocarcinoma following term delivery where there is no mole is around 1 in 50 000 pregnancies. There is no recognized geographical variation.

Aetiology

Hydatidiform mole is more common in pregnancies in women under 20 and over 40. Past history of a mole predisposes to subsequent mole pregnancies.

Pathology

Macroscopically, choriocarcinoma arises within the uterus following normal pregnancy, ectopic pregnancy, spontaneous abortion or hydatidiform mole. It is characteristically a haemorrhagic tumour with no detectable placental remnant.

Microscopically, the distinction between a benign mole and choriocarcinoma is made by the absence of villi in the choriocarcinoma with areas of necrosis and haemorrhage. The cells of the trophoblast have malignant features with many mitoses and pleomorphic cells with multiple nucleoli.

Natural history

Local invasion involves the uterine wall at an early stage. Lymph node metastases are rare. Early blood-borne dissemination occurs to lungs, liver and the central nervous system. Other common distant sites involved are skin, bowel and spleen. Bone metastases are rare.

Symptoms

These include:

- vaginal bleeding within 1 year of pregnancy
- abdominal or pelvic discomfort.

Up to one-third of patients may present with symptoms of metastatic disease such as cough, haemoptysis, weight loss, headache or fits.

Signs

The uterus can be enlarged and tender on pelvic examination or a pelvic mass palpable. Chest signs secondary to lung collapse or effusion might be present, the liver enlarged and palpable, and there might be focal neurological signs associated with brain metastases.

Differential diagnosis

Choriocarcinoma must be distinguished from hydatidiform mole. Other causes of uterine bleeding such as fibroids and cervical or endometrial carcinoma should be considered.

Investigations

Blood tests

Blood levels of human chorionic gonadotrophin (HCG) are important. This is raised in normal pregnancy but also with hydatidiform mole and choriocarcinoma. It is an important indicator of tumour bulk in choriocarcinoma and an invaluable tumour marker for monitoring treatment.

Ultrasound

Ultrasound of the uterus gives a characteristic picture in hydatidiform mole and choriocarcinoma. It can also be used to assess the extent of local invasion through the uterine wall and fallopian tube and ovarian involvement.

CT scan

CT scan of the brain, chest abdomen and pelvis is required for full staging information.

Magnetic resonance imaging

MRI will give further detailed evaluation of the uterus and local tumour infiltration within the pelvis.

Histology

The diagnosis of choriocarcinoma will be confirmed histologically on examination of the uterine contents removed at examination under anaesthetic and suction evacuation.

Staging

Choriocarcinoma is staged as follows:

- Stage 1 – Confined to the uterus
- Stage II – Early spread to vagina or ovary
- Stage III – Lung metastases
- Stage IV – Metastases outside the lungs.

A prognostic score has been described by which patients can be divided into those with a good, intermediate or poor prognosis. This uses a number of parameters including age, parity, preceding pregnancies, HCG level, number, site and size of metastases.

Treatment

Because of its rarity and the complex nature of its treatment, all patients should be referred to a major centre experienced in the management of choriocarcinoma.

Surgery

Suction evacuation of the uterus is the initial treatment in all cases.

Chemotherapy

Subsequent chemotherapy is based on close monitoring of serum HCG levels. Indications for treatment include:

- very high levels persisting after evacuation (>20 000 IU)
- rising levels of HCG
- continued uterine bleeding
- metastatic disease.

All the above are signs of active choriocarcinoma.

Low-risk patients

Low-risk patients who are young with disease restricted to the uterus and vagina or those with lung metastases account for 80 per cent; they will receive chemotherapy with methotrexate as a single agent.

Intermediate-risk patients

Intermediate-risk patients who are over 39 years with localized disease or have spleen or liver metastases receive chemotherapy with actinomycin D, vincristine and etoposide.

High-risk patients

Those with metastases in the gastrointestinal tract or liver receive more intensive chemotherapy called EMA-CO comprising etoposide, actinomycin D, methotrexate, vincristine and cyclophosphamide. Multiple drugs are used in this context to prevent resistance emerging in surviving cells.

Because of the high risk of CNS metastases, prophylactic treatment with intrathecal methotrexate is also recommended for high-risk patients and all those with lung metastases.

Established CNS metastases are treated with dexamethasone and multiple drug chemotherapy as for the high-risk group.

Tumour-related complications

Bleeding from the uterus or metastatic sites resulting in gastrointestinal, intracerebral or intrapulmonary haemorrhage may be seen. Respiratory failure can complicate multiple pulmonary metastases or be precipitated by their treatment owing to rapid tumour lysis.

Treatment-related complications

Rapid tumour destruction with chemotherapy of widespread metastases can cause not only respiratory failure but also extensive metabolic disturbance (tumour lysis syndrome; see Chapter 22).

Many patients have proceeded after successful treatment to have further pregnancies without complications. There is, however, some concern that oral contraceptive treatment in the immediate period after chemotherapy may provoke further relapse and oral contraception should be avoided for 6 months following completion of chemotherapy.

Prognosis

The outlook for patients with choriocarcinoma is extremely good. It is only those who have high-risk disease, including those over 40 years with bulky (>5 cm) metastases, multiple sites or more than a total of eight metastases, brain metastases and very high HCG levels (>10 000 IU) in whom survival of less than 100 per cent can be anticipated and, even in this group, over 85 per cent will be cured.

Screening

Routine screening of pregnant women is not indicated but high-risk patients who have had previous trophoblastic disease (mole or choriocarcinoma) should have careful monitoring of HCG following delivery.

FURTHER READING

Cannistra SA. Cancer of the ovary. *New England Journal of Medicine* 2004;**351**:2519–29

Hoskin PJ, Symonds P (eds). *Uterine Cancer*. Clinical Oncology Special Issue, Vol 20. Elsevier, London, 2008

SELF-ASSESSMENT QUESTIONS

1. Which of the following is true of cancer of the cervix?
   a. It increases in incidence with age
   b. It is related to infection with the herpes zoster virus
   c. It is more common in higher socioeconomic groups
   d. It is found in most patients at screening
   e. It is falling in incidence in the UK

2. Which of the following is true of cancer of the cervix?
   a. The common form is an adenocarcinoma
   b. Squamous cancers typically arise from the endocervical canal
   c. Surface ulceration is common
   d. The usual path of spread is into the uterine cavity
   e. Lymph node spread is rare

3. Which three of the following are recognized features of cancer of the cervix?
   a. Renal failure
   b. Constipation
   c. Dysuria
   d. Amenorrhoea
   e. Post-coital bleeding
   f. Urinary incontinence
   g. Low back pain

4. In the treatment of cancer of the cervix, which of the following is true?
   a. Surgery is preferred for stages I to III disease
   b. Chemotherapy has an important role in primary treatment
   c. Hormone replacement therapy is contraindicated
   d. Radiotherapy is indicated if lymph nodes are involved at surgery
   e. Metastatic disease may respond to anti-oestrogens

5. Which of the following is true of endometrial cancer?
   a. It is related to infection with the HPV virus
   b. It is most common in premenopausal women
   c. It can be prevented by cervical smear screening programmes
   d. It is associated with hypothyroidism
   e. It can be caused by treatment for breast cancer

6. Which three of the following are true in the treatment of endometrial cancer?
   a. Most cases are cured after radical hysterectomy
   b. Advanced disease may respond to anti-oestrogen therapy
   c. Radiotherapy is not useful as the cancer is radioresistant
   d. Chemotherapy is effective for advanced disease
   e. Hormone replacement therapy should be encouraged after treatment

7. Which of the following applies to cancer of the ovary?
   a. It is most common in women under 40 years of age
   b. It is common in Japan and the Far East
   c. It is usually diagnosed with symptoms at an early stage
   d. There is a 50 per cent risk in patients with the *BRCA1* gene
   e. It is associated with smoking

8. In cancer of the ovary which of the following is true?
   a. Common types are cystic
   b. Teratomas are usually malignant
   c. Blood-borne spread is an early feature
   d. The common histology is a squamous carcinoma
   e. The level of CEA is used to monitor response

SELF-ASSESSMENT QUESTIONS

9. Which three of the following are usually associated with cancer of the ovary?
   a. A high level of CA125
   b. Haematuria
   c. Dysmenorrhoea
   d. Abdominal distension
   e. Renal failure
   f. Ascites
   g. Constipation

10. Which of the following is true of the treatment of ovary cancer?
    a. Radical surgery is usually curative
    b. Unilateral salpingo-oophorectomy is the usual operation for stage I
    c. Chemotherapy with cisplatin and paclitaxel is standard in stage III
    d. Hormone replacement therapy is contraindicated
    e. Postoperative radiotherapy is indicated for high-risk stage I disease

11. Which of the following is true of cancer of the vagina?
    a. It is more common in women who have had previous CIN
    b. It is more common than cancer of the vulva
    c. The common form is an adenocarcinoma
    d. The usual treatment when the cancer is localized is radical surgery
    e. Adjuvant chemotherapy may have a role in high-risk cases

12. Which of the following is true of cancer of the vulva?
    a. It typically spreads to iliac lymph nodes
    b. It is more common after renal transplantation
    c. Blood-borne metastases occur at an early stage
    d. Radical radiotherapy is indicated for early disease
    e. The prognosis is related to age

13. Which of the following is true of choriocarcinoma?
    a. It occurs in 1 in 5000 live pregnancies
    b. It typically occurs in women aged 20–40 years
    c. Metastases are present in a third of women at presentation
    d. Surgical excision is the best treatment
    e. Future pregnancy is contraindicated

14. Which three of the following are true of the treatment for choriocarcinoma?
    a. Chemotherapy is indicated if there is an HCG level >20 000 IU
    b. Chemotherapy response is monitored by serial levels of HCG
    c. The most useful drug is cisplatin
    d. Intrathecal chemotherapy is required by all patients
    e. Chemotherapy is not required for low-risk patients
    f. Prophylaxis against tumour lysis is required for advanced disease
    g. Infertility is a common side-effect

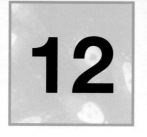

12 CNS TUMOURS

- Astrocytoma 211
- Oligodendroglioma 213
- Meningioma 213
- Pituitary tumours 214
- Craniopharyngioma 216
- Pineal tumours 216
- Germ cell tumours 216
- Ependymomas 217
- Medulloblastoma 217
- Chordoma 218
- Haemangioblastoma 218
- Lymphoma 218
- Metastases 219
- Carcinomatous meningitis 221
- Further reading 223
- Self-assessment questions 224

A discussion of the general principles will be followed by specific examples.

Epidemiology

Each year in the UK there are 4400 cases of CNS tumours, 2600 cases in men and 1800 cases in women, accounting for 1.6 per cent of all cancer cases and leading to a total of 3600 deaths per annum. One to two per cent of autopsies performed after death from other causes reveal occult brain primary tumours. There is a bimodal age incidence with peaks at 5–9 and 50–55 years, varying with the type of tumour, e.g. medulloblastomas are very rare beyond adolescence, glioblastomas are very rare in adolescents and children. There is a slight male predominance in all types except meningioma.

Aetiology

In the vast majority of cases no aetiological factors can be identified. Several associations have been identified but these conditions are themselves very rare. Genetic predisposition to CNS tumours has been identified in the following rare syndromes:

- neurofibromatosis – neurofibroma, and neurofibrosarcoma, optic nerve glioma, ependymoma, meningioma
- tuberose sclerosis – glioma and hamartoma
- Von Hippel–Lindau syndrome – cerebellar haemangioblastoma
- Li–Fraumeni syndrome – gliomas
- Gorlin's syndrome – medulloblastoma.

Industrial exposure to vinylchloride has been associated with the development of gliomas. The controversy regarding a cause and effect relationship between electromagnetic radiation and CNS tumours continues. In HIV-positive cases, primary cerebral lymphoma is associated with infection by the Epstein–Barr virus.

Pathology

Classification of tumours according to their cell of origin is outlined in Table 12.1; 80 per cent

TABLE 12.1 Classification of primary CNS tumours according to the tissue of origin

Tissue of origin	Tumour
Glial (50%)	Astrocytoma, oligodendroglioma, ependymoma
Meninges (25%)	Meningioma, meningiosarcoma
Pituitary (20%)	Craniopharyngioma, adenoma
Vascular (2%)	Angioma, haemangioblastoma
Pineal (<1%)	Pinealoma, pineoblastoma
Germ cells (<1%)	Teratoma, dysgerminoma
Miscellaneous	Chordoma, medulloblastoma, lymphoma

are intracranial and 20 per cent spinal, childhood tumours tending to be located in the cerebellum, adult tumours in the cerebral hemispheres. Highly malignant tumours will have necrosis and haemorrhage on cut section, oedema of the surrounding cerebral tissue, and may not be well circumscribed. Multifocal high-grade gliomas and lymphomas are recognized. Calcification is seen in craniopharyngiomas, oligodendrogliomas and some meningiomas, making them visible on a plain skull X-ray.

Spinal tumours can be classified further according to their origin in relation to the dural/spinal cord anatomy into three groups:

- extradural, e.g. metastases, chordoma
- intradural extramedullary, e.g. meningiomas, neurofibromas
- intramedullary, e.g. astrocytomas, ependymomas, haemangioblastomas, lipomas, dermoids.

Tumours can be subclassified into grades according to the degree of differentiation. This grading reflects the expected behaviour of the tumour and takes into account factors such as the degree of tumour cellularity, the number and appearance of mitotic figures and the presence of necrosis.

Natural history

Direct infiltration is the main mode of spread and the cause of death of the majority of patients dying from CNS tumours. All CNS tumours, even if benign, enlarge by infiltrating and/or compressing the adjacent neural tissue,

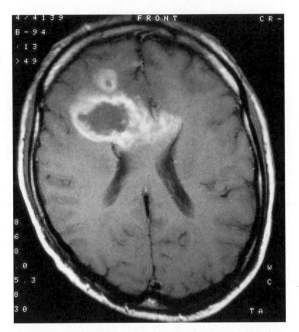

Figure 12.1 High grade glioma. MRI of the brain showing a large tumour infiltrating across the corpus callosum.

and in turn the increasing peritumoral oedema around the tumour leads to raised intracranial pressure. Raised intracranial pressure might also be due to hydrocephalus from compression of the ventricular system leading to impaired drainage of cerebrospinal fluid (CSF) and ventricular dilatation proximal to the block. Local infiltration will also lead to focal brain damage manifested as focal neurological signs, and some tumours cross the corpus callosum in the midline to involve the contralateral hemisphere (Fig. 12.1). Tumours prone to CSF seeding include medulloblastoma, ependymoma,

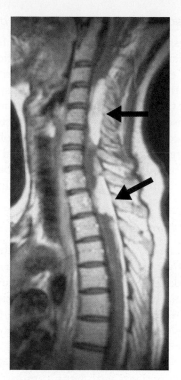

Figure 12.2 Multiple meningeal tumour deposits. Sagittal MRI of the cervicothoracic spine and spinal cord.

pineoblastoma, germ cell tumours and lymphoma. This results in meningeal deposits anywhere from the foramen magnum down to the mid-sacrum (Fig. 12.2).

Insertion of a shunt to relieve hydrocephalus can, rarely, lead to distant dissemination of tumour. Lymphatic spread is not seen as the neural tissue does not have a true lymphatic drainage system. Distant metastases are extremely rare, but are described in patients with very aggressive tumours such as glioblastomas that have invaded the dural venous sinus system, and medulloblastomas.

Symptoms and signs

Cerebral tumours

Patients with cerebral tumours usually present with one or more of the following:

- epilepsy
- raised intracranial pressure
- focal neurological deficit.

The patient may present with an epileptic fit which can be generalized, affecting the whole body, or focal, or affecting a region or single part of the body related to the anatomical origin within the brain. A cerebral tumour should be considered in any patient presenting de novo in this manner, particularly with focal epilepsy. Raised intracranial pressure can lead to headaches with an early morning predominance, nausea, vomiting, somnolence, apathy, poor concentration, memory impairment and personality change. Clinically, there may be papilloedema, upgoing plantar responses, evidence of impaired higher mental functions and impairment of consciousness. Local pressure from a tumour will lead to dysfunction of the affected tissue owing to ischaemia, which will be manifested clinically by focal neurological signs corresponding to the affected portion of the brain. These will be upper motor neurone in type, e.g. spasticity, hyperreflexia and upgoing plantar reflexes in the case of a hemiparesis.

Spinal tumours

These may present with one or more of the following:

- spinal cord compression
- cauda equina compression.

Spinal cord compression can arise when the lesion lies between the foramen magnum and the lower limit of the cord at the junction of the L1 and L2 vertebrae. There will be a pattern of upper motor neurone loss of function below the level of the block, associated with a sensory level and sphincter disturbance.

Cauda equina compression arises if the lesion is somewhere below the lower limit of the spinal cord (at approximately L1/L2 level) affecting only nerve roots, and therefore the signs are those of a lower motor neurone lesion affecting the lower limbs, i.e. hypotonia, weakness, wasting, fasciculation, hyporeflexia, downgoing plantar reflexes and a dermatomal sensory loss. The urethral and anal sphincters may also be impaired.

Investigations

Computed tomography (CT)

This will give information regarding the location, size and degree of local invasion of the tumour. The advent of spiral CT heralded an era of improved image reconstruction in planes other than the usual axial images. It is particularly good for delineating the skeletal anatomy but poor at surveying the posterior fossa owing to the thickness of the bone in this region and proximity of mastoid air cells, both of which can lead to streak artefacts. Artefacts from surgical clips and dental amalgam can also produce problems.

Magnetic resonance imaging (MRI)

MRI should be considered the investigation of choice for imaging of CNS tumours. The high lipid content of neural tissue leads to high contrast and in turn a high spatial resolution. The ability to image directly in non-axial planes (rather than reconstruct non-axial planes as in CT) lends itself to high quality images of the brain and spinal cord. These are ideal for neurosurgical planning and radiotherapy treatment planning. MRI is also vastly superior to CT in demonstrating the subtle changes of meningeal disease. However, MRI is not as useful as CT in showing the skeletal anatomy.

Magnetic resonance angiography (MRA)

This is a useful tool for delineating the arterial blood supply to a tumour, allowing optimal planning of management.

Positron emission tomography (PET)

Cerebral tissue avidly takes up glucose as a metabolic substrate. Systemic administration of the positron emitting isotope of fluorodeoxyglucose allows imaging of the brain. Tumours, particularly high-grade gliomas, will concentrate the tracer and therefore form an image against the background of the surrounding normal brain. Other metabolic substrates such as amino acids (e.g. methionine) can also be exploited for PET. Functional imaging from PET can provide useful information on tumour activity and extent complementary to that obtained from CT and MRI.

Stereotactic needle biopsy or open biopsy

This is essential to obtain a specimen for histological diagnosis. When surgical resection is not feasible, e.g. a tumour located at a critical site such as the brainstem, a needle biopsy will be the least traumatic means of sampling a tumour. Otherwise, open biopsy and tumorectomy are performed, and have the advantages of providing a larger specimen for histological analysis and potentially being of therapeutic benefit by allowing complete excision or debulking of the tumour.

Lumbar puncture

This can be of value in providing further information to assist in diagnosis and treatment, e.g. in providing CSF for cytology in carcinomatous meningitis and high-risk non-Hodgkin's lymphoma, and, in the case of germ cell tumours, allowing assay of CSF α-fetoprotein and β-human chorionic gonadotrophin. However, a lumbar puncture should not be routinely performed in patients with brain tumours because of the risk of coning (compression and herniation of the brainstem through the foramen magnum), which may be fatal. Lumbar puncture should always be preceded by fundoscopy and a CT or MRI scan of the brain to exclude raised intracranial pressure.

Myelography

This is now an obsolete investigation, having been superseded by CT and MRI. It entails the instillation of radio-opaque contrast into the subarachnoid space by either lumbar puncture or cisternal puncture.

Treatment

The skill and advice of a neurosurgeon should always be sought when investigation and treatment of such patients is planned. Ideally, this should be in the context of a multidisciplinary team comprising an oncologist, neurosurgeon and neuroradiologist.

Surgery

This is the treatment of choice for all brain and spinal tumours as most are relatively radioresistant, making them incurable by radiotherapy alone. Complete excision should be the goal of the neurosurgeon both to clear the tumour and to obtain adequate tissue for diagnosis. However, CNS tissue is not tolerant of trauma, is critical to normal body functioning and has no powers of regeneration, and so frequently the best that can be expected is surgical debulking. Tumours of the brainstem and pineal region are notoriously difficult to resect and are associated with high operative morbidity and mortality.

Radiotherapy

The CNS is not tolerant of high doses of radiation and therefore curative doses carry the risk of permanent neurological impairment. Radiotherapy has a complementary role to surgery, being ideal for eradicating small volume disease left behind after attempted surgical clearance, but can also be used to treat radiosensitive tumours arising in critical areas of the brain with a high expectation of cure, e.g. a dysgerminoma arising in the pineal region. Focused radiotherapy techniques such as stereotactic arc therapy, gamma-knife treatments and intensity-modulated radiotherapy (IMRT) permit high-dose treatment to small volumes of brain with relatively little irradiation of the surrounding normal brain. They are therefore ideally suited to the 'curative' treatment of small tumours (e.g. solitary brain metastases), boost treatments following whole brain radiotherapy or re-treatment of recurrences after radiotherapy.

Chemotherapy

Only germ cell tumours are potentially curable by chemotherapy alone. The role of chemotherapy in other CNS tumours is mainly palliative in intent. The blood–brain barrier acts as an obstacle to the free passage of chemotherapy drugs. Lipid-soluble drugs such as the nitrosoureas BCNU and CCNU, procarbazine, vincristine, cisplatin and very high doses of methotrexate enter the brain in sufficiently high concentrations. More recently, the oral agent temozolamide has been shown to be of benefit in the management of gliomas. Methotrexate and cytosine arabinoside given intrathecally by lumbar puncture or intraven- tricularly via an indwelling Ommaya resevoir are of value as regional chemotherapy in the management of meningeal deposits from lymphoma, leukaemia and solid tumours.

Supportive therapy

Dexamethasone 4–16 mg daily is very effective at relieving raised intracranial pressure. Prolonged usage does, however, lead to symptoms and signs of Cushing's syndrome, oral candidiasis and proximal myopathy, which may exacerbate neurological deficits. Mannitol intravenously is useful as an adjunct in an acute exacerbation of raised intracranial pressure. Anticonvulsants should be given only for documented fits and patients with epilepsy or recent craniotomy should be advised not to drive until fit free according to national guidelines. Many patients will have problems with the activities of daily living from neurological deficit, and referral to a neurophysiotherapist, occupational therapist and social worker is very important.

ASTROCYTOMA

These arise from astrocytes in the brain or spinal cord, and are most common in adults but arise also during childhood. They are divided histologically into low grade (Grades 1 and 2) and high grade (Grades 3 and 4), which correlate with prognosis. Grade 4 tumours are termed glioblastoma multiforme. These constitute 50 per cent of astrocytomas, arising in adults with a peak incidence of 50 years. They are usually found in cerebral hemispheres, especially the frontal and temporal lobes, are extensively necrotic (Fig. 12.3) and haemorrhagic, and are often associated with oedema of the adjacent brain. Tumours close to the midline can spread to the contralateral hemisphere via the corpus callosum or basal ganglia. Glioblastomas are occasionally multifocal (Fig. 12.4). Spinal cord astrocytomas are very rare (Fig. 12.5).

Surgery should be performed with the aim of complete macroscopic and microscopic resection, although this goal is not often attained owing to the diffusely infiltrative nature of the tumour and its position within the brain. Postoperative radiotherapy will not be necessary for

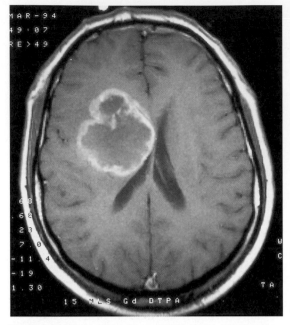

Figure 12.3 High grade glioma. MRI of the brain showing a large tumour with a necrotic centre and compressing the adjacent ventricle.

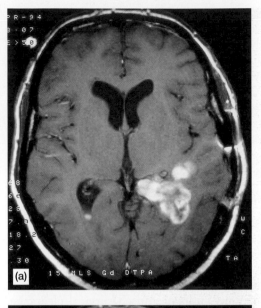

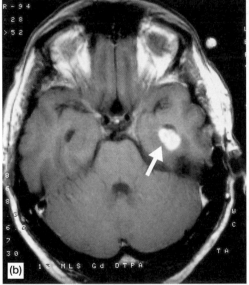

Figure 12.4 Multifocal high grade glioma. MRI of the brain. (a) Several foci are seen in the parieto-occipital lobe. (b) Further focus in the temporal lobe.

Grade 1 tumours that have been completely resected. All other grades and incompletely resected Grade 1 tumours (in practice the vast majority) should receive postoperative radiotherapy to maximize local control and in turn prolong survival.

One newer strategy for high-grade gliomas has been to implant up to eight carmustine-implanted biodegradable copolymer wafers (Gliadel®) into the tumour cavity at the time of surgery. When combined with radiotherapy, carmustine wafers, compared with placebo wafers, significantly improved 1-year survival from 50 to 59 per cent, and 3-year survival from 2 to 9 per cent. This strategy is most effective if 90 per cent or more of the tumour has been resected

Poor prognostic factors include high-grade tumours, advanced age, poor neurological performance status, limited surgical resection and a presentation other than epilepsy. Five-year survival for Grade 1 tumours is about 60 per cent, but high-grade tumours have an extremely poor prognosis, with a median survival of 3 months when biopsy alone is performed, 8 months when treated with radiotherapy, and a 1-year survival of 30 per cent. Apart from demonstrating innate radioresistance, gliomas are also relatively resistant to chemotherapy. This is not helped by the sanctuary effect conferred by the

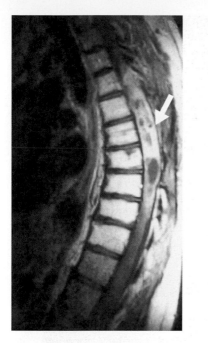

Figure 12.5 Spinal astrocytoma. Sagittal MRI of the thoracic spine. There is a part solid, part cystic mass arising from the spinal cord.

blood–brain barrier. Meta-analysis of individual randomized trials demonstrates a 5 per cent absolute survival advantage at 2 years for chemotherapy, equating to an increase in 2-year survival from 15 to 20 per cent. Patients with a good performance status should be considered for chemotherapy to prolong symptom-free survival and overall survival. Active drugs include the nitrosoureas BCNU and CCNU, vinca alkaloids, procarbazine and cisplatin. The combination PCV (procarbazine, CCNU, vincristine) is widely used, has been shown to be superior to single-agent BCNU, and has been particularly active in anaplastic astrocytomas.

Temozolomide has superseded other drugs and combinations. It undergoes hydrolysis to monomethyl triazenoimidazole carboxamide (MTIC) and this readily crosses the blood–brain barrier. It is moderately active, and has the advantage of being an oral agent. It is usually given concurrently with cranial radiotherapy (60 Gy in 30 fractions over 6 weeks) at a dose of 75 mg/m^2/day for 42 consecutive days and then continued as monotherapy for 5 out of every 28 days for 6 cycles over 6 months. With this approach, median survival is increased from 12 months to 15 months corresponding to an improvement in 2-year survival from 10 per cent to 27 per cent. Temozolomide is also a useful as first-line treatment for those failing primary surgery/radiotherapy. In a randomized trial in patients with recurrent, pretreated glioblastoma multiforme, temozolomide was superior to procarbazine with a 6-month survival of 60 per cent versus 44 per cent for procarbazine. The partial response rate is low at around 5 per cent, but disease stabilization occurs in around a third, and response rates are higher for lower grade gliomas.

OLIGODENDROGLIOMA

These constitute only 5 per cent of gliomas, arising exclusively in adults with a mean age of 40 years. They are usually found in the cerebral hemispheres, particularly in the frontal lobes (50 per cent) and adjacent to the ventricles, and 20 per cent are bilateral. They are slow-growing, well-circumscribed tumours; 40 per cent have foci of calcification and, unlike gliomas, there is little associated oedema for their size. Patients often have a history of epilepsy or gradual deterioration in higher mental functions. Low-grade tumours are compatible with a long survival after surgery alone, which can be curative. The principles of management mirror those for astrocytomas.

MENINGIOMA

These constitute 15 per cent of intracranial tumours, are most common in adults and are the only CNS tumours that are more common in females. They arise from the arachnoid mater, adjacent to the major venous sinuses, the most common sites being the parasagittal region, olfactory groove, sphenoidal ridge and suprasellar region, and sometimes arise as an intradural extramedullary spinal tumour. They are usually benign, slow growing and well circumscribed, may erode overlying skull, and 20 per cent are partly calcified. More locally invasive maligant variants are occasionally seen. Primary treatment is surgery, although their proximity to the venous sinuses can lead to perioperative problems so careful case selection is important. Radiotherapy is considered after incomplete surgical excision without which approximately 50 per cent of patients will sustain a recurrence. Radiotherapy will reduce the risk of recurrence by half in this context but is also used for inoperable cases or recurrence after surgery. Focused radiotherapy techniques such as multiple arc roatations, gamma-knife radiosurgery, tomotherapy or intensity-modulated radiotherapy (IMRT) are ideal for treating well-circumscribed, spheroidal, benign tumours of this nature. The prognosis is very good as the natural history is measurable in years and decades. Some cases can be managed with observation alone. Chemotherapy has no defined role in this disease.

PITUITARY TUMOURS

The vast majority are benign adenomas, with a tiny minority seen as metastases (breast and lung primary cancers) or true primary carcinomas. Pituitary adenomas can be classified according to the staining characteristics of the cell of origin into three groups:

- Chromophobe adenomas (50 per cent) are often large, forming the bulk of non-secretory tumours but might secrete prolactin.
- Eosinophil adenomas (40 per cent) are much smaller than chromophobe adenomas and might secrete growth hormone or prolactin.
- Basophil adenomas (10 per cent) are usually small, and might secrete ACTH, rarely TSH, LH or FSH.

They can also be divided according to their macroscopic diameter into microadenomas (<10 mm) – the majority, or macroadenomas (>10 mm).

Adenomas present with vague symptoms such as headache or with more specific abnormalities. The optic chiasm is a close anatomical relation of the pituitary fossa below and therefore suprasellar extension can lead to chiasmal compression and visual disturbance. Testing of the visual fields to confrontation and perimetry typically reveals a bitemporal hemianopia, although occasionally lateral extension involves the cavernous sinuses resulting in a palsy of the 3rd, 4th and 6th cranial nerves and in turn ocular palsies leading to diplopia. Examination of the fundi can reveal a pale disc consistent with optic atrophy. Hypopituitarism can result from compression of the pituitary gland adjacent to the tumour or pressure on the hypothalamus. Growth hormone secretion is the first to be impaired followed by the gonadotrophins. Diabetes insipidus indicates superior extension into the supra-optic nuclei. Pituitary apoplexy is a rare, acute presentation of pituitary failure owing to haemorrhage or infarction of the pituitary. Hypothalamic pressure can also lead to a loss of hypothalamic regulation and in turn disturbances in homeostasis such as loss of temperature regulation and disturbance of appetite and sleep.

Eighty per cent of pituitary adenomas are hormonally active. Prolactin may be elevated in half the cases from loss of the inhibitory hormone produced by the hypothalamus or direct secretion by the eosinophilic or chromophobe adenoma cells. This can present as galactorrhoea, amenorrhoea, lack of libido or erectile dysfunction. Eosinophilic adenoma can also produce growth hormone, manifest as acromegaly, and basophilic adenomas can secrete ACTH leading to Cushing's disease or Nelson's syndrome. Less than 1 per cent secrete TSH producing hyperthyroidism. Plurihormonal adenomas have been seen. Many of the so-called non-functioning adenomas actually produce the gonadotrophins LH and FSH but do not produce a clinically detectable syndrome until they expand the pituitary fossa and compress surrounding structures.

Investigations

Referral to an endocrinologist

An expert baseline endocrine assessment to evaluate hypothalamic and pituitary function is mandatory before surgery and after treatment the patient will require lifelong follow-up and hormone replacement therapy.

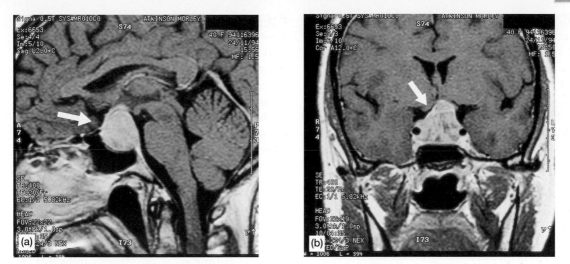

Figure 12.6 Pituitary adenoma. (a) Sagittal MRI of the brain showing an enhancing tumour that occupies the pituitary fossa and extends into the suprasellar region. (b) Coronal MRI from the same patient. Note the proximity of the tumour to the cavernous sinuses.

Visual field perimetry

This is the most objective means of documenting visual field defects, and gives a hard copy, which can be stored in the patient's notes for comparison at a later date.

Plain radiographs

AP and lateral skull X-ray will document any bony expansion of the pituitary fossa.

Magnetic resonance imaging (MRI)

MRI, particularly sagittal views of the pituitary fossa, provides a detailed assessment of the pituitary itself and potential sites of local tumour spread (Fig. 12.6).

Computed tomography (CT)

Reconstructed coronal CT images can be complementary to MRI for difficult cases requiring surgery.

Treatment

Surgery

This is preferred if there is significant, progressive visual impairment. Trans-sphenoidal microsurgical hypophysectomy provides a tissue diagnosis, instant decompression of the optic chiasm and other adjacent structures, and a cessation of hormone hypersecretion. Complete resection of the pituitary tumour and its extensions or substantial debulking will provide optimum long-term local control for macro-adenomas, but partial removal of the pituitary may suffice for a micro-adenoma. If there is much suprasellar or lateral extension of a large adenoma, a frontal (transcranial) approach will give greater access.

Radiotherapy

This is preferred as primary treatment when the risks of surgery are considered high. There is a high recurrence rate after surgery alone for macro-adenomas, but the addition of postoperative radiotherapy increases 10-year disease-free survival from 10 to over 80 per cent. Radiotherapy alone is successful in the long-term control of hormone hypersecretion, although the maximum benefit is expressed after some years. In acromegalics, there is a 20 per cent per annum decline in growth hormone levels, but normalization might never occur, particularly if pretreatment levels were very high. Similar results are seen in prolactin- and ACTH-secreting tumours. There is a 30 per

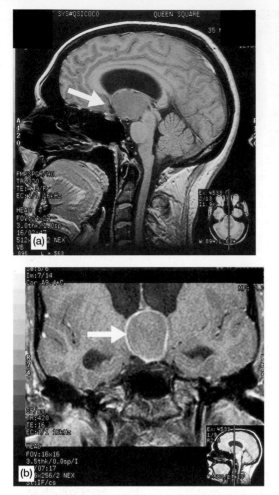

Figure 12.7 Craniopharyngioma. (a) Sagittal MRI of the brain showing a solitary, well-circumscribed, cystic mass in the suprasellar region. (b) Coronal MRI from the same patient.

cent 10-year risk of hypopituitarism after radiotherapy. Focused radiotherapy techniques (see Meningioma section above) are being increasingly used to avoid irradiation of the surrounding normal brain and optic chiasm.

Dopamine agonists

Bromocriptine and cabergoline mimic the prolactin inhibitory hormone produced by the hypothalamus, and are of value in the treatment of prolactinoma when they can induce dramatic tumour regression and thereby defer the need for surgery or radiotherapy.

CRANIOPHARYNGIOMA

This is very rare, usually arising in children, and constitutes 10 per cent of all childhood intracranial tumours. It is most common in Japan but rare in the US and Western Europe. It is a suprasellar tumour arising from nests of epidermoid cells in the pars tuberalis (Rathke's pouch), slow growing, benign, three-quarters being partly cystic and calcified (Fig. 12.7).

Presentation is as for pituitary adenomas and surgery is the treatment of choice, with radiotherapy having the same role as for pituitary tumours, i.e. after incomplete excision or for inoperable cases. Historically, the cystic nature of these tumours made them amenable to instillation of radio-isotopes such as yttrium-90 and phosphorus-32. Prognosis is very good with an 80 per cent 5-year survival and 70 per cent 5-year disease-free survival.

PINEAL TUMOURS

These are rare. Characteristically they present with obstructive hydrocephalus owing to their proximity to the CSF ventricular outflow pathway, or ocular palsies, especially paralysis of upward gaze (Parinaud's syndrome). Surgery is particularly difficult and hazardous in this region. A ventriculoperitoneal shunt may be required. Germinomas and astrocytomas are the commonest tumours in the pineal region. Rarer, intrinsic tumours of the pineal gland include:

- *Pinealoma*: this is very rare, but is the most common pineal tumour with a peak incidence at 15–25 years. It is slow growing, well circumscribed, non-invasive, and treated by surgical excision.
- *Pineoblastoma*: this is even rarer and much more aggressive than pinealoma, CSF dissemination being a frequent complication.

GERM CELL TUMOURS

Teratomas and dysgerminomas (analogous to seminoma) may arise from islands of ectopic germ cells in the suprasellar region (Fig. 12.8)

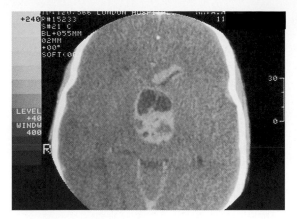

Figure 12.8 Suprasellar teratoma. Transverse CT image of the brain of a young child showing a complex cystic lesion arising in the suprasellar region.

or pineal. Patients with confirmed CNS disease should be referred to a regional centre specializing in the treatment of germ cell tumours. The tumours are radiosensitive and chemosensitive but the prognosis is not as good as for their testicular counterparts. Serum and CSF α-fetoprotein and β-human chorionic gonadotrophin measurements are useful to confirm diagnosis and monitor response to treatment.

EPENDYMOMAS

These constitute 10 per cent of childhood intracranial tumours with a peak incidence during the first decade of life. They arise throughout the CNS from cells lining ventricles, central canal of the spinal cord and choroid plexus, although the vast majority arise near the 4th ventricle, 40 per cent being supratentorial and 60 per cent infratentorial. They are well circumscribed, usually well differentiated, slow growing, and may be calcified (Fig. 12.9). Spread via CSF is well recognized, particularly if high grade and infratentorial.

Combined surgery and radiotherapy give the greatest chance of local control, selected patients at high risk of CSF dissemination receiving radiotherapy to the craniospinal axis. The prognosis is a 5-year survival of about 50 per cent falling to 40 per cent at 10 years.

MEDULLOBLASTOMA

This is the most common intracranial tumour in children (see Chapter 18), accounting for 20 per cent of intracranial tumours in the under-16s with 80 per cent arising in those under 15

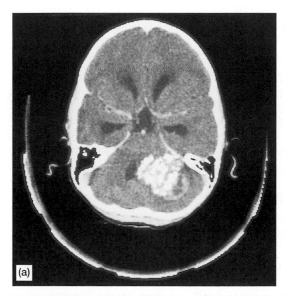

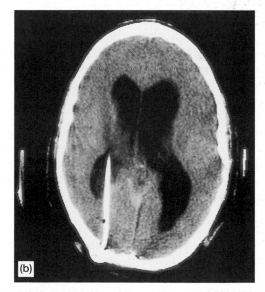

Figure 12.9 Ependymoma. (a) Seen on CT there is a heavily calcified mass arising from the posterior fossa of a child. (b) CT image from the same child showing obstructive hydrocephalus leading to massive ventricular dilatation. A shunt has been inserted to relieve this.

years of age, most during the first decade. The cells of origin are fetal elements of the external granular layer of the cerebellum, and it is found centrally in the vermis in children and more laterally in the hemispheres in young adults. There is a high risk of spread via CSF (one-third of cases) and it occasionally metastasizes outside the CNS, usually to bone. It presents with cerebellar ataxia and/or obstructive hydrocephalus.

Patients require a posterior fossa craniotomy and tumorectomy, a shunt being inserted to relieve raised intracranial pressure. Medulloblastoma is one of the most radiation-sensitive CNS tumours. Radiotherapy to the craniospinal axis is invariably indicated and the 5-year survival is approximately 50 per cent. Trials comparing chemotherapy (vincristine and CCNU) and radiotherapy with radiotherapy alone have not shown a substantial advantage for the combined modality treatment. A major issue is the impaired growth development and neuropsychiatric consequences of CNS irradiation in infants and young children.

CHORDOMA

This is a very rare tumour that presents in adult life, arising from notochord remnants in the axial skeleton anywhere from the sella turcica to the sacrum. In adults, these remnants persist in the nucleus pulposus of the intervertebral disc. Fifty per cent are sacrococcygeal, 35 per cent arise in the spheno-occipital region and 15 per cent in the vertebral column. They are slow growing, well circumscribed, gelatinous, extradural tumours with areas of haemorrhage and necrosis, often reaching a large size and causing compressive symptoms. A characteristic histological finding is the so-called 'physaliferous' cells. They are locally invasive and can be confused with metastatic adenocarcinoma or chondrosarcoma, with less than 10 per cent metastasizing to distant sites.

Radical excision should be attempted, although it is rarely possible, and postoperative radiotherapy is necessary in the majority, giving a 50 per cent 5-year survival falling to 20 per cent at 10 years. There are few pub-lished data regarding the use of chemotherapy, which is not particularly effective. A sarcoma-style protocol (e.g. doxorubicin and ifosfamide) can be used for palliation of symptoms refractory to radiotherapy or to control distant metastatic disease. Recent data suggest a possible role for imatinib (Glivec®) which acts on tumours like chordomas over-expressing platelet derived growth factor receptor B (PDGFRB).

HAEMANGIOBLASTOMA

These are more common in children and form part of the von Hippel–Lindau syndrome. They are usually cerebellar in origin with the hemispheres affected more than the vermis. The tumour is slow growing, well circumscribed, and associated with polycythaemia owing to ectopic secretion of erythropoietin.

LYMPHOMA

(See also Chapters 16 and 20.) Primary cerebral lymphoma is very rare, and extracerebral involvement raises the possibility of secondary involvement of the brain. It is associated with AIDS but also occurs sporadically. It presents with symptoms of global cerebral dysfunction such as epilepsy, cognitive impairment and somnolence, or focal neurological signs. Standard lymphoma chemotherapy penetration is hindered by the blood–brain barrier (BBB) and the tumour is too bulky to make intrathecal treatment feasible. High-dose ($5\ \text{g/m}^2$) methotrexate is used to circumvent the BBB and osmotic disruption of the BBB has also been used. Chemotherapy is usually integrated with whole brain radiotherapy. CNS toxicity is a concern with such protocols. There is a tendency for CSF spread leading to involvement of the spinal cord and retina. In these circumstances, craniospinal irradiation can be of benefit. As with high-grade gliomas, long-term survivors are exceptional. It has a very poor prognosis, even in non-AIDS patients, with a median survival untreated of 3–4 months rising to 15 months after cranial radiotherapy.

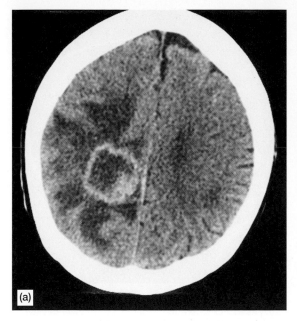

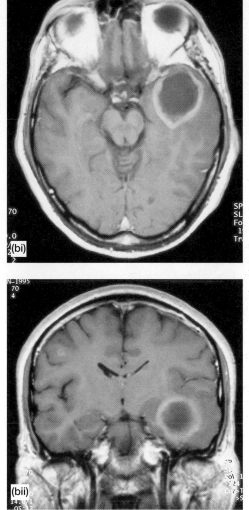

Figure 12.10 Solitary brain metastasis. (a) Contrast-enhanced CT image of the brain showing a solitary metastasis arising in the right parietal region. This is typically well circumscribed and hypodense with ring enhancement, and associated with oedema of the surrounding brain. (b) MRI of the brain demonstrating a solitary brain metastasis. i: Transverse view. ii: Coronal view. There is no associated cerebral oedema in contrast to Figure 12.11.

METASTASES

These usually originate from cancers of the lung, breast, kidney, colon, pancreas and melanoma. Lung cancer is the most common primary (50 per cent), particularly small cell and large cell variants, where one-quarter to one-half of patients will have cerebral metastases at autopsy. They are most frequent in the frontal and parietal lobes, usually rounded, well circumscribed, and enhance on CT and MRI with intravenous contrast (Fig. 12.10). They are often associated with cerebral oedema (Fig. 12.11) and can occasionally be confused with a cerebral abscess.

One-third to one-half of such individuals will die as a result of the cerebral component of their disease, and therefore attaining local control is a priority. The majority of patients will present with multiple cerebral/cerebellar metastases (Fig. 12.12). In these circumstances, radiotherapy is the most appropriate treatment. It is important to achieve neurological stability prior to proceeding with treatment. Judicious use of dexamethasone to treat raised intracranial pressure is essential, as radiotherapy can

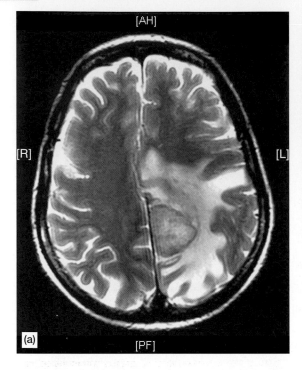

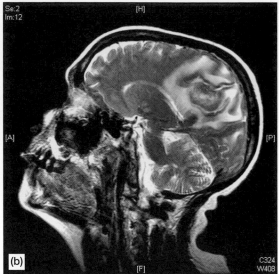

Figure 12.11 Solitary brain metastasis. MRIs. There is much associated cerebral oedema. (a) Transverse view. (b) Sagittal view.

exacerbate any pre-existing cerebral oedema. Radiotherapy fields are designed to treat the whole brain with the use of a pair of opposed lateral fields, with an inferior baseline running from the superior orbital ridge through the tragus of the ear. Evidence from well-conducted randomized trials indicates a response rate for most symptoms such as headache, epilepsy and neurological disability in the order of 80 per cent. The net result is an improvement in functional independence for the majority of treated patients. Cranial nerve palsies are often less responsive. In approximately two-thirds of responders, the improvement will be sustained for more than 12 months.

Potentially curable tumours such as germ cell tumours are managed aggressively, even if there are multiple sites of metastatic disease. Craniotomy and biopsy can be considered for the more common solid tumours if there is no known primary and no other malignant tissue to biopsy. Excision should be considered for a solitary brain metastasis in selected patients with solid tumours if they are of good perform-

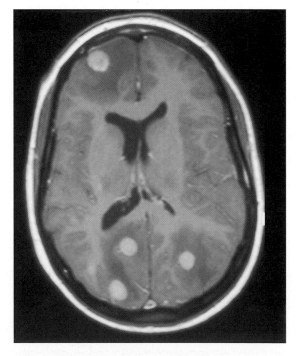

Figure 12.12 Multiple cerebral metastases. Transverse MRI of the brain.

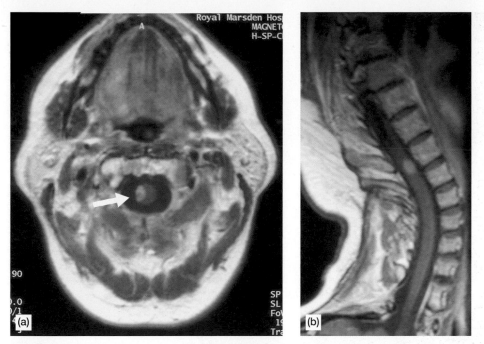

Figure 12.13 Intramedullary metastasis. (a) MRI of base of skull. There is an eccentric area of contrast enhancement within the cervical spinal cord corresponding to a metastasis. (b) Sagittal MRI showing a metastasis within the spinal cord.

ance status and there is no evidence of distant metastases elsewhere, or in a patient with previous cancer after a prolonged disease-free period. Excision of a solitary metastasis should be followed by radiotherapy to the whole brain and a boost to the site of excision.

Newer radiotherapy techniques such as stereotactic radiotherapy (SRT) using multiple non-coplanar arcs of radiation delivery, gamma-knife, tomotherapy and intensity-modulated radiotherapy (IMRT) allow dose escalation by virtue of their superior radiation dosimetry. Their role is this context is still being explored, but they hold much promise, particularly for treatment of one or several metastases. Evidence already suggests that in selected patients with solitary metastases, SRT yields 2-year actuarial control rates of 60–70 per cent.

Intramedullary metastases present with characteristic sensory dissociation and upper motor neurone signs. They are comparatively rare (Fig. 12.13).

CARCINOMATOUS MENINGITIS

Tumour spread to the CNS can manifest as diffuse involvement of the meninges around the brain (Fig. 12.14) and/or spinal cord. This is particularly seen in haematological malignancies (e.g. non-Hodgkin's lymphoma), breast cancer, lung cancer and melanoma. It can present with non-specific symptoms such as headache, vomiting, meningism, lethargy, confusion, or more focal neurological deficit, typically cranial nerve palsies. Such patients might have disease that extends along the optic nerves to involve the optic disc (Fig. 12.15) or peripheral retina (Fig. 12.16). Its onset and presentation is insidious, and it is easy to mistake some of the symptoms for other conditions, e.g. opiate toxicity. Diagnosis can be made from typical appearances on a double-dose contrast-enhanced MRI, although lumbar puncture is often necessary to obtain CSF for cytology and

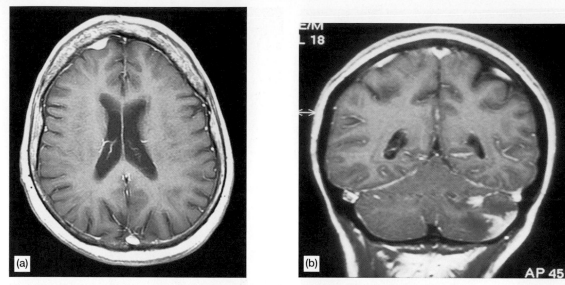

Figure 12.14 Meningeal carcinomatosis. MRI of the brain. (a) Transverse view. (b) Coronal view.

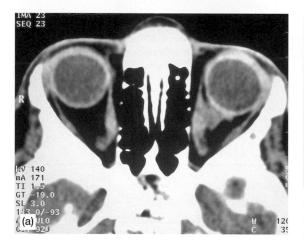

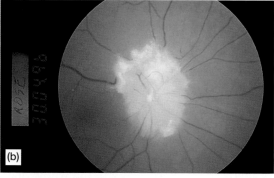

Figure 12.15 Optic nerve metastases. (a) Transverse CT image showing irregular thickening of the optic nerve. (b) Fundoscopy showing irregular, pale plaque of tumour at optic disc.

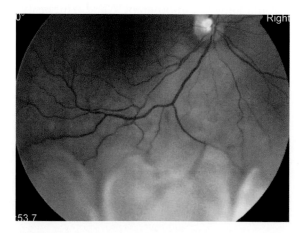

Figure 12.16 Choroidal metastasis. Fundoscopy showing a secondary retinal detachment and subretinal effusion.

confirm the diagnosis. The diagnosis can sometimes remain elusive owing to negative imaging and cytology, in which case further cytological sampling is indicated. Treatment options include intrathecal instillation of chemotherapy agents, such as methotrexate, at twice weekly intervals via lumbar puncture or an Ommaya intraventricular catheter, and/or cranial/craniospinal radiotherapy. The outlook for solid tumour carcinomatous meningitis is extremely poor, many patients dying within weeks of their diagnosis. Newer treatments such as intrathecal liposomal cytarabine (Depoocyt®) are yet to be proven for this indication.

FURTHER READING

Bernstein M, Berger MS. *Neuro-Oncology: the essentials*. Thieme, New York, 2008

DeMonte F, Gilbert MR, Mahajan A, McCutcheon IE. *Tumours of the Brain and Spine*. Springer, New York, 2007

Schiff D, O'Neill DP. *Principles of Neuro-Oncology*. McGraw-Hill, London, 2005

Tonn JC, Westphal M, Rutga JT *et al. Neuro-Oncology of CNS Tumours*. Springer, Berlin and Heidelberg, 2005

SELF-ASSESSMENT QUESTIONS

1. Which three of the following are common features of CNS tumours?
   a. Hypothyroidism
   b. Cranial nerve palsy
   c. Raised intracranial pressure
   d. Epilepsy
   e. Taste disturbance
   f. Insomnia
   g. Mania

2. Which one of the following is true about pituitary tumours?
   a. Blindness is frequent
   b. Olfactory disturbance is frequent
   c. Binasal hemianopia is the commonest form of visual disturbance
   d. Epilepsy is rare
   e. Hemiparesis is sometimes seen

3. Which three of the following statements are true regarding the treatment of gliomas?
   a. Surgical excision is indicated for multifocal tumours
   b. Complete surgical excision is rarely achieved
   c. All types have a high mortality within 5 years of diagnosis
   d. They are very sensitive to radiotherapy
   e. Temozolomide crosses the blood–brain barrier
   f. Nitrosoureas are active drugs
   g. Chemotherapy leads to response rates of 30–50 per cent

4. Which one of the following is true about meningiomas?
   a. They are not well visualized by computed tomography
   b. They are readily identified by magnetic resonance imaging
   c. The majority are malignant in their behaviour
   d. Radiotherapy is used routinely after surgery
   e. Active treatment is always advisable

5. Which three of the following statements best describe brain metastases?
   a. Best seen by PET imaging
   b. Can be confused with cerebral abscesses
   c. Never treated surgically as they represent disseminated disease
   d. Usually multiple rather than solitary
   e. Produce symptoms distinct from those of a primary brain tumour
   f. Chemotherapy has no significant role in their management
   g. They usually lead to the death of the patient

6. Which one of the following is true about carcinomatous meningitis?
   a. Behaves more favourably than cerebral metastatic disease
   b. Associated with ocular spread of malignant disease
   c. Treated by systemic chemotherapy
   d. Usually seen with computed tomography images
   e. Intrathecal chemotherapy with cisplatin is a useful treatment

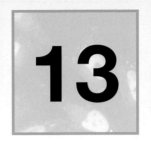

13

HEAD AND NECK CANCER

- Carcinoma of the oral cavity — 225
- Carcinoma of the oropharynx — 232
- Carcinoma of the larynx — 232
- Carcinoma of the hypopharynx — 233
- Carcinoma of the nasopharynx — 234
- Carcinoma of the paranasal sinuses — 235
- Salivary gland tumours — 235
- Orbital tumours — 237
- Further reading — 237
- Self-assessment questions — 238

Each year in the UK there are 8000 cases of head and neck cancer leading to a total of 2500 deaths per annum. Nearly 90 per cent arise in the over-50s, the incidence increasing with age, and there is a strong male predominance with a male to female ratio of 2:1 for oral cancer and 5:1 for laryngeal cancer. Incidence rates vary greatly from region to region within each country, and the incidence and mortality rates are increasing. Worldwide, the highest incidence is in India and Sri Lanka where in some areas they are the most common cancers, constituting up to 40 per cent of the total. Other pockets of high incidence include South America and the Bas-Rhin region of France (oral cancer), and Newfoundland (lip). The head and neck contain the origins of the respiratory and gastrointestinal tracts, both of which are exposed to environmental carcinogens through the air we breathe and the food and drink we ingest. Each site will be dealt with individually, although cancer of the oral cavity will be described in detail as many of the basic principles are applicable to head and neck cancer in general. As a general rule, the prognosis worsens as the tumour site moves further down the aerodigestive tract from the lips.

CARCINOMA OF THE ORAL CAVITY

The oral cavity extends from the skin–vermilion junction of the lips to the junction of the hard and soft palates above and to the line of circumvallate papillae on the tongue below. This includes carcinoma of the lip, anterior two-thirds of tongue, floor of mouth, buccal mucosa, hard palate, retromolar trigone and lower alveolus.

Aetiology

Tobacco accounts for 90 per cent of oral cavity cancers. Inhalation of tobacco smoke from cigarettes, pipes and cigars is the major cause of cancer of the floor of the mouth. As with lung cancer, the greater the amount smoked and the higher the tar content, the higher the risk. Chewing tobacco and betel nut carry a particularly high risk of carcinoma of the buccal mucosa and cancers arising in the retromolar trigone. Heavy alcohol consumption is a major risk factor and high-alcohol mouthwashes have also been implicated. Alcoholics also tend to have poor nutrition, and their low intake of vitamins A and C might add to their risk of developing cancer. Carcinoma of the lip is more common in those with outdoor occupations where ultraviolet exposure is greater, and this accounts for the predominance of this tumour on the lower lip. Physical trauma from poor dentition can lead to malignant transformation at the site of trauma, usually the lateral border of the tongue. Chronic heat trauma from clay-pipe smoking can lead to carcinoma of the lip. Asians frequently chew betel nut to relieve indigestion and as a social habit, but this substance also contains carcinogens. It is easily detected by the dark brown staining between the teeth. During the nineteenth century, chronic syphilitic glossitis was a major cause of carcinoma of the tongue. This has declined with the advent of effective antibiotic treatment against syphilis at an early stage and it is no longer justified to check routinely the syphilis serology in all patients with oral cavity cancer. In recent years, a role for human papilloma virus (HPV), especially HPV 16, has emerged.

Pathology

The tumours can be frankly ulcerated, with raised, everted, nodular edges, or papilliform, or appear as subtle areas of superficial denudation of the mucosa. Synchronous primaries sometimes occur either in the oral cavity or elsewhere in the aerodigestive tract. The tumour can be secondarily infected, and there may be surrounding white plaques – leukoplakia – which are premalignant (Fig. 13.1). Ninety per cent are squamous carcinomas, the remainder being adenocarcinomas, mucoepidermoid carcinomas, adenoidcystic carcinomas, lymphomas and melanomas. In situ carcinoma and/or dysplasia might be seen in the surrounding mucosa.

Natural history

The tumours spread to adjacent subsites of the oral cavity and invade the deeper layers of the mucosa, reaching muscle in the case of the tongue and cheek, and even the underlying bone of the maxilla or mandible. Tumours of the lower alveolus tend to spread along the

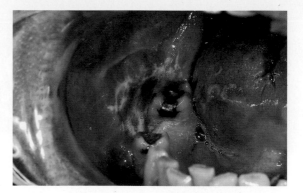

Figure 13.1 Leucoplakia. The retromolar region has a white, superficial, lace-like appearance. This may lead to the development of a squamous carcinoma.

alveolus by insidious submucosal spread, so that their microscopic extent can be much greater than appreciated macroscopically. A high proportion of tumours spread to the regional lymph nodes even when they are not palpable, e.g. 70 per cent in carcinoma of the tongue, the incidence being greater with increasing tumour size and increasingly undifferentiated tumours. Tumours adjacent to the anatomical midline can spread to lymph nodes bilaterally. First station lymph nodes include those in the jugulodigastric, submandibular, and submental groups. Second station lymph nodes are those of the jugular, and the upper and lower posterior cervical groups. Haematogenous spread is uncommon at diagnosis and usually seen in the terminal phase of the disease, the lungs being the most common site, followed by bone.

Symptoms

Many patients are asymptomatic, the tumour having been noticed at a routine dental examination (Fig. 13.2), but some complain of soreness at the site of the tumour owing to chronic superficial ulceration, and occasionally the presentation is due to cervical lymph node enlargement. In locally advanced cases, pain might be more marked and radiate to the ear, while a fungating tumour will lead to halitosis. Bulky tumours of the tongue (Fig. 13.3) will interfere with mastication and swallowing and lead to difficulty with speech.

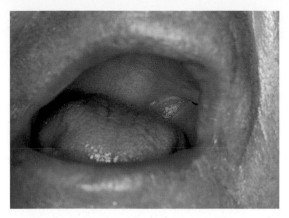

Figure 13.2 T1 squamous carcinoma arising from the left side of the palate.

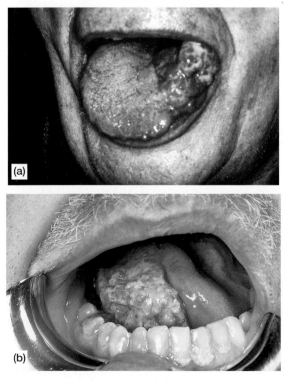

Figure 13.3 (a) A large carcinoma of the tongue. Such tumours will interfere with speech and swallowing. (b) Further example.

Signs

Patients frequently have physical signs consistent with heavy smoking and alcohol intake. Oral hygiene is often poor with an increased incidence of dental decay and gum disease, and this should be noted as it is relevant to the planning of radiotherapy. A thorough ENT examination is mandatory, preferably by an ENT surgeon. The primary tumour should be described in detail with respect to its position (preferably supplemented by a drawing), size and depth of invasion. Areas of leukoplakia should be sought and care taken to exclude another primary tumour. The tumour should be palpated with a gloved finger to complement inspection, feeling for induration and mucosal irregularity. All patients should have an indirect laryngoscopy. If available, direct fibreoptic endoscopy of the nasal fossa, nasopharynx, oropharynx, hypopharynx and larynx will give vital information regarding the site of origin and local tumour spread. The neck should be palpated very carefully to detect enlarged lymph nodes, recording their distribution (preferably with a diagram), size, number, consistency, degree of tenderness and fixation to surrounding structures. Small tender lymph nodes are frequently due to associated infection in the region of the tumour rather than lymph node metastases.

Differential diagnosis

Other causes of oral ulceration should be considered including:

- simple aphthous ulceration
- lichen planus
- herpes simplex
- syphilis.

Investigations

Biopsy

A biopsy is essential in order to obtain tissue for histological analysis, and can be performed in an outpatient setting, by an ENT/oral surgeon.

Examination under general anaesthetic

This allows detailed palpation of the tumour to define its precise size, position and extent of local invasion.

Oral pantogram (OPG)

This is good for excluding invasion of the mandible or maxilla, and provides a detailed survey of the teeth, which will help plan any dental procedures that may be necessary prior to radiotherapy.

Fine needle aspirate of any enlarged lymph nodes

This should be performed in the outpatient clinic and the specimen sent for immediate cytology. As the result may make a substantial difference to the proposed treatment, it is worth repeating the aspiration if a negative lymph node is still clinically suspicious.

Chest X-ray

This should be performed in all cases to exclude obvious lung metastases, although suspicious areas should be reassessed by a CT scan of the chest.

Computed tomography or magnetic resonance imaging of the oral cavity and neck

CT and MRI are useful for defining the local extent of the tumour, particularly when it arises from a site that is difficult to visualize or palpate, e.g. subglottic larynx. They also have an important role in visualizing lymph node metastases, which may be impalpable or inaccessible, e.g. retropharyngeal lymph nodes. Identification of bone invasion is of particular importance with respect to staging and planning of treatment and this is an area where CT is superior to MRI. Soft tissue and anatomical definition is greater with MRI. The head and neck CT protocol can be extended to include the thorax and to exclude pulmonary metastases.

Staging

The TNM staging is used:

- Tis – Carcinoma in situ
- T0 – No evidence of primary
- TX – Primary cannot be assessed
- T1 – 2 cm or less in greatest dimension
- T2 – >2 but not >4 cm in greatest dimension
- T3 – >4 cm in greatest dimension
- T4 – Invasion of deep (extrinsic) muscle of tongue, skin, cortical bone or maxillary sinus
- N0 – No regional lymphadenopathy
- N1 – Single ipsilateral node 3 cm or less in greatest dimension
- N2 – Single ipsilateral node >3 but not >6 cm in greatest dimension or multiple ipsilateral nodes not >6 cm or bilateral/contralateral nodes not >6 cm in greatest dimension
  - N2a – Single ipsilateral node >3 but not >6 cm in greatest dimension
  - N2b – Multiple ipsilateral nodes none >6 cm in greatest dimension
  - N2c – Bilateral/contralateral node(s) >6 cm in greatest dimension
- N3 – Any node >6 cm in greatest dimension
- M0 – No distant metastases
- M1 – Distant metastases.

Treatment

Patients should ideally be seen at a joint clinic attended by a clinical oncologist and a head and neck surgeon. Patients should be advised to stop smoking and drinking alcohol to lessen the risk of mucositis during radiotherapy or chest infections after an anaesthetic. Advice should be sought from a dietitian, as patients are frequently malnourished at presentation owing to neglect, oral soreness or dysphagia and are therefore unlikely to tolerate either radical radiotherapy or surgery well. The patient might require a softer consistency of diet or liquid supplements. A liquidizer can be very useful. Patients having radiotherapy should be referred to a dentist to have mild degrees of dental decay immediately dealt with by conservative measures, e.g. filling, while any teeth with serious decay can be extracted prior to radiotherapy.

Radical treatment

Surgery

The aim of surgery is to remove the primary tumour with a margin adequate to encompass all microscopic spread, and if necessary include an excision of the regional lymph nodes and reconstruct any major tissue deficits. Surgery can be used as the sole primary treatment, combined with radiotherapy or as salvage for local recurrence following radical radiotherapy. Surgery is sometimes the treatment of choice for locally advanced tumours, i.e. T3 and T4 tumours, as these are bulky tumours that may invade adjacent bone when they are particularly difficult to eradicate by radiotherapy alone. There is also an increased risk of osteonecrosis after radiotherapy when the bone is invaded and this is a particularly difficult management problem. However, radical surgery can involve a major resection of tissue, leading to severe functional morbidity. For example, resection of part of the tongue will result in some degree of dysarthria and possibly difficulty in mastication of food and swallowing, and such symptoms can severely compromise the patient's quality of life. Therefore, T1, T2 and small bulk T3 tumours are usually best treated by radiotherapy with surgery reserved for local recurrence.

The surgeon can also elect to perform a radical dissection of the cervical lymph nodes when these are involved. This is a major procedure involving removal of the ipsilateral nodes en bloc together with the internal jugular vein (IJV) and some other tissues such as the sternocleidomastoid and accessory nerve. The IJV cannot be sacrificed bilaterally, although a modified radical dissection can be performed on the contralateral side if necessary (IJV preserved). It can also be a curative procedure and provides valuable staging and prognostic information. Radiotherapy is advisable after neck dissection if three or more nodes are involved or if there is any evidence of extracapsular spread outside a lymph node.

Improvements in surgical techniques have resulted in more patients being able to benefit from reconstructive procedures after radical cancer surgery. This has lessened considerably the functional morbidity experienced after major resections of the tongue and other structures of the oral cavity.

Speech therapy is of value after major resections in the oral cavity, particularly of the

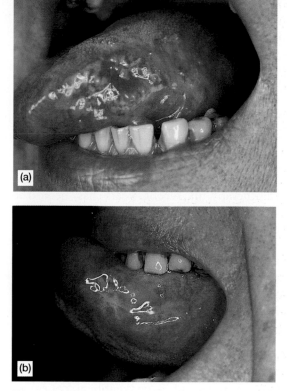

Figure 13.4 T1 squamous carcinoma arising from the lateral edge of the tongue. (a) Before treatment and (b) 6 months after interstitial implant. Tongue function, speech and swallowing have been fully preserved.

tongue, floor of mouth and lips, which might result in speech and swallowing difficulties.

Radiotherapy

As with surgery, radiotherapy can be used as the sole primary treatment, combined with surgery or for salvage of local relapse after surgery, and to treat all stages of local disease. It has the advantage of preserving the voice, speech, swallowing and tissues that surgery would sacrifice, and is therefore the treatment of choice for T1 and T2 tumours.

Historically, brachytherapy using radioactive needles (e.g. caesium), wire (e.g. iridium) or grains (e.g. gold) was superior to external beam radiotherapy in terms of local control and cosmetic outcome for small primary tumours with no lymph node involvement (Fig. 13.4).

External beam radiotherapy is routinely used in current clinical practice. It has the advantage of including the first station lymph nodes adjacent to the primary tumour as a prophylactic measure to eradicate subclinical tumour deposits, and facilitates treatment of the whole cervical lymph node chain at risk if there are palpable lymph node metastases. Radiotherapy gives poor local control when used alone for bulky T3 and T4 tumours, and therefore forms part of a combined modality approach with surgery. The most significant advance for radiotherapy in recent years has been the development of CHART – continuous, hyperfractionated, accelerated radiotherapy. This regimen involves rapid completion of treatment combined with avoidance of breaks in radiotherapy owing to weekends. CHART involves treatment three times daily, 7 days a week for 2.5 weeks (54 Gy in 36 fractions). The rationale is that it does not allow the tumour to repopulate, as can occur when the tumour has a short potential doubling time and treatment is protracted and interrupted over the 6–7 weeks of a conventional course of radiotherapy. A large, well-conducted randomized trial comparing CHART with a conventional course of radiotherapy has confirmed superiority of CHART for advanced laryngeal cancers. Unfortunately, the logistic difficulties inherent in CHART have precluded its widespread acceptance and implementation. Further trials are in progress. Advances in the technology of radiation delivery such as intensity-modulated radiotherapy (IMRT) will undoubtedly play a role in these diseases. IMRT allows the high-dose radiation envelope to be matched in three dimensions to the shape of the volume of tissue containing the tumour. It therefore spares the surrounding organs at risk such as the spinal cord and parotid salivary glands. Apart from reduced morbidity from standard dose/fractionation schedules, IMRT allows significant dose escalation for what is essentially a highly sensitive cancer to radiotherapy. Alternatively, IMRT allows re-treatment following failure of a previous course of radiotherapy, and also faciltates safe delivery of concurrent chemoradiotherapy (CRT).

Chemotherapy

The most active agents are 5FU and cisplatin, which in combination will give an objective response rate of 60–80 per cent. Chemotherapy alone cannot be used with expectation of cure, and adjuvant/neoadjuvant chemotherapy has no proven survival benefit. For more locally advanced tumours, meta-analysis of over 60 trials suggests an 8 per cent absolute survival advantage for the subgroup receiving CRT. Preoperative or postoperative chemotherapy seems less efficacious. CRT is therefore a current standard of care in many countries. Severe mucositis is a common side-effect of CRT.

An alternative strategy is to combine radiotherapy with the monoclonal antibody cetuximab (Erbitux®). This inhibits the epidermal growth factor receptor (EGFR) which is often overexpressed in head and neck cancer. In the pivotal phase 3 study, weekly cetuximab and radiotherapy, when used for locally advanced head and neck cancer (particularly oropharyngeal cancers – see below), increases locoregional control and progression-free survival. Median overall survival was prolonged to 49 months compared with 29 months for radiotherapy alone, corresponding to 3-year survivals of 55 per cent and 45 per cent respectively. The frequency of severe grades of mucositis is comparable, unlike CRT. The *K-ras* oncogene is involved in the growth of head and neck cancers and evidence is emerging that, if this mutates, the response to cetuximab is decreased compared with tumours with 'wild-type' *K-ras*.

Palliative treatment

Surgery

Major resection is not justified for the palliation of symptoms in incurable cases owing to the trauma sustained and the possibility of major postoperative morbidity with loss of function, but debulking might be necessary to avert respiratory obstruction or dysphagia. Tracheostomy could be indicated if there is upper airway obstruction as this is a particularly distressing symptom.

Radiotherapy

Radiotherapy can be used in cases of locally advanced disease even when the prospect of cure is low, as it is of value in relieving obstructive symptoms.

Chemotherapy

The combination of 5FU and cisplatin has been a standard treatment for some years. Median survival time is typically around only 6 months. The addition of the cetuximab (see above) to standard chemotherapy increases median survival by 2–3 months.

Tumour-related complications

Locally advanced tumours are often necrotic and infected, which can lead to embarrassing halitosis, an unpleasant taste and local discomfort. A course of the appropriate antibiotic (usually metronidazole) and chlorhexidine mouthwash can help. Obstruction of the aerodigestive tracts is very distressing and warrants urgent consideration for a tracheostomy. Trismus, dysphonia, dysphagia and salivary fistulae are all seen.

Treatment-related complications

Surgery

Difficulty in mastication, swallowing, dysarthria and dysphonia result from surgical resection of structures involved in these processes. Poor healing is a particular problem following extensive surgery when the vascularity of the tissue has been compromised, especially if the tissues have been previously irradiated. Osteomyelitis can complicate surgery when there has been a resection of bone (e.g. mandibulectomy), which has become secondarily infected. Treatment is with high doses of the appropriate antibiotic and further surgery might be required to remove the sequestrum.

Radiotherapy

The oral mucosa is very sensitive to radiation, the reaction beginning during the second week of radiotherapy as erythema and soreness, progressing to severe discomfort manifested as a fibrinous mucositis leading to dysphagia and difficulty in mastication. This can be lessened by advising patients to use a very soft toothbrush to avoid gingival trauma, regular mouthwashes to prevent secondary infection, avoiding smoking, alcohol, spicy foods, and food or drink that is very hot or very cold. Soluble aspirin 600 mg gargled and swallowed four times a day can relieve oral and oropharyngeal discomfort, while Mucaine 10 mL four times a day sipped slowly can also help the latter. Oral candidiasis should be treated promptly with a topical or systemic antifungal. Local anaesthetic lozenges are also useful. A dry mouth is very common during radiotherapy and might recover only partially or not at all. It results from radiation damage to the parotids and minor salivary gland(s) at the site of radiation beam entry and/or exit from the oral cavity, predisposing the patient to dental caries, making swallowing difficult and exacerbating any radiation mucositis. Artificial saliva sprays are the treatment of choice but oral hygiene is also important. Careful monitoring or nutrition is necessary and many patients will require nutritional support with some form of enteral nutrition.

Trismus is a late complication of both surgery and radiotherapy and is due to fibrosis in and around the temporomandibular joint leading to restriction of jaw opening and closing. Osteonecrosis is a late complication of radiotherapy, usually affecting the mandible as the maxilla has a better blood supply. It can be precipitated by a dental infection or extraction many years after radiotherapy.

Prognosis

The prognosis varies greatly with site of origin, TNM stage and histological grade, and the reader should refer to a more specialized text for more detailed data. In general there is a high expectation of cure for all T1 and T2 tumours with a 5-year survival of 60–90 per cent, falling to less than 30 per cent for T4 tumours.

Screening/prevention

Dentists play a vital part in screening as they have the opportunity to inspect the oral cavity in many people on a regular basis, but unfortunately the people most at risk of cancer tend to be those who are least likely to attend a dentist. Long-term survivors should be kept under close surveillance in the clinic as many will develop second primaries, usually in the head and neck region but also in the lung and gastrointestinal tract.

Many cases of oral cavity cancer could be prevented by better patient education, i.e. by reducing tobacco smoking, chewing tobacco and betel nut. It is reasonable to presume that reducing alcohol consumption would lessen the incidence of cancers of the oral cavity. There is some evidence that fenretinide could prevent the development of leukoplakia in a high-risk population. Similarly, a diet rich in fruit and vegetables might be protective.

Rare tumours of the oral cavity

Other rare carcinomas

The palate and oral mucosa contain a number of minor salivary glands, which can develop mucoepidermoid carcinomas, adenocarcinomas and adenoid cystic carcinomas, treated by surgery with radiotherapy after incomplete excision or for inoperable tumours.

Kaposi's sarcoma

The oral cavity, particularly the palate, is a common site for this disease and it should prompt serological testing to exclude AIDS (see Chapter 20).

Soft tissue and bone sarcomas

These are exceptionally rare but include leiomyosarcoma, rhabdomyosarcoma, fibrosarcoma, malignant fibrous histiocytoma, osteosarcoma and Ewing's sarcoma.

Metastases

Tumour cells can spread via the blood to the gingiva or lower alveolus, from which they can erode the overlying mucosa and mimic a primary carcinoma of the oral cavity. The lung is a common source of such metastases.

CARCINOMA OF THE OROPHARYNX

Each year in the UK there are 900 cases of oropharyngeal cancer, 650 cases in men and 250 cases in women, leading to 350 deaths per annum. The oropharynx comprises the tonsils, posterior third of the tongue, soft palate and posterior wall of the oropharynx down to the level of the hyoid bone. As the oropharynx is a direct extension of the oral cavity, tumours arising in this region are similar in their epidemiology, presentation and pathology. Of those developing oropharyngeal cancer, one-third have evidence of prior infection with HPV, especially type 16, rising to one-half of those developing tonsillar cancer. Such individuals are less likely to smoke or drink alcohol in excess, and much more likely to have had multiple oral sex partners. Indeed, the relative risk for developing oropharyngeal cancer is around 3 for each of smoking and alcohol, but around 30 for HPV infected individuals. The structures comprising the oropharynx have a bilateral pattern of lymphatic drainage to the neck, which should be considered when planning treatment. Radiotherapy is the preferred treatment for all but the earliest tumours as radical resection of the tumour is likely to produce functional compromise greater than that from radiotherapy alone. It should be noted that the oropharynx is a site where lymphoid tissue is concentrated and where lymphoma occasionally arise. HPV-associated cancers have a much better prognosis.

CARCINOMA OF THE LARYNX

Each year in the UK there are 2200 cases of laryngeal cancer, 1800 cases in men and 400 cases in women, accounting for 0.8 per cent of all cancer cases and leading to a total of 800 deaths per annum. These tumours are much more common in men with a male-to-female predominance of 10:1, predisposed to by smoking, and 95 per cent are squamous carcinomas. All patients complaining of a hoarse voice that has persisted longer than a month should undergo indirect laryngoscopy to visualize directly the vocal cords. Glottic tumours arise on the vocal cords and present at an early stage, as distortion of the vocal cords is rapidly manifest as dysphonia noted by both patients and physicians alike. Tumours can arise above the cords (supraglottic) or below the cords (subglottic). These non-glottic tumours present later in their natural history as they grow insidiously and have to reach a large size before the patient presents with dysphagia, stridor or symptoms from direct invasion of the glottis. A tumour in the supraglottic larynx can lead to referred pain in the ipsilateral ear. The vocal cords have a poor lymphatic drainage and therefore lymph node metastases are less common at this site compared with a 70 per cent incidence from supraglottic tumours, as the supraglottis has a rich lymphatic drainage. The TNM staging system is used for laryngeal tumours, the T stage is outlined below (N staging is the generic head and neck version cited above):

- Tis – Carcinoma in situ
- T0 – No evidence of primary tumour
- TX – Primary tumour cannot be assessed

Supraglottis
- T1 – Tumour limited to one subsite of supraglottis with normal vocal cord mobility
- T2 – Tumour invades mucosa of more than one adjacent subsite of supraglottis or glottis or region outside the supraglottis (e.g. mucosa of base of tongue, vallecula, medial wall of pyriform sinus) without fixation of the larynx
- T3 – Tumour limited to larynx with vocal cord fixation and/or invades any of the following: postcricoid area, pre-epiglottic tissues
- T4 – Tumour invades through the thyroid cartilage, and/or extends into soft tissues of the neck, thyroid and/or oesophagus

Glottis
- T1 – Tumour limited to vocal cord(s) (might involve anterior or posterior commissure) with normal mobility

– T1a – Tumour limited to one vocal cord
– T1b – Tumour involves both vocal cords
- T2 – Tumour extends to supraglottis and/or subglottis, and/or with impaired vocal cord mobility
- T3 – Tumour limited to the larynx with vocal cord fixation
- T4 – Tumour invades through the thyroid cartilage and/or to other tissues beyond the larynx (e.g. trachea, soft tissues of neck, including thyroid, pharynx)

Subglottis
- T1 – Tumour limited to the subglottis
- T2 – Tumour extends to vocal cord(s) with normal or impaired mobility
- T3 – Tumour limited to larynx with vocal cord fixation
- T4 – Tumour invades through cricoid or thyroid cartilage and/or extends to other tissues beyond the larynx (e.g. trachea, soft tissues of neck, including thyroid, oesophagus).

Laryngeal tumours can be treated by surgery or radiotherapy. A partial or total laryngectomy will have the disadvantage of changing the quality of the voice, and therefore radiotherapy is preferred for T1, T2 and small bulk T3 tumours. The prognosis from glottic tumours is excellent, reflecting their early presentation and low rate of lymphatic spread. Although there is a strong rationale for its use, neoadjuvant chemotherapy has not been shown to confer a survival advantage in locally advanced laryngeal cancer, although it could facilitate laryngeal preservation in a higher proportion of patients.

CARCINOMA OF THE HYPOPHARYNX

The hypopharynx extends from the level of the tip of the epiglottis to the lower border of the cricoid and comprises the pyriform fossae, posterior pharyngeal wall and postcricoid region. The tumours are squamous carcinomas that tend to present late with dysphagia. There is an association with iron deficiency (Plummer–Vinson syndrome). Pharyngolaryngectomy has historically been the treatment of choice but with inevitably a significant degree of functional compromise. Combined modality treatment with chemotherapy and radiotherapy is now an established alternative, particularly for locally advanced disease.

CARCINOMA OF THE NASOPHARYNX

Each year in the UK there are 220 cases of nasopharyngeal cancer, 150 cases in men and 70 cases in women, leading to a total of 100 deaths per annum. This disease has a marked geographical variation, being more common in the Far East, particularly Southern China where it is endemic. There is very strong evidence that in areas of high incidence the disease is related to infection with the Epstein–Barr virus (EBV). In endemic areas it has a peak incidence at a younger age (15–25 years versus 40–60 years in developed countries) and a predominance of anaplastic tumours (squamous in developed countries). There is a lesser association with excess alcohol and tobacco consumption compared with other head and neck sites. Routes of spread include:

- nose – produces epistaxis, nasal discharge and blockage
- orbit – produces diplopia
- eustachian tube – blockage produces deafness
- cavernous sinus – causes palsies of cranial nerves 3, 4, 5 and 6
- cribriform plate – produces loss of smell
- pterygoid muscles and parapharyngeal space – produces inability to open jaw fully (trismus).

The TNM staging is employed (generic N-staging):

- Tis – Carcinoma in situ
- T0 – No evidence of primary tumour
- TX – Primary tumour cannot be assessed
- T1 – Tumour confined to the nasopharynx
- T2 – Tumour extends to soft tissues of oropharynx and/or nasal fossa
  - T2a – Without parapharyngeal extension
  - T2b – With parapharyngeal extension
- T3 – Tumour invades bony structures and/or paranasal sinuses

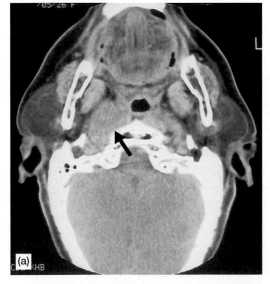
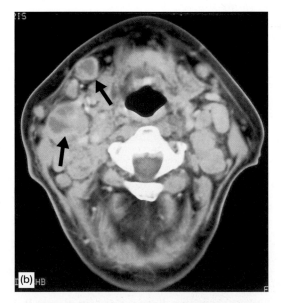

Figure 13.5 Nasopharyngeal carcinoma. (a) Transverse CT image of the base of skull. There is soft tissue within the nasopharynx, particularly on the right side. (b) Same patient. CT image of the neck showing multiple enlarged, necrotic lymph nodes consistent with nodal metastases.

■ T4 – Tumour with intracranial extension and/or involvement of cranial nerves, infratemporal fossa, hypopharynx, or orbit.

CT or MRI are the investigations of choice for delineating the locoregional extent of the tumour (Fig. 13.5), CT being superior with respect to delineation of the skeletal anatomy, which is frequently involved by the tumour. Seventy per cent will have overt or occult lymph node metastases with a tendency to bilateral involvement. The treatment of choice is chemoradiotherapy, typically using cisplatin. The prognosis for squamous carcinoma is poor with a 5-year survival of less than 20 per cent versus up to 50 per cent for other histological types. The advent of IMRT will make re-treatment of this particular site to high doses a real possibility.

CARCINOMA OF THE PARANASAL SINUSES

These are rare: sites of origin include the frontal, ethmoid, maxillary and sphenoid sinuses. The maxillary sinus is the most frequently affected. They are usually squamous carcinomas, frequently presenting late as the symptoms are mistaken for those of chronic sinusitis. All too often, by the time of diagnosis, they have spread beyond the bony walls of the sinus and have led to other symptoms owing to local invasion of adjacent structures, such as diplopia from orbital involvement (Fig. 13.6), or epistaxis from nasal cavity involvement. They can also invade the cranial cavity. Radical surgery is hazardous owing to adjacent vital organs and therefore radiotherapy is the treatment of choice. Approximately 40 per cent will survive 5 years after treatment. It should be noted that the sinuses are a potential site of extranodal lymphoma.

SALIVARY GLAND TUMOURS

The parotid gland forms the vast bulk of salivary gland tissue and therefore is the most

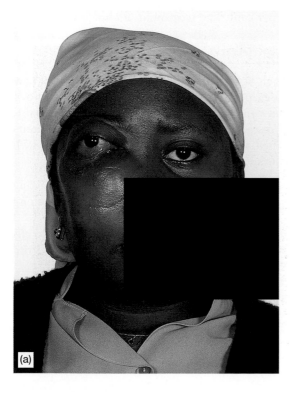

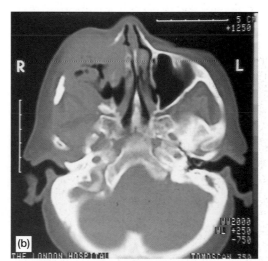

Figure 13.6 Carcinoma of the maxillary antrum. (a) Frontal view of face. Note the swelling of the right cheek owing to anterior spread from the antrum. Superior spread into the orbit has led to proptosis of the right eye. (b) CT image of the base of skull from the same patient showing destruction of the facial bones on the right side.

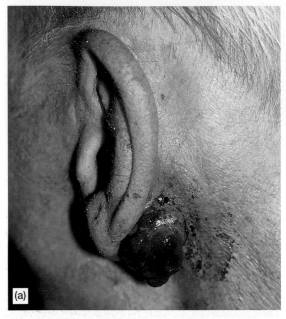

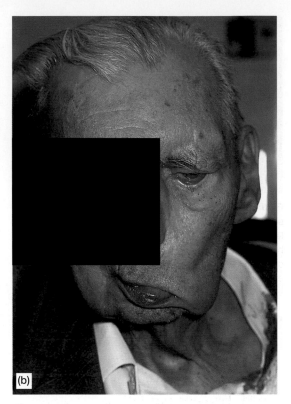

Figure 13.7 Adenoid cystic carcinoma of the parotid. (a) Tumour fungation through the skin posterior to the left ear. (b) Same patient. Dense left lower motor neurone facial nerve palsy characteristic of a malignant parotid tumour.

common site for tumours, while the sublingual, submandibular and smaller glands distributed throughout the oral cavity are rarely involved. There are several variants described below.

Pleomorphic adenoma

This is the most common salivary gland tumour constituting 75 per cent, with a peak incidence at 30–50 years. It usually arises in the superficial lobe of the gland, is a benign tumour and therefore slow growing. There is never any associated facial nerve weakness – this feature should always suggest carcinoma or lymphoma. All cases are treated by superficial parotidectomy. Postoperative radiotherapy is indicated if there is capsular rupture at the time of surgery or incomplete microscopic clearance. There is a small risk of transformation of a recurrence into a carcinoma.

Adenolymphoma

This is a benign, slow-growing tumour most commonly arising in the lower pole of the

superficial lobe of the parotid, and is bilateral in 5 per cent. The treatment of choice is surgery.

Carcinoma

Each year in the UK there are 500 to 600 new cases per annum. This usually arises de novo but can develop in a pleomorphic adenoma. It is distinguished clinically from benign tumours when a facial nerve palsy is present (Fig. 13.7). Variants include:

- adenoid cystic carcinoma – slow-growing and has a tendency for invasion along nerves and into the cranial cavity
- acinic cell carcinoma arising from serous cells
- mucoepidermoid carcinoma arising from mucin cells
- adenocarcinoma
- squamous carcinoma – must be distinguished from a metastasis
- undifferentiated carcinoma.

The treatment of choice is resection of the lobe of origin followed by radiotherapy to the

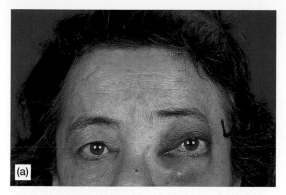

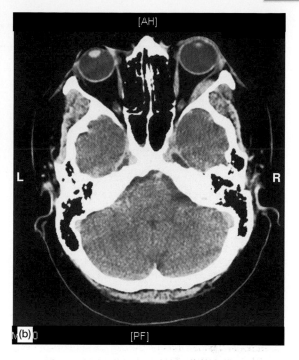

Figure 13.8 Orbital metastasis. This is most commonly seen in cancers of the breast, prostate and lung. (a) The left eye demonstrates non-axial proptosis. The patient has severe diplopia. (b) CT image through the orbits showing abnormal tissue in the lateral aspect of the left eye, pushing it forward.

parotid. Five-year survival varies between 20 and 80 per cent depending on tumour type and histological grade.

Lymphoma

The parotid is a common site of extranodal non-Hodgkin's lymphoma. Localized disease can be treated by radiotherapy, with chemotherapy used for more advanced disease.

ORBITAL TUMOURS

These are all very rare, presenting because of a mass effect leading to proptosis and diplopia. Benign tumours include haemangioma, leiomyoma, rhabdomyoma, hypoma, fibroma, meningioma, neurofibroma, schwannoma, pseudotumour and 'malignant' granuloma, e.g. Wegener's granulomatosis. Malignant tumours include gliomas, rhabdomyosarcoma, leiomyosarcoma, malignant fibrous histiocytoma, fibrosarcoma, osteosarcoma, chondrosarcoma, Ewing's sarcoma, lymphoma, Langerhans' cell histiocytosis, melanoma, nephroblastoma, plasmacytoma and metastases, particularly from breast and lung cancers (Fig. 13.8).

Tumours within the eye itself are also very rare, presenting with visual loss and strabismus. Benign tumours include naevi, leiomyoma, haemangioma and hamartoma. Malignant tumours include retinoblastoma, medulloepithelioma, melanoma and metastases.

With both sites, optimum management will preserve vision in the affected eye as much as possible, and usually comprises radiotherapy alone, surgery alone or combined modality treatment.

FURTHER READING

Genden EM, Varvares MA. *Head and Neck Cancer – an evidence-based team approach*. Thieme, New York, 2008

Harrison LB, Hong WK, Sessions RB. *Head and Neck Cancer – a multidisciplinary approach*. Lippincott Williams and Wilkins, London, 2008

Myers EN, Suen JY. *Cancer of the Head and Neck*. Saunders, Philadelphia, 2003

Werning JW. *Oral Cancer*. Thieme, New York, 2007

SELF-ASSESSMENT QUESTIONS

1. Which three of the following statements are true for head and neck cancers?
   a. Account for 10 000 deaths per annum in the UK
   b. Overall they are more frequent in men
   c. Laryngeal cancer is more frequent in women
   d. Associated with chronic gum disease
   e. Associated with human papilloma virus infection
   f. Associated with gonorrhoea
   g. High incidence in Asia

2. Which one of the following is not true about head and neck cancer?
   a. May be preceded by leucoplakia
   b. Lymph node involvement is more likely with increasing size of primary tumours
   c. Adenocarcinoma is rare
   d. Three-quarters are squamous carcinomas
   e. The pattern of lymph node spread is predictable

3. Which three of the following statements are common presentations for head and neck cancers?
   a. Oral candidiasis
   b. Headache
   c. Enlarged cervical lymph node(s)
   d. No symptoms
   e. Diplopia
   f. Chronic mucosal ulcer
   g. Loss of taste

4. Which one of the following best describes the role of radiotherapy in head and neck cancer?
   a. Protons are the treatment of choice
   b. Only suitable for those where surgery is contraindicated
   c. Cannot be used to treat lymph gland areas
   d. Leads to permanent voice loss
   e. Has a high cure probability for small tumours

5. Which three of the following statements best describe CHART?
   a. Involves treatment over weekends
   b. Utilizes multiple fractions per day
   c. Radiotherapy is delivered in a shorter overall time
   d. Given concurrently with accelerated chemotherapy
   e. There is less acute toxicity
   f. Cetuximab is part of the protocol
   g. Is considered standard practice

6. Which one of the following best describes the role of chemotherapy in head and neck cancer?
   a. Cisplatin is the mainstay of treatment
   b. Chemotherapy does not add to the toxicity of radiotherapy
   c. Adjuvant chemotherapy is given to most patients
   d. Cannot be given with cetuximab
   e. K-ras oncogene expression predicts for response to chemotherapy

7. Which three of the following are important prognostic factors for head and neck cancer?
   a. Lymph node involvement
   b. Hepatitis seropositivity
   c. Depth of invasion
   d. Alcohol consumption
   e. Size of tumour
   f. Tobacco consumption
   g. Trismus

8. Which one of the following best describes the role of radiotherapy in head and neck cancer?
   a. Best outcome attained when given as single modality treatment
   b. The main toxicity is mucositis
   c. Has low probability of local control of tumour
   d. Unsuitable for treating involved lymph nodes
   e. Can only be used for tumours of oral cavity

14 ENDOCRINE TUMOURS

■ Thyroid cancer   239
■ Tumours of the parathyroid gland   246
■ Tumours of the adrenal glands   246
■ Carcinoid tumours   248

■ Multiple endocrine neoplasia (MEN)   251
■ Further reading   252
■ Self-assessment questions   253

THYROID CANCER

Epidemiology

Each year in the UK there are 1650 cases of thyroid cancer, 450 cases in men and 1200 cases in women, accounting for 2.9 per cent of all cancer cases and leading to a total of 350 deaths per annum. Well-differentiated thyroid cancer has a high survival rate but accounts for 75 per cent of thyroid cancer deaths. The overall incidence increases with age, papillary and medullary types typically arising in young adults, while follicular carcinomas and anaplastic cancers are usually seen in later adult life. There is a female predominance of 4:1 and a particularly high incidence in Iceland, Israel and Hawaii.

Aetiology

Ionizing radiation is a recognized aetiological agent. Radiation-induced cancers have a latency of 5–40 years, with a peak at 15 years after exposure. Radiation induces papillary cancer, which has been described following childhood irradiation for thymic hyperplasia, ringworm and cervical lymphadenitis, and in atomic bomb survivors. A higher incidence of follicular cancer has been noted in endemic goitre areas where there is a dietary deficiency of iodine, while a higher incidence of papillary cancer is seen in areas where there is an excess of iodine in the diet. Multiple endocrine neoplasia (MEN – see end of this chapter) is a dominantly inherited condition, type 1 being occasionally associated with differentiated thyroid cancer while type 2 is associated with medullary cancer, which is more often multifocal and presents at a younger age than its sporadic counterpart.

Other rare associations include:

■ Pendred's syndrome (goitre and nerve deafness at birth)
■ Gardener's syndrome (polyposis of the bowel, osteomas and sebaceous cysts)
■ Cowden's disease (multiple hamartomas).

Pathology

The tumour usually appears as a firm, well-circumscribed lump, often with a pseudocapsule of compressed thyroid tissue at its periphery. The cut surface will have a characteristic glistening appearance of colloid if there is a significant follicular element. There can be haemorrhage and necrosis in anaplastic tumours, and it is sometimes multifocal. Follicular, papillary and medullary cancers tend to grow very slowly over many years, while anaplastic cancers are usually fast growing and locally invasive. Tumours may arise in ectopic thyroid tissue in the tongue, a thyroglossal cyst, sublingual, infrahyoid, pretracheal, mediastinal and pericardial regions.

Microscopically, thyroid cancer is characterized by invasion of the capsule and/or thyroid vasculature. There are four main types:

- follicular carcinoma (50 per cent)
- papillary carcinoma (20 per cent)
- anaplastic carcinoma (25 per cent)
- medullary carcinoma (4 per cent).

The presence of papillary structures is diagnostic of papillary carcinoma, although these tumours frequently contain a follicular component also. Follicular carcinoma must be distinguished from an adenoma. It is usually well differentiated with colloid held within follicles and there are no papillary elements. Anaplastic carcinoma is very poorly differentiated, usually with no identifiable follicular elements. Medullary carcinoma arises from the parafollicular ('C') cells, with the inherited form often multifocal in origin. Amyloid might be identified within the stroma and immunocytochemistry will be positive for the hormone calcitonin. *RET* gene testing can show a characteristic mutation in familial cases. Squamous carcinoma, clear cell carcinoma and Hurthle cell carcinoma are also recognized.

Natural history

The tumour initially spreads within the lobe of origin, contained by the capsule, but can then invade the contralateral lobe via the isthmus. Capsular invasion will lead to infiltration of surrounding structures such as the trachea, larynx, recurrent laryngeal nerves and skin. Papillary and medullary carcinomas have a propensity to metastasize to lymph nodes, the affected groups comprising the deep cervical, supraclavicular and paratracheal chains. All may give rise to distant metastases, the lung being the most common site, followed by the skeleton, liver, skin, brain and kidney. Lung metastases are often very numerous and small, sometimes giving a 'snowstorm' appearance. Follicular and anaplastic variants are the types most often associated with distant metastases.

Symptoms

The most common presentation is with a painless solitary lump in the neck (Fig. 14.1). Some patients complain of a hoarse voice, which raises the suspicion of extracapsular extension leading to pressure on one or both of the recurrent laryngeal nerves innervating the vocal cords. Dysphagia is noticed if the tumour is very large and causing extrinsic compression of the pharynx or upper oesophagus, and could suggest retrosternal extension if the neck mass is small. Patients with medullary carcinoma sometimes complain of diarrhoea, which is thought to be due to secretion of prostaglandins by the tumour.

Signs

The patient will be euthyroid. The thyroid lump is usually confined to one side of the neck, moving with swallowing and protrusion of the tongue, non-tender, firm/hard in consistency and well circumscribed. Stridor might be heard owing to either recurrent laryngeal nerve involvement or extrinsic tracheal compression. Vocal cord

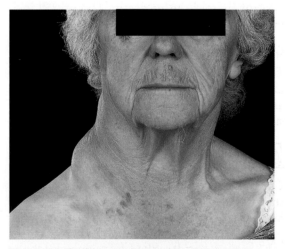

Figure 14.1 Papillary carcinoma of the thyroid. The tumour is arising from the right lobe of the thyroid and has spread to lymph nodes on the same side of the neck.

palsy can be confirmed by indirect laryngoscopy (IDL). Extracapsular invasion can lead to loss of the normal laryngeal mobility. Lymphadenopathy can be palpable in the deep cervical and supra-clavicular regions, while anaplastic tumours sometimes invade the overlying skin to produce induration, erythema and nodularity.

Differential diagnosis

This includes:

- benign tumours of thyroid, e.g. adenoma
- other malignant tumours of thyroid, e.g. lymphoma, fibrosarcoma
- metastases, e.g. carcinoma of the lung, hypernephroma, melanoma.

Investigations

Serum markers

Thyroglobulin is a useful marker of differenti-ated thyroid cancer after ablation of normal thyroid tissue. Calcitonin should be measured in any patient suspected of having medullary carcinoma, e.g. if there is a family history of thy-roid carcinoma at a young age or associated diarrhoea. These patients should also be screened for other MEN type 2 tumours, i.e. parathyroid adenomas (parathyroid hormone level), phaeochromocytoma (blood cate-cholamine levels, urinary vanillylmandelic acid, bilateral adrenal MRI).

Chest X-ray

This should be performed in all patients to exclude obvious pulmonary metastases. These are usually small and numerous giving a 'snow-storm' appearance (Fig. 14.2).

Thyroid ultrasound and fine needle aspiration (FNA)

Carcinoma will give rise to a solid nodule rather than a cystic one and in either case FNA should be performed to obtain a cytological diagnosis.

FNA of enlarged lymph nodes

This is essential to distinguish reactive lymph node enlargement from metastatic infiltration.

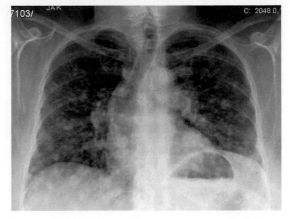

Figure 14.2 Multiple small lung metastases typical of thyroid cancer.

Open thyroid biopsy

This is required only in inoperable tumours when an FNA has proven negative or given an equivocal histological diagnosis.

Isotope thyroid scan

In the case of thyroid cancer, administration of a tracer dose of technetium-99 or iodine-131 will give rise to a cold spot relative to the surround-ing functioning thyroid tissue, giving useful information to the surgeon regarding its loca-tion and extent. Functioning adenomas will produce a hot spot.

CT scan of the neck and chest

This can be of value in assisting the surgeon to make a decision regarding operability of a large mass, particularly when retrosternal extension is suspected (Fig. 14.3), or for radiotherapy planning at a later date. CT is also the most sen-sitive means of detecting small pulmonary metastases, which might be below the spatial resolution of a radioiodine whole body scan.

Staging

- TX – Primary tumour cannot be assessed
- T0 – No evidence of tumour
- T1 – Tumour 1 cm or less in greatest dimension, limited to thyroid
- T2 – Tumour >1 cm but not >4 cm in greatest dimension, limited to thyroid

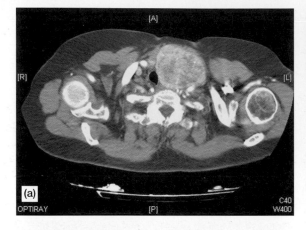

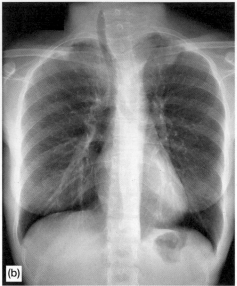

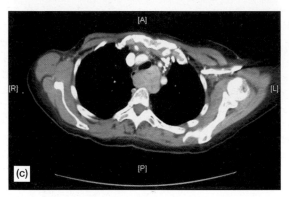

Figure 14.3 Medullary carcinoma of the thyroid. (a) CT scan of the neck showing a massive tumour arising from the left lobe of the thyroid, pushing the trachea to the right side of the neck. (b) Chest radiograph from the same patient. Note the soft tissue mass in the neck and tracheal deviation. (c) CT scan of the thorax showing retrosternal extension of tumour that had not been appreciated from the chest radiograph.

- ▪ T3 – Tumour >4 cm in greatest dimension, limited to thyroid
- ▪ T4 – Tumour of any size extending beyond thyroid capsule
- ▪ NX – Lymph nodes cannot be assessed
- ▪ N0 – No nodes involved
- ▪ N1 – Regional nodes involved
  - N1a – Ipsilateral cervical nodes
  - N1b – Bilateral, midline or contralateral cervical nodes or mediastinal nodes.

Note: All 'T'categories can be subdivided into 'a' (solitary) and 'b' (multiple).

Treatment

All patients should have some form of thyroid ablation followed by physiological hormone replacement therapy to prevent hypothyroidism and maintain thyroid stimulating hormone (TSH) at very low ('suppressed') levels to minimize the likelihood of recurrence of a TSH-dependent tumour.

Radical treatment

Surgery

This can be curative when used alone, all patients requiring a total thyroidectomy with the aim of removing all thyroid tissue and any extracapsular extension, with care taken to preserve the parathyroid glands and recurrent laryngeal nerves if possible. A cervical lymph node dissection should be undertaken when there is overt lymph node invasion.

Unsealed source brachytherapy and external beam radiotherapy

Radioiodine is concentrated in the thyroid gland and can therefore be used for the diagnosis of locoregional and metastatic disease, for

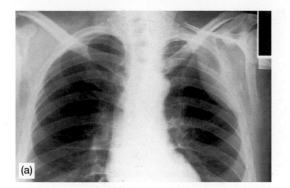

Figure 14.4 Metastatic follicular carcinoma of the thyroid. (a) Plain chest radiograph showing a left upper lobe pleural metastasis. (b) Iodine-131 uptake scan showing increased activity (dark) in the corresponding region. (c) Whole body iodine-131 uptake scan demonstrating widespread metastatic disease.

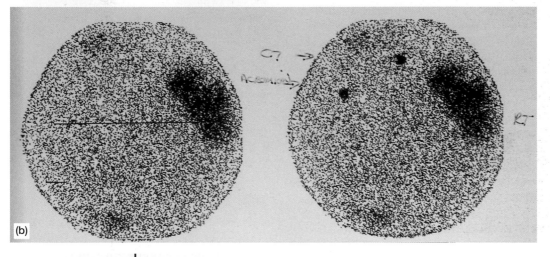

the ablation of a thyroid remnant and/or tumour persisting after surgery, and as a means of detecting early relapse. It is concentrated not only by normal thyroid tissue, but also by 70–80 per cent of well-differentiated thyroid carcinomas and their metastases (Fig. 14.4). Radioiodine is given as an oral preparation using strict radiation protection procedures, with the large doses used for ablation of thyroid and tumour being given in an inpatient setting. Patient selection is important, as those with claustrophobia might not be suited to long periods left alone in a protected room. Urinary incontinence or dementia can pose a risk of contamination to staff, visitors or other patients on the ward. It emits β-particles (electrons) with a tissue range of only 2 mm, and it is these that ablate the thyroid/tumour. It also emits low-energy γ-photons, which are a radiation hazard to staff and visitors but allow external monitoring of the distribution, concentration and excretion of the isotope.

Radioiodine (e.g. 3.7Gbq activity) is given after thyroid surgery to destroy any remaining normal thyroid tissue after total or near total thyroidectomy. There are several reasons to ablate the thyroid remnant:

- it can obscure occult disease in the neck or upper thorax on a whole body radioiodine scan
- it may prevent a physiological rise in TSH on hormone therapy withdrawal and can therefore make follow-up thyroglobulin assays and whole body radioiodine scans less sensitive
- it may be a source of new primary cancer or local recurrence.

If whole body scans at any time demonstrate any evidence of distant metastases, much higher therapeutic doses (e.g. 5.5 GBq activity) are given. Most patients will require one to three such treatments. The success of the treatment is determined by the avidity of the metastases for iodine.

External beam irradiation to the neck is used when there is residual papillary or follicular carcinoma in the neck that is not concentrating iodine-131, and is necessary in all cases of anaplastic carcinoma and incompletely excised medullary carcinomas.

Palliative treatment

Surgery

Tracheostomy is occasionally necessary, particularly with anaplastic tumours causing tracheal compression (Fig. 14.5) and when there are bilateral recurrent laryngeal nerve palsies leading to total vocal cord paralysis and upper respiratory airway obstruction.

Radiotherapy

Death from asphyxiation owing to a rapidly growing anaplastic carcinoma is particularly unpleasant and distressing for all concerned and under such circumstances, even if the patient has distant metastases, radiotherapy to the neck is justified.

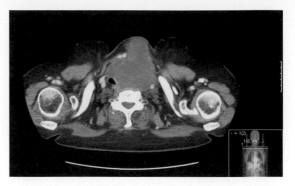

Figure 14.5 Anaplastic cancer of the thyroid. CT image of the lower neck showing a large mass on the left side pushing the trachea to the right.

Chemotherapy

This has no role in the curative treatment of thyroid cancer. Patients with anaplastic carcinoma and symptoms refractory to all other treatments can be considered for palliative chemotherapy. Adriamycin is the most active agent. Responses are infrequent and short-lived.

Hormone therapy

Elderly patients unfit for surgery with small, well-differentiated tumours can be treated by thyroxine alone at a dose sufficient to suppress TSH, as the natural history of the disease is likely to exceed the patient's natural life expectancy.

Tumour-related complications

Respiratory obstruction is seen with anaplastic carcinomas owing to extrinsic compression of the trachea or bilateral damage to the recurrent laryngeal nerves, while dysphagia can result from extrinsic compression of the cervical oesophagus and/or retrosternal extension. Superior vena cava obstruction is a rare complication associated with a large retrosternal tumour.

Treatment-related complications

Surgery

Specific complications include risk of secondary haemorrhage during the postoperative period, laryngeal oedema, hypoparathyroidism (hypocalcaemia leading to perioral paraesthesia, tetany, Trousseau's sign, Chvostek's sign) and vocal cord palsy from damage to the recurrent laryngeal nerves leading to dysphonia and respiratory obstruction.

Radiotherapy

External beam irradiation to the neck will result in an acute radiation laryngitis characterized by sore throat, dysphagia and dysphonia. Late complications include chronic laryngeal oedema, intense subcutaneous fibrosis leading to restricted neck movements and radiation chondritis of the tracheal cartilage rings.

Radioiodine

Severe adverse reactions to radioiodine are rare. Possible complications include nausea, acute parotitis, sore throat from radiation laryngitis, acute pneumonitis if there are miliary lung metastases, myelosuppression, leukaemogenesis and induction of cancer elsewhere (there is some uptake in the salivary glands, stomach, colon and bladder). Acute thyroiditis is also recognized – this may cause temporary upper airway obstruction in severe cases. It settles quickly with corticosteroids. Radiation protection protocols should prevent radiation exposure to staff and relatives of those receiving high doses of radioiodine.

Hormone replacement therapy

Inappropriate dosage or poor patient compliance can lead to either hypothyroidism or hyperthyroidism. Hypothyroidism leads to a physiological rise in TSH, which may be detrimental if there is any occult residual disease.

Prognosis

Differentiated thyroid cancer has a very good prognosis. Papillary carcinoma has the best prognosis of all with a long-term (40-year) survival of more than 90 per cent, followed by follicular carcinoma (80–90 per cent) and medullary carcinoma (60–70 per cent). Of those with differentiated thyroid cancer, one-third will sustain a relapse after initial therapy. Two-thirds of such relapses will occur within

the first decade of follow-up, and of those with distant metastases half will be cured by salvage therapy. Most patients with anaplastic carcinoma will die within 6 months after diagnosis. Children have an extremely good prognosis, young adults fare better than the elderly and women fare better than men, again reflecting the incidence of differentiated thyroid cancer in these groups. For differentiated thyroid cancer, age <15 or >45 years, male gender, tumour >4 cm, bilobar disease, extracapsular invasion, lymphatic invasion, non-iodine concentrating tumour, and distant metastases at diagnosis are poor prognostic factors.

Screening/prevention

Patients treated for differentiated thyroid cancer require life-long follow-up. This usually involves regular thyroglobulin measurements with or without whole body iodine uptake scans after endogenous or exogenous TSH stimulation. Thyroid hormone replacement therapy is usually withdrawn 2–6 weeks before such investigations. This precipitates acute hypothyroidism, a physiological rise in TSH, and therefore acts as a provocation test to facilitate detection of occult disease. In recent years, recombinant thyrotropin-α (Thyrogen®) given by intramuscular injection has been used for those individuals who do not have an adequate TSH response to hormone withdrawal, and for those where the transient myxoedema of hormone withdrawal is intolerable. A thyroglobulin level of >2 ng/mL 72 hours after TSH provocation usually warrants further investigation (neck ultrasound/MRI, CT scan of the thorax, whole body radioiodine scan) to exclude local relapse and/or distant metastatic disease.

Patients developing medullary carcinoma of the thyroid have a significant risk of having MEN type 2, particularly if aged 20–40 years with a multifocal carcinoma. A calcium provocation level of calcitonin (measured before, 2 and 5 minutes after intravenous calcium) might unmask an otherwise borderline level and is useful for screening members of MEN 2 families who might have occult medullary carcinoma. Alternatively, risk-reducing thyroidectomy at an early age can be appropriate for those with familial medullary carcinoma even if calcitonin levels are normal.

Rare tumours

Lymphoma

This constitutes less than 2 per cent of extranodal lymphomas, with a median age at presentation of 65 years and a female predominance. It is invariably a non-Hodgkin's lymphoma, usually diffuse high grade, and could be preceded by Hashimoto's thyroiditis. It is staged and treated using the same principles as for lymphoma elsewhere and has a 5-year survival of about 40 per cent.

TUMOURS OF THE PARATHYROID GLAND

These are rare and are sometimes part of MEN types 1 or 2. Adenomas are usually impalpable and solitary, and present with hyperparathyroidism (high serum calcium, low serum phosphate, hyperchloraemic metabolic acidosis, evidence of subperiosteal bone resorption on plain radiographs, e.g. of phalanges, nephrolithiasis). The glands can be imaged by radioisotope imaging using a technetium-99 scan (images the thyroid) followed by a thallium-201 scan (images both the thyroid and the parathyroids), subtraction of the two images giving an image of the parathyroids alone. Ultrasound or MRI of the neck are alternatives, and venous sampling for parathyroid hormone is useful for tumours that cannot be visualized. Parathyroidectomy is the sole treatment. Carcinoma is extremely rare.

TUMOURS OF THE ADRENAL GLANDS

Tumours of the adrenal gland are rare, accounting for approximately 100 deaths per annum in the UK.

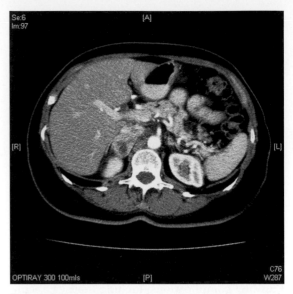

Figure 14.6 Phaeochromocytoma. CT image of the abdomen showing a heterogeneous mass arising above the upper pole of the right kidney.

Phaeochromocytoma

This is a very rare tumour arising from the autonomic cells of the adrenal medulla, with a peak incidence at 35–55 years but can occur from infancy to old age. Recognized associations include:

- multiple endocrine neoplasia type 2 (*RET* gene mutation)
- neurofibromatosis I
- Von Hippel–Lindau syndrome
- Sturge–Weber syndrome
- tuberose sclerosis.

Ninety-nine per cent are found in the abdomen or pelvis, 90 per cent of these in the adrenal medulla (Fig. 14.6), the most common extra-adrenal site being adjacent to the aortic bifurcation. Other sites include the sympathetic chain, bladder, thorax (usually paravertebral) and carotid arch. The tumours can be very small or weigh several kilograms, are well circumscribed and slow growing, with 10 per cent bilateral (70 per cent of those arising in familial cases), 90 per cent benign and 10 per cent malignant (more likely for extra-adrenal tumours). They are rich in lipid and therefore yellow in cut section. Phaeochromocytomas arise from chromaffin cells of neural crest origin. The cells therefore stain with chrome salts and enzymes such as dopa decarboxylase and contain neurosecretory granules. As most tumours are benign, local invasion is unusual, although malignant tumours can infiltrate the underlying kidney and retroperitoneum. Lymphatic spread is unusual but malignant tumours can spread to lung, bone and liver. The classic presentation is with paroxysms of headache, postural dizziness, feelings of apprehension and fear, pallor, sweating, tremor, chest pain and palpitations. Attacks last minutes to hours and are followed by a feeling of exhaustion and muscle pain, and can be precipitated by emotion, exertion, posture, bending, pressure on tumour, foods or handling of tumour at operation. Thyrotoxicosis should be excluded as it might present in a similar manner. Half the patients have sustained hypertension, which may be difficult to control with conventional antihypertensive agents, while 70 per cent have postural hypotension. Investigations include:

- urinary vanillylmandelic acid (VMA)
- meta-iodobenzyl guanidine (mIBG) imaging
- MRI scan of adrenals
- selective venous sampling
- selective angiography.

VMA and catecholamines are measured using a 24-hour urine collection, and are useful screening tests during investigation of malignant hypertension. Urinary VMA is elevated in phaeochromocytoma, while high levels of adrenaline suggest an adrenal origin, high levels of noradrenaline suggest an extra-adrenal tumour, and high levels of dopamine suggest a malignant phaeochromocytoma. CT is the best investigation for delineating site and size of primary and excluding gross tumour in the contralateral adrenal, but is limited by its resolution of 0.5–1 cm, which will miss some tumours.

Selective venous sampling is used to localize radiologically occult tumours, identifying their venous drainage using multiple venous samples that are tested for catecholamines. Selective arteriography is also of value when surgery is planned, as phaeochromocytomas have a rich vascular supply, but it may precipitate a hypertensive crisis.

Imaging with mIBG is useful for malignant tumours as part of staging or in the context of MEN 2 when a multiplicity of tumours is possible. The compound is taken up by adrenergic tissue. It is of particular benefit in staging patients with malignant tumours, the iodine moiety being radioactive iodine-131 and therefore detectable by a gamma camera to give a whole body image. Uptake of mIBG opens up an additional therapeutic option for malignant tumours.

Laparoscopic unilateral adrenalectomy is the treatment of choice for those with a contralateral normal adrenal as it reduces the small but potentially fatal risk of acute adrenal insufficiency later in life associated with bilateral adrenalectomy. Adrenal cortex-sparing bilateral adrenalectomy is preferable to sacrificing both adrenals in their entirety for those with proven bilateral disease. Whatever surgery is planned, expert anaesthetic advice and preoperative alpha and beta blockade (e.g. phenoxybenzamine with propranolol or labetolol alone) is necessary as the tumour will be handled leading to a release of catecholamines. At laparotomy it is important to inspect the contralateral adrenal for a second primary. In inoperable cases, phenoxybenzamine is a useful medical therapy, being an α-adrenergic receptor blocker. Alpha-methyltyrosine inhibits hydroxylation of tyrosine to dopa, an intermediate compound in the synthesis of catecholamines and is a more toxic alternative. External beam radiotherapy and chemotherapy have no role in the curative treatment of these tumours, although the former is of value in palliating local symptoms from metastases. mIBG scan be used to treat metastatic disease if the tumour concentrates enough of it. Only one-third of patients will concentrate mIBG to an adequate degree within their tumours and of these only one-third will show evidence of an objective response. With regard to prognosis, the vast majority will be cured by surgery alone. Even patients with malignant tumours can survive for many years, death often resulting from cardiovascular complications (e.g. myocardial infarction, cerebrovascular accident) rather than from metastatic disease. Annual biochemical screening, with MRI of the adrenals if it is abnormal, is recommended in asymptomatic MEN 2 individuals or those who have previously undergone unilateral adrenalectomy.

Adrenal cortex tumours

Benign tumours are common at autopsy in the general population, but may be part of MEN 1 disease. Most are non-functioning, the majority of functioning tumours arising in females. Of functioning tumours, those arising in prepubertal patients are virilizing, while those in postpubertal patients tend to produce Cushing's syndrome, although Conn's syndrome (primary hyperaldosteronism) may also result. A CT scan will delineate the primary tumour if greater than 1 cm in diameter, although angiography is more sensitive, and treatment is by adrenalectomy.

Malignant tumours are rare, with a slight female predominance, arising at a younger age than most other carcinomas (median 35–55 years). Half are functioning and as with benign tumours are more frequent in females. Presentation is with vague abdominal symptoms, and up to one-third have signs of endocrine dysfunction, usually a combination of Cushing's syndrome and virilism. Half have metastatic disease at presentation, haematogenous spread occurring to lung and liver. Investigation and treatment is as for benign tumours. In advanced disease metyrapone (250 mg–1 g qds) is useful for palliation of Cushing's syndrome by inhibiting 2β-hydroxylase, but it might exacerbate virilism and physiological glucocorticoid replacement is necessary. Aminoglutethimide can be added if control is insufficient. An alternative is mitotane (o,p'-DDD), which causes necrosis and atrophy of normal adrenal tissue and differentiated carcinoma cells, reducing steroid output in 70 per cent and giving objective tumour regression in one-third, although response is slow and glucocorticoid cover necessary.

CARCINOID TUMOURS

Carcinoid tumours form one of several types of gastroenteropancreatic (GEP) neuroendocrine tumours (see Chapter 9), although distinguished by their appearance, albeit rare, at sites outside the gastrointestinal tract

Epidemiology

These are rare tumours arising at a younger age than carcinomas, with a peak incidence at about 50 years. There is no significant sex predominance or geographical pattern.

Aetiology

It can be a feature of multiple endocrine neoplasia type 1.

Pathology

They usually arise submucosally and appear as a nodule, often red/brown in colour, yellow in cut section; they can be multifocal, and, unlike in carcinomas, ulceration is uncommon. Carcinoid is most common in the small bowel – 90 per cent arise in the ileum, particularly the terminal segment, 7 per cent in the jejunum, 2 per cent in the duodenum and 2 per cent in a Meckel's diverticulum, but can arise elsewhere in the gastrointestinal tract, e.g. stomach, colon, rectum and other midline structures, such as thyroid, lung, bladder, testes, ovaries, common bile duct and pancreas. An encasement reaction characterized by a massive fibrous stroma can occur when the tumour reaches the mesentery and this predisposes to bowel obstruction. Carcinoids arise from APUD (amine precursor uptake and decarboxylation) cells, which are derived from the neural crest cells. Midgut-derived carcinoids characteristically stain with and reduce silver salts (argentaffin reaction), others stain with silver but cannot reduce it (argyrophilic reaction, e.g. gastric and bronchial carcinoids), while hindgut-derived carcinoids do not take up silver at all. Immunocytochemistry indicates staining for chromogranin, which is useful when the diagnosis is in doubt.

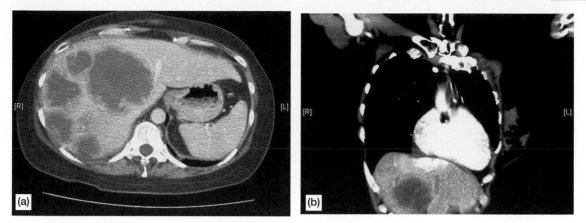

Figure 14.7 Carcinoid tumour with multiple liver metastases. (a) Transverse CT image. (b) Coronal CT image.

Natural history

The tumours are frequently slow growing and local infiltration of surrounding tissues is unusual. In contrast to a carcinoma, lymphatic spread is uncommon. Haematogenous spread is more common with larger primary tumours and is usually to the liver (Fig. 14.7) as most tumours will arise in the portal circulation. The primary tumour is often small compared with the bulk of liver metastases and symptoms of the carcinoid syndrome. Ileal tumours frequently metastasize, especially if more than 2 cm in diameter, while appendiceal, rectal and bronchial carcinoids rarely metastasize. The metastases are characteristically multiple and bulky compared with the primary, and can undergo spontaneous necrosis. The skeleton is sometimes a site of distant metastases and these may be osteoblastic.

Symptoms

Symptoms depend on the site and size of the tumour. Asymptomatic carcinoids are often found incidentally at appendicectomy, when they are almost invariably benign and therefore very rarely metastasize to the liver. The patient might notice an abdominal mass if the tumour is large and superficial, or experience colicky abdominal pain if there is significant stenosis of the bowel lumen. Ultimately there could be symptoms of subacute small bowel obstruction. Bronchial carcinoids present with haemoptysis or bronchial obstruction leading to recurrent chest infections. Carcinoid syndrome arises when there are liver metastases, so that the vasoactive tumour products, particularly 5-hydroxytryptamine (5-HT; serotonin), reach the systemic circulation. The syndrome can also arise in tumours originating outside the portal circulation (e.g. lung) or spreading outside it (e.g a heavy burden of skeletal metastases). It comprises:

- flushing – distribution may vary with site of primary
- weals – from release of histamine
- lacrimation
- facial oedema
- tachycardia, hypotension
- wheezing
- diarrhoea, borborygmi, abdominal colic and weight loss.

A given patient with liver metastases will not necessarily have all these symptoms and might complain of hepatic pain if a large subcapsular metastasis infarcts. Attacks can be precipitated by alcohol, stress, emotion, ingestion of food, infusion of calcium, noradrenaline or pentagastrin. Carcinoid syndrome can occur without liver metastases if there is a large burden of disease outside the portal circulation territory, e.g. lung, bone.

Signs

The patient with advanced disease often looks remarkably well bearing in mind the bulk of liver metastases. The patient can appear malnourished if diarrhoea has been a particular problem, an abdominal mass might be palpable or there might be signs in the chest of pulmonary collapse/consolidation depending on the site of the primary tumour. Hepatomegaly is expected in patients with carcinoid syndrome. Auscultation of the heart can reveal tricuspid or pulmonary valve disease, although left-sided cardiac lesions have been described with bronchial carcinoids, and there might also be signs of heart failure.

Differential diagnosis

Other tumours arising at the site of the carcinoid should be considered, although none produces a syndrome akin to carcinoid when there are liver metastases. It should be noted that carcinomas at other sites can produce a carcinoid syndrome from 5-HT production, e.g. medullary carcinoma of the thyroid, small cell lung cancer.

Investigations

Urinary 5-hydroxyindoleacetic acid (5-HIAA)

Twenty-four hour urinary 5-HIAA is elevated in those with carcinoid syndrome, reflecting metabolism of 5-HT. A false positive result can be obtained if the diet at the time of urine collection is rich in bananas, pineapples, avocados or walnuts. Malabsorption syndromes (e.g. coeliac disease) can also cause modest elevations in 5-HIAA. Apart from 5-HT, carcinoids can produce histamine, kallikrein, motilin, enteroglucagon, neurotensin, substance P, prostaglandins, insulin, ACTH, glucagon, parathyroid hormone and calcitonin, most of which can be assayed if clinically relevant.

Chromogranin A

This is the only applicable serum marker.

Computed tomography/magnetic resonance imaging

CT/MRI scan of the liver and site of primary tumour defines the locoregional extent of the primary tumour and will exclude liver metastases.

Hepatic angiography

This is of value if resection of liver metastases or embolization is planned.

Staging

There is no formal staging system in routine clinical use.

Treatment

Radical treatment

Surgery

The primary tumour should be completely excised as this offers the only chance of long-term cure, with 5-year survival of 90 per cent. Radical lymph node resection is unnecessary, although obviously enlarged nodes should be cleared to ensure a complete resection of the tumour or at least significant cytoreduction.

Palliative treatment

Dietary advice

Referral to a dietitian may help the patient to avoid ingestion of substances which may precipitate an attack of flushing and permit modification of the diet to lessen diarrhoea and protein-losing enteropathy.

Surgery

In patients with symptoms from one large liver metastasis or multiple metastases confined to one lobe of the liver, resection could be justified to reduce tumour bulk, thereby reducing secretion of vasoactive peptides and therefore palliating symptoms. Careful supervision is essential during the perioperative period to avert a hypotensive crisis when the tumour is handled. Bypass of an intestinal obstruction might also be necessary.

Radiotherapy

Carcinoids are not sensitive to radiation, although low doses of radiation are useful for the palliation of skeletal metastases. Isotope therapy using mIBG (see Phaeochromocytoma section above) is worth considering if a preliminary scan shows uptake by the metastases.

Pharmacological measures

Codeine phosphate (30–60 mg tds) or loperamide (up to 16 mg daily) are both useful for the treatment of diarrhoea. Historically, drugs used for the palliation of symptoms refractory to more conventional measures include:

- parachlorophenylalanine – blocks conversion of tryptophan to 5-HT
- cyproheptadine – blocks action of 5-HT on its receptors
- ketanserin – a 5-HT2 receptor antagonist.

However, these have been superseded by the somatostatin analogue octreotide (Sandostatin®) which is a potent inhibitor of the physiological effects of carcinoid tumours and should be considered the treatment of choice. The treatment can also have an antiproliferative effect on the tumour leading to disease stabilization. α-Interferon occasionally yields useful responses and can be combined with octreotide.

Hepatic arterial embolization

This can benefit up to 80 per cent of patients with symptomatic hepatic metastases, with palliation lasting up to 3 years. This procedure can be repeated as necessary.

Chemotherapy

Streptozotocin, cisplatin and etoposide, and other combinations of drugs, have been used but with a partial response rate of 30 per cent or less.

Tumour-related complications

As with any other gastrointestinal tumour, perforation, obstruction or intussusception can all occur. Ectopic hormone production is seen, the tumour producing growth hormone-releasing hormone leading to acromegaly or ACTH leading to Cushing's syndrome. Pellagra is a rare syndrome characterized by glossitis, dermatitis in sun-exposed areas, diarrhoea and dementia, and is due to the tumour consuming tryptophan, which is a precursor for nicotinic acid. Heart failure might ensue in advanced cases owing to damage to the pulmonary and tricuspid valves.

Treatment-related complications

All cytoreductive treatments can release large amounts of vasoactive substances and therefore patients with bulky tumours should be pretreated with parachlorophenylalanine and cyproheptadine to avoid a serotonergic crisis.

Prognosis

Carcinoid tumours are usually very slow-growing so that even patients with heavy metastatic burdens could survive for many years. Appendiceal carcinoids have an excellent prognosis as they are small, easily removed and rarely metastasize.

MULTIPLE ENDOCRINE NEOPLASIA (MEN)

Type 1

Described by Werner, it is dominantly inherited. It is caused by a mutation of the *MEN 1* gene on chromosomal region 11q13. Involved glands include:

- parathyroids (90 per cent) – hyperplasia or adenoma; usually the presenting feature
- pancreatic islets (80 per cent) – adenoma, carcinoma or more rarely diffuse hyperplasia
- anterior pituitary (65 per cent) – adenoma
- adrenal cortex (40 per cent) – hyperplasia or adenoma
- carcinoid tumours and lipomata – rare occurrences.

Type 2

Originally described by Sipple, it has an autosomal dominant inheritance owing to a 10q11 chromosome region mutation affecting the *RET* gene. Involved glands include:

- parafollicular cells of thyroid – medullary carcinoma (>95 per cent); usually the presenting feature
- adrenal medulla – phaeochromocytoma (50 per cent)
- parathyroids – hyperplasia or adenoma (<25 per cent).

Subtype A (the commonest) has no mucocutaneous features while subtype B (5 per cent) is characterized by multiple small subcutaneous or submucosal neuromas of the oral cavity and lips, autonomic ganglioneuromatosis, and Marfanoid habitus. Familial medullary carcinoma of the thyroid forms a third subtype.

Mixed MEN

This demonstrates features of both types 1 and 2, usually pituitary adenomata and phaeochromocytoma.

FURTHER READING

Hay I, Vass JAH. *Clinical Endocrine Oncology*. Blackwell, Oxford, 2008

Mazzaferri EL, Harmer C. *Practical Management of Thyroid Cancer*. Springer, New York, 2005

McDougall IR. *Thyroid Cancer in Clinical Practice*. Springer, New York, 2007

Yao JC, Hoff PM. *Neuroendocrine Tumours*. Saunders, Philadelphia, 2007

SELF-ASSESSMENT QUESTIONS

1. Which three of the following statements are true for thyroid cancer?
   a. Commoner in men
   b. Accounts for more than 5000 cases per annum in the UK
   c. Medullary subtype is rare
   d. May be caused by exposure to ionizing radiation
   e. May be caused by thyroxine replacement therapy
   f. May be part of an inherited cancer syndrome
   g. Associated with prostate cancer

2. Which one of the following best describe follicular carcinoma of the thyroid?
   a. Associated with MEN type 2
   b. Rapidly growing
   c. Best treated with surgery and radio-isotope therapy

   d. High risk of spread to liver
   e. Associated with a poor prognosis

3. Which three of the following statements are applicable to medullary carcinoma of the thyroid?
   a. Associated with MEN type 2
   b. May lead to a high serum calcium
   c. A high serum thyroglobulin is typical
   d. Associated with phaeochromocytoma
   e. It is a highly chemosensitive cancer
   f. It is a highly radiation-sensitive cancer
   g. Surgery is the mainstay of treatment

4. Which one of the following is not true about carcinoid?
   a. Often metastasizes to the liver
   b. May be slow growing
   c. 5-HIAA is a useful marker
   d. Is incurable
   e. Is not sensitive to radiation

■ Soft tissue sarcomas 254
■ Osteosarcoma 259
■ Ewing's sarcoma 263
■ Other bone tumours 265
■ Further reading 265
■ Self-assessment questions 266

SOFT TISSUE SARCOMAS

Epidemiology

Soft tissue sarcomas are rare tumours with around 1000 cases reported in the UK each year divided equally between men and women. In children the predominant tumour is a juvenile rhabdomyosarcoma, which will be considered in the section on paediatric tumours. It has very different characteristics to the soft tissue sarcomas of adults. In adults these tumours can occur at any age, the incidence being slightly more common in the 50–70 year age group.

Aetiology

Usually there is no identifiable cause but the following factors may be of importance:

■ chronic mechanical irritation – sarcomas can be induced in animal models but this does not appear important in humans
■ radiation – a small number of sarcomas are undoubtedly related to previous therapeutic irradiation with tumours developing several years after exposure
■ familial – these sarcomas form part of the Li–Fraumeni syndrome where they are associated with tumours of breast, brain, adrenal cortex and leukaemias in close relatives under the age of 45 years. They are also seen in patients with von Recklinghausen's syndrome of familial neurofibromatosis when malignant change occurs within a pre-existing neurofibromata
■ chemical – angiosarcoma is associated with vinyl chloride exposure.

Pathology

Sites for soft tissue sarcomas include:

■ limbs (upper 15 per cent; lower 40 per cent)
■ retroperitoneum (20 per cent)
■ viscera (bladder, bowel, uterus – 10 per cent)
■ trunk (10 per cent)
■ head and neck (4 per cent).

Macroscopically, soft tissue sarcomas are often large, fleshy tumour masses with associated haemorrhage and necrosis. They invade local soft tissues, nerves and blood vessels.

Microscopic classification of soft tissue sarcomas is based on the finding of recognizable connective tissue elements within the tumour. The basis of the diagnosis is the finding of malignant

TABLE 15.1 Classification of soft tissue sarcomas

Sarcoma subtype	Tissue type	Features
Fibrosarcoma	Fibrous tissue	Most common type, typically found in thigh
Liposarcoma	Fat	Lower extremity and retroperitoneum
Rhabdomyosarcoma	Skeletal muscle	Adult forms are alveolar or pleomorphic
Leiomyosarcoma	Smooth muscle	Uterus and gastrointestinal tract common, also limbs and retroperitoneum
Malignant fibrous histiocytoma (MFH)	Histiocytes	Especially legs, buttocks and retroperitoneum
Neurogenic sarcoma (neurofibrosarcoma)	Neural tissue	Arise within large nerves, e.g. sciatic, median, spinal roots
Synovial sarcoma	Uncertain	Arise around joints, especially thigh, foot, knee
Angiosarcoma	Blood vessels	Scalp, breast, liver
Lymphangiosarcoma	Lymph vessels	Sites of chronic lymphoedema, e.g. postmastectomy arm

spindle cells, which may form characteristic patterns as in a fibrosarcoma when a 'herringbone' pattern is described, and malignant fibrous histiocytoma when a 'cartwheel' pattern may be seen. A classification of the soft tissue sarcomas is shown in Table 15.1.

Histological grade is an important prognostic feature of sarcomas and a three-point scale is used to describe the degree of differentiation. This must, however, be interpreted in the light of the cell type. For example, angiosarcoma will usually appear well differentiated but is usually a highly malignant tumour. Similarly, virtually all synovial sarcomas can be regarded as high-grade tumours irrespective of their grading.

Natural history

There is extensive local growth with infiltration of surrounding structures including blood vessels and nerves, and early blood-borne spread to lungs is the most common distant site.

Lymph node spread is relatively uncommon except for synovial and epithelioid sarcomas, alveolar rhabdomyosarcoma and angiosarcoma.

Symptoms

Peripheral sarcomas present as a lump which may be present for some time before it becomes symptomatic. Retroperitoneal sarco-

mas can grow to a large size before causing symptoms, the most common of which is backache. Rapid increase in size of a pre-existing neurofibroma should alert to the possibility of malignant change to a neurofibrosarcoma.

Signs

At presentation, peripheral sarcomas are often large masses within soft tissue. Figure 15.1 shows a large soft tissue sarcoma arising in the lower limb. Movement can become limited, particularly when close to joints. Retroperitoneal masses can be palpable per abdomen.

Differential diagnosis

Other benign soft tissue masses should be considered, such as a neurofibroma, lipoma or fibroma.

Investigations

Routine investigations such as full blood count and blood biochemistry are usually unremarkable.

Radiography

Chest X-ray might show pulmonary metastases (Fig. 15.2). If normal, a CT scan of the chest should be performed to further exclude metastases.

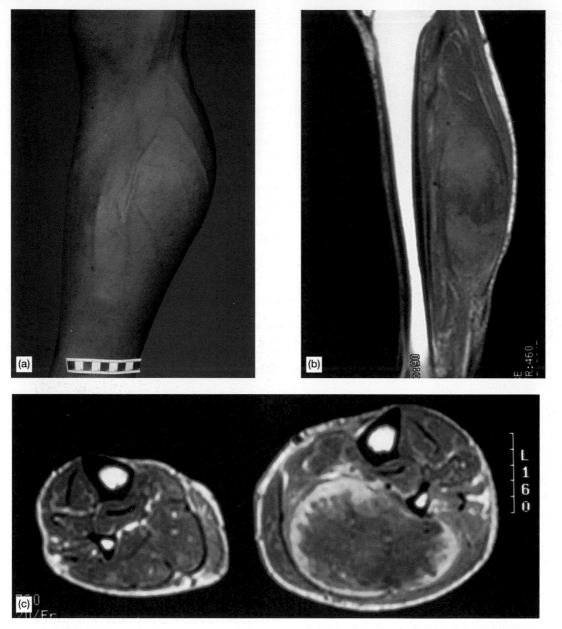

Figure 15.1 Soft tissue sarcoma (liposarcoma of the lower limb) seen (a) clinically and (b and c) on MR scan, demonstrating the extensive involvement of the muscle compartment.

CT scan or MRI

MRI of the primary site will give most precise definition of the soft tissue extent and involvement of local structures as shown in Figure 15.3.

CT scan of the lungs is essential to exclude small volume lung metastases before considering radical treatment.

PET scan is increasingly used in the staging of soft tissue sarcoma and can also predict tumour grade related to the glucose uptake rates (SUV).

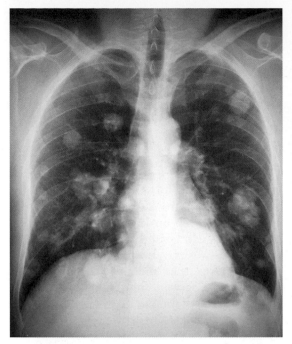

Figure 15.2 Chest X-ray demonstrating multiple pulmonary metastases from a soft tissue sarcoma.

Biopsy

Biopsy of the primary lesion is essential to confirm the diagnosis and the type of sarcoma. Definition of a sarcoma can be difficult and, if needle biopsy is not sufficient, an open biopsy is needed. It is important that this is performed in consultation with the surgeon who will perform the definitive resection as implantation at the biopsy site can occur and this should be included in the resection.

Staging

Staging is based on the size of the primary tumour as follows:

- Tl – Tumour <5 cm max. diameter
- T2 – Tumour >5 cm max. diameter
- N0 – No nodes
- NI – Regional nodes

Grade is classified as follows:
- Gl – Low grade
- G2 – Intermediate grade
- G3 – High grade.

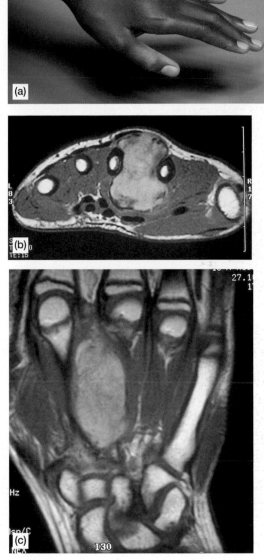

Figure 15.3 (a) Fibrosarcoma arising on dorsum of the hand and (b and c) MRIs to show detail of precise anatomical location.

Treatment

Sarcoma management is complex and these tumours are relatively rare. They should therefore be treated by specialized multidisciplinary teams incorporating surgical and oncological expertise in this field.

Local treatment

Wide surgical resection including excision of any previous biopsy scar, combined with radiotherapy, which may be given pre- or postoperatively, enables conservation of the affected limb. Amputation is avoided if at all possible but may be necessary for locally advanced tumours or those that progress despite radiotherapy.

Retroperitoneal tumours present a more difficult surgical problem and resection might not be possible. High-dose irradiation is required, delivering doses of at least 60 Gy in 6 weeks.

Radiation alone might control a soft tissue sarcoma but is inferior to the combination of surgery with irradiation.

The role of adjuvant chemotherapy remains under investigation. Soft tissue sarcoma is not a particularly chemosensitive tumour but meta-analyses suggest that there may be a small benefit for local and distant relapse-free survival, but not overall survival, from intensive adjuvant chemotherapy.

Isolated limb perfusion with drugs such as melphalan might benefit locally advanced, unresectable limb tumours.

Metastatic disease

Chemotherapy has only limited activity. Responses are seen with cisplatin and Adriamycin or epirubicin and ifosfamide but long-term remissions are few and the toxicity of treatment is considerable.

Surgical resection (metastatectomy) is the most successful treatment of lung metastases if feasible.

Tumour-related complications

Local effects owing to tumour size are the main problem associated with soft tissue sarcomas. In general, paraneoplastic effects and systemic complications such as hypercalcaemia are not features of these tumours, although hypoglycaemia has been described as a rare association with massive retroperitoneal sarcomas.

Treatment-related complications

The emphasis of modern treatment is towards limb preservation. However, the effects of extensive resection and radiotherapy can lead to functional deficits in the limb with joint stiffness, loss of muscle power and limb oedema.

Prognosis

The prognosis for peripheral limb tumours is better than that for sarcomas affecting the retroperitoneum, trunk or internal organs. With conservative limb-preserving treatment local control rates will be in the order of 80 per cent with 5-year survival around 60 per cent depending on the tumour stage and grade. Patients with operable lung metastases have a 5-year survival of around 30 per cent following metastatectomy.

Future developments

The major change in the management of soft tissue sarcomas has been in the development of limb-preserving treatment in the place of amputation. The main difficulty now lies in the management of systemic disease for which there is no satisfactory treatment. Adjuvant chemotherapy has been proposed as a possible way of reducing systemic relapse but trials to date demonstrate only small benefits.

Rare tumours

Extraosseous Ewing's and primitive neuroectodermal tumours (PNET)

These are rare soft tissue tumours characterized by small round cells rich in glycogen morphologically identical to the classical Ewing's tumour of bone (see below). Extraosseous Ewing's is most common on the trunk and extremeties, arising in soft tissue, distinct from bone, whilst PNET is most common in the chest, when it may be termed 'Askin's tumour', and also the abdomen and pelvis. Management and prognosis follows that of classical Ewing's tumour of bone (see below).

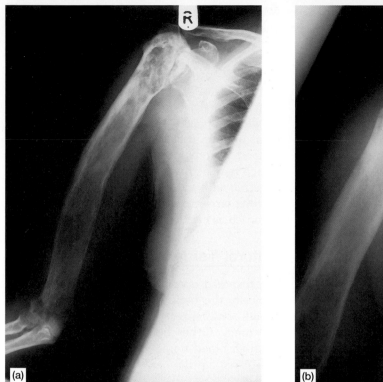

Figure 15.4 X-rays showing (a) pre-existing Paget's disease of bone in a humerus within which (b) an osteosarcoma has subsequently developed.

Desmoid tumours

These classically arise in the abdominal wall in women postpartum but can occur at any site, presenting as a diffuse fibrous infiltrative tumour which, while pathologically benign, can cause serious effects by virtue of its relentless local growth. Surgical resection is the treatment of choice but when inoperable, slow regression is achieved following a radical dose of radiotherapy.

Stewart–Treves tumour

This is the name given to the rare development of a lymphangiosarcoma in the upper limbs of women with chronic lymphoedema secondary to the treatment of breast carcinoma. Treatment can be difficult owing to the pre-existing oedema and associated postoperative and postradiotherapy changes. Amputation might be necessary.

Dermatofibroma

This is a benign tumour of the skin presenting as a fibrous nodule typically on the limbs, distinct from simple fibromas by the presence of histiocytes on microscopy. Its malignant counterpart is dermatofibrosarcoma protuberans, so called because of its macroscopic appearance with an hour-glass shape pushing the epidermis outwards. It is usually found on the trunk and histologically it is essentially a fibrosarcoma.

OSTEOSARCOMA

Epidemiology

Osteosarcoma is the most common malignant tumour of the bone, although it is rare in relation to other malignancies. It occurs mainly in adolescents, particularly during periods of active bone growth with a second peak of incidence in those over 60 years when it is related to Paget's disease. It is almost twice as common in males as females.

Aetiology

No recognizable aetiological agent is present for the majority of cases. Paget's disease can be a pre-existing feature in adult osteosarcoma, as shown in Figure 15.4.

Osteosarcoma is a rare late effect following therapeutic irradiation. Historically it is associated with radium dial painting and the use of thorium-based contrast agents, e.g. thorotrast, as contrast medium in diagnostic radiology.

It can occur as a component of the rare Li–Fraumeni syndrome in which bone or soft tissue sarcomas are associated with a familial pattern of breast, brain and adrenal cortex tumours, and leukaemia. In these cases germline mutations of the *P53* gene are found. An association with deletions in the retinoblastoma gene on the long arm of chromosome 13 is seen in 70 per cent and other genetic changes including loss of heterozygosity on chromosomes 3q, 17q and 18p have also been described. Survivors of hereditary retinoblastoma have a relative risk of up to 500 for developing osteosarcoma with a latency of 10 years or more. It is seen in 15 per cent of patients with bilateral retinoblastoma.

Pathology

The most common site for osteosarcoma is in a long bone, particularly around the knee, 30 per cent arising from the lower femur and 15 per cent in the upper tibia; 10 per cent arise in the humerus and the remainder can affect any bone, including the axial skeleton. Two principle groups are described, 'central (medullary)' and 'surface (peripheral)' tumours. The classical osteosarcoma is a central tumour and accounts for 95 per cent of those seen.

Macroscopically, the tumour arises in the metaphysis and grows both eccentrically, expanding the cortex and raising the periosteum at its edges, and also along the medulla.

Within the tumour will be areas of haemorrhage and necrosis together with new bone formation in the subperiosteal regions to form the classic Codman's triangles and sunray spicules seen on X-ray.

Pathological fracture through the tumour-bearing bone can occur.

Microscopically, there are two main populations of cells: a background stroma of spindle-shaped sarcomatous cells containing a matrix, which may be myxoid, cartilaginous or osteoid, together with multinucleate giant cells. Grading of osteosarcoma is not usual, all tumours being regarded as high grade.

Natural history

Local spread occurs within the bone of origin, typically the bone medullary cavity, and early blood-borne spread can occur, particularly to the lungs. Other bones may also be affected through blood-borne spread. Lymph node disease is not a prominent feature.

Symptoms

There is usually pain in the bone and there may be a lump around the site of origin. There is sometimes a history of preceding trauma although no causal relationship exists. Symptoms from metastases include cough and haemoptysis but other features of malignant disease such as anorexia and weight loss are infrequent unless very advanced.

Signs

Swelling and deformity of the bone are seen. The area is often hot and red and an audible bruit might be heard. Thinning of the periosteum can result in a characteristic crackling on palpation and there may be crepitus if fracture has occurred. There is often an associated fever.

Differential diagnosis

Other causes of bone swelling should be considered, including benign tumours such as osteochondromas and other malignant tumours.

Investigations

Routine investigations are often unremarkable, although there could be leukocytosis, and the alkaline phosphatase will be inappropriately raised. (Remember that in growing children and adolescents the normal range for alkaline phosphatase is increased during bone growth.)

Radiography

Plain X-ray of the affected bone will show local destruction of bone with areas of new bone formation, which may form the classic Codman's triangles and sunray spicules but more often are less well demarcated. There will be periosteal elevation and pathological fracture might be seen. In adults, coexisting Paget's disease might be present, as illustrated in Figure 15.4 (see above).

CT or MRI scan

Further detail of the precise extent of bone destruction and spread within the medullary cavity will be found on CT or MRI scan, the latter being the investigation of choice.

CT scan of the lungs is important to identify pulmonary metastases.

Isotope bone scan

This will give further information on the extent of local bone involvement and also identify any bone metastases.

PET scanning might play a role in intital staging and response assessment, in particular distinguishing residual tumour from postoperative change.

Staging

The TNM staging for bone tumours is shown below:

- TX – Primary cannot be assessed
- T0 – Primary tumour not identified
- T1 – Tumour ≤8 cm in maximum dimension
- T2 – Tumour >8 cm in maximum dimension
- T3 – Discontinuous tumours in the primary bone site.

Treatment

The mainstay of modern treatment for osteosarcoma is a course of intensive chemotherapy together with local removal or irradiation of the site of origin.

Chemotherapy

Schedules based on the use of combination chemotherapy containing cisplatin, ifosfamide and Adriamycin have been shown to be as effective as the original multidrug chemotherapy regimens that used high-dose methotrexate in doses of between 8 and 12 g/m^2 of body surface area in combination with other drugs such as Adriamycin, bleomycin, vincristine, cyclophosphamide and dactinomycin.

Local treatment

Following induction chemotherapy with satisfactory response, conservative limb-preserving resection of the bone is undertaken. This might entail the use of an appropriate prosthesis or excision of the entire bone if expendable as in the case of a rib or the fibula. In children a prosthesis that can be expanded to accommodate growth can be used as shown in Figure 15.5.

For surgically unresectable disease, local radiotherapy will be given with the aim of delivering a dose of up to 60 Gy in 6 weeks. In certain sites, particularly in the spine close to the spinal cord, the dose can be limited by the tolerance of CNS tissue. Following local treatment chemotherapy will be continued for a total of around 20 weeks.

Metastases

Patients presenting with lung metastases will be treated by metastatectomy if resectable alongside local surgery for the primary tumour.

Palliation

Palliative treatment might be required for relapsed disease. Local irradiation could be valuable for local pain and to arrest tumour growth through the skin. Amputation can be considered for recurrent disease but only when there is thought to be a realistic chance of long-term salvage.

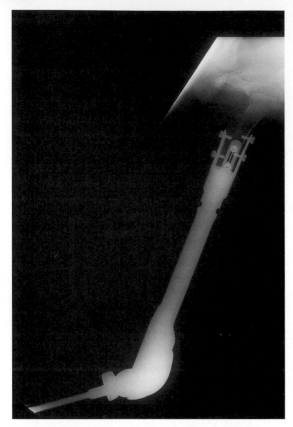

Figure 15.5 X-ray of extendable prosthesis used following resection of tumour from the lower femur.

Metastatic disease might require further chemotherapy and limited pulmonary metastases can be resected.

Tumour-related complications

The principal complication is pathological fracture.

Treatment-related complications

The affected limb might have limitation of movement and muscle strength. Prostheses fitted to young patients who have not completed their growth will require revision from time to time. Following amputation, which might still be needed by a small number of patients, specific problems can include phantom limb pain and stump ulceration and chafing. Thoracotomy can result in limited respiratory reserve depending on the extent of resection required, and postoperative pain in the thoracotomy scar is a well-recognized problem.

Chemotherapy will have considerable acute morbidity including nausea, vomiting, alopecia and mucositis. Longer term problems arise from nephrotoxicity related to the use of methotrexate or cisplatin, and neurotoxicity from cisplatin or vincristine. In children growth retardation is sometimes seen with effects on subsequent maturation and fertility.

Prognosis

Overall, with the use of modern chemotherapy-based schedules for treatment, the 5-year survival for non-metastatic osteosarcoma is between 40 and 50 per cent. Prognosis is related to size of primary tumour and response to neoadjuvant chemotherapy. In patients presenting with lung metastases, up to 20 per cent could become long-term survivors and as many as 40 per cent of those relapsing with pulmonary metastases can be salvaged. Elderly patients have a worse prognosis partly owing to the limitations of delivering intensive chemotherapy to this group. Those with tumours secondary to Paget's disease have a 5-year survival of only 4 per cent.

Rare tumours

Parosteal sarcoma

This typically occurs in young adults, and is a peripheral tumour arising from the juxtacortical part of the bone metaphysis growing concentrically around the bone. The lower femur and upper tibia are the usual sites. Surgical excision is the treatment of choice. This is a low-grade malignancy with a low risk of metastases. Prognosis is better than that for an osteosarcoma, with 5-year survival figures of 50–70 per cent. Occasionally transformation into a high-grade osteoarcoma can be seen.

EWING'S SARCOMA

Epidemiology

Ewing's sarcoma is the third most common sarcoma of bone affecting predominantly children and young adults, the maximum incidence being between the ages of 10 and 20 years. A rare extra-osseous form of Ewing's is also recognized. The incidence of Ewing's in the UK is 0.6 in 100 000 and males are affected more than females. It is relatively rare in black populations.

Aetiology

There is no recognized aetiological agent but a specific chromosomal translocation in Ewing's has been shown between chromosomes 11 and 22, and other similar translocations between chromosome 22 and chromosomes 21, 7 and 17 have also been described.

Pathology

Ewing's can affect any bone and is found in long bones, vertebrae and limb girdles, especially the pelvic bones where over 20 per cent are found. Macroscopically, it arises in the diaphysis of the bone, growing subperiosteally. Periosteal reaction as it traverses the length of the bone can give rise to the characteristic onion peel appearance of the bone on X-ray. To the naked eye the tumour contains areas of necrosis, and haemorrhage and cystic regions have also been seen.

Microscopically, Ewing's is composed of sheets of small round cells rich in glycogen. Ewing's is now considered to be one of the tumours in the group of PNET. The surface marker CD99 is characteristic for these tumours.

Natural history

There is local growth, the primary often reaching a considerable size, and blood-borne dissemination with metastases to lungs in particular. Lymph node metastases are not usually a major feature.

Symptoms

Ewing's is typically painful and characteristically pain is intermittent in the early development of the tumour mass. There might be a preceding history of trauma but no causal relationship is recognized. Pathological fracture can occur. Lung metastases can cause cough or haemoptysis.

Signs

The tumour mass will be apparent as a palpable mass often tender to palpation. Associated fever, particularly in advanced cases, can be noted. Spinal Ewing's can result in neurological deficits.

Differential diagnosis

Ewing's must be differentiated from other primary tumours of bone. Other round cell tumours that can affect bone should also be excluded, in particular lymphoma, neuroblastoma and anaplastic carcinoma.

Investigations

Blood cell count

A full blood count can demonstrate a raised white cell count and occasionally a mild anaemia might also be present.

Biochemistry

Biochemical tests can be normal or show an inappropriately raised alkaline phosphatase.

Radiography

X-ray of the affected bone will show thinning of the diaphysis and in later stages extensive bone destruction (Fig. 15.6). The characteristic onion peel appearance of successive layers of periosteal reaction can also be seen.

Chest X-ray and, if normal, CT scan of the lungs should be performed to evaluate the possibility of lung metastases.

CT scan or MRI

MRI will show greater detail of the tumour mass, in particular soft tissue invasion, and

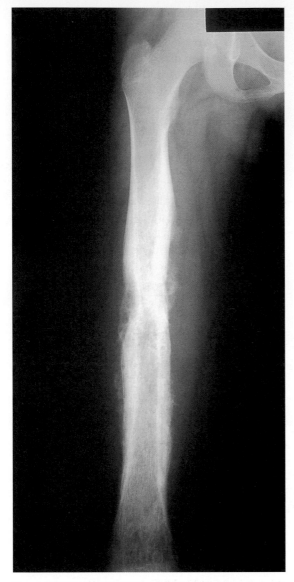

Figure 15.6 X-ray of Ewing's sarcoma in the femur.

spread along the marrow cavity of the bone. Spiral CT of the lungs is essential to exclude small volume lung metastases.

Biopsy

Biopsy of the primary lesion is essential to confirm the diagnosis.

Staging

There is no recognized staging system for Ewing's sarcoma.

Treatment

Chemotherapy

The common chemotherapy schedule used is based on the use of VAC (vincristine, Adriamycin and cyclophosphamide); more intensive schedules alternating VAC with ifosfamide and etoposide can also be used.

Local treatment

After 2–3 months of chemotherapy, radiotherapy will be the treatment of choice for most patients to deliver a total dose of between 50 and 60 Gy in 5–6 weeks.

Surgery can be used instead, particularly for bones such as rib and fibula, which can be removed in toto. Chemotherapy is then continued for several months following local treatment.

Palliative treatment

Standard chemotherapy as described above is appropriate for widespread symptomatic metastases. Local symptoms of pain or bleeding can be better dealt with by local radiotherapy. In selected patients high-dose chemotherapy with autologous marrow transplant could be an option.

Tumour-related complications

These include pathological fracture and spinal cord compression from rapid growth of spinal tumours.

Treatment-related complications

Chemotherapy can result in acute nausea, vomiting and alopecia. In the longer term, vincristine can be associated with a peripheral neuropathy and, in high doses, Adriamycin is cardiotoxic. For this reason actinomycin D is substituted once a tolerance dose has been reached.

High-dose radiotherapy to a limb can result in joint stiffness, skin changes and lymphoedema.

Prognosis

The overall 5-year survival for patients without metastases treated with modern chemotherapy-based regimens is around 50 per cent. This is determined particularly by tumour size ranging from 70 per cent in tumours <500 cm³ to 35 per cent in tumours >500 cm³.

Local control rates can approach 90 per cent and are greater in long bones than in the pelvis.

OTHER BONE TUMOURS

Chondrosarcoma

This is the second most common bone tumour after osteosarcoma, typically affecting the pelvic bones, although it can also occur in the femur, humerus and scapula. It is a tumour of adults and usually slow growing. A primary might arise de novo from apparently normal bone, or a secondary when it arises within a pre-existing chondroma. Rarely (<5 per cent) chondrosarcoma can be extraskeletal.

Initial treatment is radical surgical resection or, if it is inoperable, radiotherapy.

Well and moderately differentiated forms have a good prognosis and only metastasize late, if at all. There is, however, a high-grade variant, which has an aggressive course, and these patients can be selected for treatment with early chemotherapy using drugs similar to the osteosarcoma schedules. The overall 5-year survival is around 35 per cent.

Osteoclastoma (giant cell tumour)

This is a tumour arising in adults usually between the ages of 30 and 50, the most common sites being the long bones around the knee, radius and humerus. There is a character-istic 'soap bubble' appearance on X-ray with eccentric thinning of the cortex. Clinically this can be demonstrated, albeit rarely, by 'eggshell crackling' on palpation.

It is composed of two populations of cells, a background stroma of spindle cells, the differentiation of which defines the activity of the tumour, and scattered multinucleate giant cells. The majority are of low-grade malignancy and present a problem of local control rather than disseminated disease.

Wide surgical excision is the treatment of choice. Around one-third will recur locally and a further one-third will be high-grade tumours, which ultimately metastasize. Local irradiation can be of value for local recurrence; chemotherapy is not usually successful in metastatic disease. The overall 5-year survival is around 65–70 per cent.

Spindle cell sarcoma

Tumours histologically identical to fibrosarcoma or malignant fibrous histiocytoma of soft tissue might be found as primary bone tumours. They are usually tumours of adults in the 30–60-year age group. Treatment is radical surgical excision. There has been some interest in giving adjuvant chemotherapy in this group of patients but to date there is no evidence that this improves survival. Overall 5-year survivals are in the range of 25–40 per cent.

Angiosarcomas also arise in bone and will be treated in the same way as the other spindle cell sarcomas of bone.

FURTHER READING

Clark MA, Fisher C, Judson I, Thomas JM. Soft tissue sarcomas in adults. *New England Journal of Medicine* 2005;**353**:701–11

Grimer RJ. Surgical options for children with osteosarcoma. *Lancet Oncology* 2005;**6**:85–92

Singer S, Demetri GD, Baldini EH, Fletcher CDM. Management of soft tissue sarcomas: an overview and update. *Lancet Oncology* 2000;**1**:75–85

SELF-ASSESSMENT QUESTIONS

1. Which of the following is true of soft tissue sarcomas?
   a. They arise from epithelial cells
   b. They are common tumours arising equally in men and women
   c. They may be associated with the Li–Fraumani syndrome
   d. In children the common form is an angiosarcoma
   e. The most common site is the upper limb

2. Which of the following is true of the pathology of soft tissue sarcomas?
   a. Blood-borne spread is rare
   b. Synovial sarcomas are always high-grade tumours
   c. Angiosarcomas are usually well differentiated
   d. Radiation-induced sarcomas are usually well differentiated
   e. Synovial sarcomas arise from joint cartilage

3. Which three of the following apply to the presentation of soft tissue sarcomas?
   a. Pain is a common feature of peripheral sarcomas
   b. Retroperitoneal sarcoma may present with chronic back pain
   c. Lung metastases may be the first manifestation
   d. Regional lymphadenopathy is common
   e. Rapid growth in a neuroma can be due to sarcomatous change
   f. Excision biopsy is the diagnostic procedure of choice
   g. May present with sudden pain due to intratumoral haemorrhage

4. In the treatment of soft tissue sarcoma which of the following is true?
   a. Large tumours are best managed with initial chemotherapy
   b. Wide local excision should be followed by radiotherapy
   c. Angiosarcomas are best treated with radiation alone
   d. Metastatic disease will respond to cisplatin-based chemotherapy
   e. Radioisotope therapy has a role in selected cases

5. Which of the following is true of osteosarcoma?
   a. It is most common over 60 years of age
   b. The most common site for distant metastases is the liver
   c. In children it is usually associated with the Li–Fraumani syndrome
   d. On X-ray it appears as a lucent defect in the cortex
   e. The most common site is in the long bones around the knee

6. In the treatment of osteosarcoma which of the following is true?
   a. Amputation is required for long bone tumours
   b. Chemotherapy is only used in the palliation of metastatic disease
   c. Resection of lung metastases can be curative
   d. Chemoradiation is given for unresectable primary sites
   e. High-dose methotrexate is the chemotherapy of choice

7. Which three of the following are true of Ewing's sarcoma?
   a. It arises from osteoclasts
   b. It is most common in the under 10 years age group
   c. Lymph node metastases are common
   d. Painless swelling is the common presentation
   e. It is composed of small round cells rich in glycogen

SELF-ASSESSMENT QUESTIONS

f. X-ray shows a characteristic 'onion peel' appearance

g. Prognosis is worse if the tumour volume is >500 cm^3

8. Which three of the following are true of bone tumours?

a. Chondrosarcoma is most common in the spine

b. Chondrosarcoma may arise within a pre-existing chondroma

c. Lung metastases are frequent in osteoclastoma

d. Characteristic giant cells are found in the stroma of osteoclastoma

e. Liposarcoma may arise within bone

f. Malignant fibrous histiocytoma of bone is usually seen in childhood

g. Primary angiosarcoma of bone is well recognized

■ Hodgkin's lymphoma   268   ■ Further reading   285
■ Non-Hodgkin's lymphoma (NHL)   275   ■ Self-assessment questions   286

Malignancies of the lymphoproliferative system can be broadly classified into Hodgkin's lymphoma and all other lymphomas, which are termed the non-Hodgkin's lymphomas. The classification of these is complex and many different systems have been described of which the WHO REAL classification has now gained international acceptance. A simplified clinical view is shown in Figure 16.1; a summary of the WHO classification is found later in this chapter.

HODGKIN'S LYMPHOMA

Epidemiology

Each year in the UK there are 1500 cases of Hodgkin's lymphoma, 850 cases in men and 650 cases in women leading to a total of 350 deaths per annum. There is a bimodal age distribution, the two peaks of incidence occurring in young people aged 20–30 years and in later life over 70 years. Overall it is almost twice as common in men as it is in women. In children the sex difference is even more extreme, occurring almost exclusively in boys under the age of 10 years. It is rare in the Japanese and in the US black population, and particularly high in the Jewish populations of the US and the UK.

Aetiology

There is no proven aetiological agent responsible for the development of Hodgkin's lymphoma.

Nodular sclerosing Hodgkin's is more common in more affluent households and the reverse is seen for other subtypes, which are more common in less affluent households.

There is a strong association with infection with Epstein–Barr virus (EBV); EBV-associated Hodgkin's seems particularly prevalent in those under 10 years and over 60 years and in this group viral DNA can be identified in the cells in up to 50 per cent.

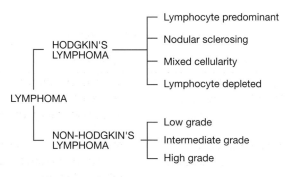

Figure 16.1 Clinical types of lymphoma.

Hodgkin's is increased in patients with HIV infection although it is less common than non-Hodgkin's lymphoma in this group.

There is a 99-fold risk in identical twins where one twin has Hodgkin's, but no increased risk in non-identical twins.

Pathology

Macroscopically, Hodgkin's lymphoma is usually found in lymph nodes, the spleen and liver. More, rarely infiltration of the lungs, bone marrow, skin or central nervous system can occur. Typically the nodes are relatively soft and uniformly enlarged. The spleen and liver appearances are of multiple nodules within their substance, the cut surface of which has been likened to that of a German sausage.

Microscopically, the diagnostic feature is the presence of binucleate cells called Reed–Sternberg cells. In addition a wide variation of other cells including lymphocytes, neutrophils, plasma cells, eosinophils, histiocytes and fibroblasts are also found infiltrating the node or affected organ. There are four major histological subclassifications, as shown in Table 16.1. Characteristically the cells are of B-cell type and the cell surface markers CD15 and CD30 can be identified on immunohistochemistry.

Natural history

Typically, stepwise involvement of adjacent node groups occurs. The most common nodes involved are those in the neck. In this situation spread is to adjacent nodes in the supraclavicular fossa, the axillae and the mediastinum before involving para-aortic nodes below the diaphragm. Extranodal involvement as a sole manifestation is rare and usually occurs in the context of extensive or bulky node disease.

Symptoms

Typically the patient is aware of a painless enlarged node in the neck. This might have been present for many weeks or months but can develop more rapidly.

'B' symptoms are characteristic of lymphomas and are:

- fever >38°C often with typical remittent pattern (Pel–Ebstein fever)
- weight loss of >10 per cent body weight
- night sweats.

Other uncommon but characteristic symptoms include generalized and often intractable itching and alcohol-induced pain in the enlarged nodes. Although the lymph nodes themselves are usually painless there might be some backache from para-aortic nodes and left-sided abdominal pain from splenic enlargement.

Signs

Enlarged lymph nodes can be present in any site, but most commonly in the neck. Typically the nodes of Hodgkin's disease are described as firm and rubbery as opposed to the hard craggy nodes of carcinoma. Palpable hepatosplenomegaly or an abdominal mass owing to para-aortic or mesenteric nodes might also be present. Inguinal and pelvic lymphadenopathy

TABLE 16.1 Histological subtypes of Hodgkin's disease

Subclass	Features	Prognosis
Lymphocyte predominant	Infiltrate of many small lymphocytes	Good
Nodular sclerosis	Node divided by fibrous bands. Cells may be rich in lymphocytes (type 1) or be of mixed type (type 2)	Type 1 – good Type 2 – moderate
Mixed cellularity	Mixed population of cells	Moderate
Lymphocyte-depleted	Fibrous node with Reed–Sternberg cells but few other cells seen	Poor

can be associated with oedema of the lower limbs, although arm oedema is an unusual complication of axillary lymphadenopathy from lymphoma. Mediastinal lymphadenopathy might present with the signs of superior vena cava obstruction.

Differential diagnosis

The main differential diagnosis is between Hodgkin's lymphoma and non-Hodgkin's lymphoma. Other causes of lymphadenopathy will also be considered including infection, which can be either pyogenic, tuberculous or viral, e.g. EBV or CMV (cytomegalovirus), toxoplasmosis and other neoplastic conditions such as leukaemia or carcinoma.

Investigations

Blood count

A full blood count may show mild anaemia and leukocytosis with a raised lymphocyte count but is frequently normal.

ESR

ESR can be raised, particularly in more aggressive forms of the disease.

Biochemistry

Serum lactate dehydrogenase is a sensitive index of disease activity and of prognostic importance.

Routine biochemical blood tests can show evidence of hepatic infiltration with raised alkaline phosphatase and γ-glutamyl transferase. More profound hepatic disturbance is rare. Obstruction of the renal tracts by enlarged nodes can cause renal failure. Hypercalcaemia is a recognized but rare finding in Hodgkin's disease.

Bone marrow examination

Unlike non-Hodgkin's lymphoma bone marrow involvement is unusual in the absence of other soft tissue involvement, i.e. stage 4 disease. Bone marrow examination is no longer routine for those patients presenting with stage 1 to 3 nodal disease in the absence of B symptoms.

Radiography

Chest X-ray can show widened mediastinal shadow owing to enlarged nodes or, more rarely, lung parenchymal infiltration. Pleural effusion is also a recognized finding.

CT and MRI

CT scan of the chest. abdomen and pelvis will give the most accurate assessment of internal lymphadenopathy and has now superseded the use of bipedal lymphangiography as the imaging of choice for staging in lymphoma. There is less experience of MRI in Hodgkin's lymphoma but wider availability and the use of new contrast agents could broaden its role in the future.

PET/CT scan

Additional staging information can be seen on fluorodeoxyglucose PET scans with normal size nodes demonstrating increased uptake indicative of lymphoma. PET can also have an important role in response assessment and follow-up.

Biopsy

A tissue diagnosis is mandatory to confirm the diagnosis and define the histological subtype of Hodgkin's lymphoma. This will usually take the form of an open lymph node biopsy where there is an accessible node in the neck, axilla, supraclavicular fossa or groin. Mediastinoscopy or laparoscopy could be required where there are no other sites accessible for biopsy.

Staging

The staging of Hodgkin's lymphoma follows the Ann Arbor classification:

- Stage 1 – Involved lymph nodes limited to one node area only
- Stage 2 – Involved lymph nodes involving two or more adjacent areas but remaining on one side of the diaphragm only
- Stage 3 – Involved lymph nodes on both sides of the diaphragm
- Stage 4 – Involvement of extranodal organs denoted by the following suffixes:

M – bone marrow
D – skin
H – liver
S – spleen.

Each stage is further subclassified 'A or 'B' according to the absence or presence, respectively, of B symptoms (see above).

Treatment

Hodgkin's lymphoma is both radiosensitive and chemosensitive and most patients can expect to be cured of their disease. Because this is a disease frequently affecting young people who will live for many years after successful treatment, there is now considerable emphasis not only on the efficacy of treatment but also on achieving cure with minimal long-term morbidity.

Localized disease (stages 1A and 2A)

The standard approach to early localized disease is for treatment to comprise:

■ short course chemotherapy, typically three or four cycles of ABVD (Adriamycin, bleomycin, vinblastine, dacarbazine) followed by
■ 'involved field' irradiation treating a volume including only those areas initially affected.

Hodgkin's lymphoma is much more sensitive to radiation than the common epithelial cancers and requires only 30 Gy given over 3 weeks (compared with 60–70 Gy for a squamous carcinoma).

Relapse in these patients can in most cases be salvaged using chemotherapy.

Advanced disease (stages 1B, 2B, 3 and 4)

Although there may be only limited nodal disease apparent, the presence of B symptoms is a poor prognostic feature and implies more widespread disease. For this reason stages 1B and 2B disease are included in this category together with those patients who have widespread node disease or involvement of systemic organs. Chemotherapy is given to these patients.

Prior to starting chemotherapy male patients should have the opportunity to consider sperm banking as subsequent fertility cannot be guaranteed after chemotherapy.

All patients having chemotherapy should be well hydrated and started on allopurinol to prevent tumour lysis syndrome (see Chapter 22). Response can be dramatic and rapid; an example of a chemotherapy response on treating bulky mediastinal nodes from Hodgkin's lymphoma is shown in Figure 16.2.

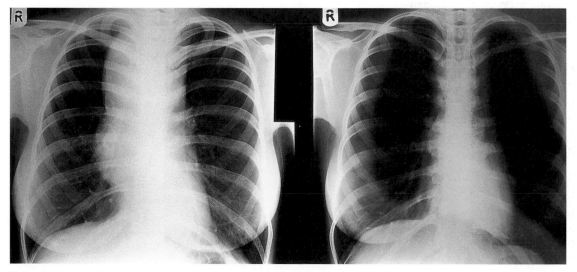

Figure 16.2 Chest X-ray before and after four cycles of chemotherapy for bulky mediastinal Hodgkin's lymphoma.

CASE HISTORY: HODGKIN'S LYMPHOMA

A 23-year-old man presented to his GP with a 1-month history of an enlarging lump in the left side of his neck. On examination he was found to have a 3 cm enlarged gland in the left deep cervical region with a further 2 cm node in the left supraclavicular fossa. These were non-tender and there were no associated foci of infection to find. On further questioning, however, he admitted to episodes of fever and several nights when he awoke drenched with sweat. A biopsy of the lymph node was undertaken and this showed nodular sclerosing Hodgkin's lymphoma. Further investigations showed a normal full blood count but an ESR of 53 mm/hour, normal biochemistry but, on CT scan, other areas of enlarged lymph nodes in the anterior mediastinum and para-aortic region with marked splenomegaly. A bone marrow examination was clear. A diagnosis of stage IIIB Hodgkin's lymphoma was made. He was recommended to receive combination chemotherapy. Prior to starting chemotherapy he was counselled with regard to future fertility and, an initial sperm count being normal, semen was taken for cryopreservation.

He underwent combination chemotherapy using Adriamycin, bleomycin, vinblastine and dacarbazine (ABVD) for which he attended the hospital outpatient chemotherapy unit on a fortnightly basis. After each visit he had 24 hours of nausea, which was controlled by taking ondansetron 4 mg twice daily for the first 2 days after chemotherapy. By the fourth week of chemotherapy his hair was thinning and he needed to shave only once every other day.

One week after the third chemotherapy injection he developed a high fever and felt generally unwell. As instructed by the chemotherapy unit he attended there for a blood count, which showed that he had had a haemoglobin of 10.3, a total white count of 0.9 with a neutrophil count of 0.2 and a platelet count of 73. Admission to the oncology ward was arranged that day and he was treated with intravenous gentamicin and tazocin. Within 24 hours his temperature had settled. He was treated with 5 days of high dose intravenous antibiotics by which time his neutrophil count had risen to 1.3 and he could be safely discharged from hospital. He proceeded with his next course of chemotherapy uneventfully.

After his fourth course of ABVD chemotherapy, a further CT scan was undertaken. This showed that the enlarged lymph nodes in the neck had disappeared but there was a residual abnormality 2 cm in size in the mediastinum and a 1.5 cm node remaining in the para-aortic region. He continued with two more courses of ABVD chemotherapy. This was followed by CT PET scan, which showed that the residual abnormalities in the mediastinum and para-aortic region persisted but that there was no FDG uptake at those sites. He was therefore considered to be in complete remission and recommended to receive 2 further months of treatment to complete his programme. His further chemotherapy was completed uneventfully. On completion of chemotherapy he noted that his nails had developed marked changes with loosening of the nail bed and a brownish discoloration. He was reassured that these were normal reactions to the bleomycin drug in the chemotherapy and over the next few months these changes grew out as new nail advanced. His hair regrew normally but it was some months before his energy levels returned and he was able to resume a normal lifestyle.

A repeat CT PET scan 3 months after completion of his chemotherapy showed that he was still in remission. He continued to attend the oncology clinic initially at 3-monthly intervals but later at less frequent intervals. Five years later he remains fit and well with no signs of active disease. He is seen at the clinic on an annual basis. He has recently married and his wife is pregnant with their first child, his fertility having been preserved despite his chemotherapy.

Specific chemotherapy

Early schedules used were based upon MOPP (mustine, vincristine, procarbazine and prednisolone). While effective in giving complete remission rates of up to 80 per cent, there is significant toxicity and modifications have been developed to minimize this morbidity.

LOPP or ChlVPP replaces the mustine by chlorambucil and in the case of ChIVPP, vincristine is replaced by vinblastine.

Anthracycline-based (i.e. Adriamycin or its analogues) schedules such as ABVD (Adriamycin, bleomycin, vincristine and dacarbazine) are also highly active and are now recognized as the chemotherapy of choice for Hodgkin's lymphoma. These schedules are associated with less long-term toxicity and randomized trials have shown cure rates to be at least equivalent to earlier schedules. Most patients will receive six to eight courses of standard chemotherapy.

For patients who have a number of adverse risk factors more intensive schedules can be advantageous; an example is the BEACOPP schedule.

Radiotherapy is only indicated in this group of patients where complete remission is not achieved at the end of chemotherapy; in this setting involved field radiotherapy delivering 30 Gy in 3 weeks will improve the prognosis of partial responders up to those who achieve a complete response with chemotherapy.

Treatment for relapse

Of those patients given initial chemotherapy for advanced disease around 40 per cent will either relapse or fail to achieve a sustained complete remission. Retreatment with the same or alternative chemotherapy regimens can result in further regression of disease for around 50 per cent but of these only 15–20 per cent will achieve long-term remission. It is therefore in this group of patients that more intensive treatment using high-dose chemotherapy and bone marrow autograft or peripheral blood progenitor cells (PBPC) (see below) is indicated. With such techniques long-term survival might be achieved in over 30 per cent of patients relapsing after conventional chemotherapy for Hodgkin's lymphoma.

Tumour-related complications

Massive lymphadenopathy can have consequences as a result of local pressure, although in general lymphoma tends to grow around structures rather than directly invade them. In the mediastinum dysphagia and superior vena cava obstruction can occur. In the abdomen renal failure from ureteric obstruction and lower limb oedema from pelvic node enlargement are seen.

Treatment-related complications

Radiotherapy

For most patients there are few if any sequelae; however, long-term effects are now seen as patients cured in their 20s and 30s are followed for several decades. Potential problems are shown in Table 16.2. An example of mediastinal fibrosis following mantle radiotherapy is shown in Figure 16.3.

TABLE 16.2 Late effects of radiotherapy for Hodgkin's disease

Site	Late radiation effects
Neck	Hypothyroidism, laryngeal oedema or fibrosis
	Treatment in puberty may induce thyroid cancer, loss of muscle and soft tissue bulk causing asymmetry
Mediastinum	Pneumonitis and lung fibrosis
	Pericarditis
Spinal cord	Myelitis
Abdomen	Increased incidence of peptic ulceration
Pelvis	Amenorrhoea in women and sterility if gonads included in radiation field

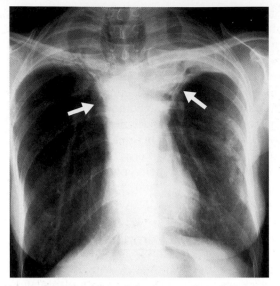

Figure 16.3 Chest X-ray following mantle radiotherapy (as demonstrated in Figure 16.2) showing post-radiation fibrosis in the mediastinum and lung apices.

Chemotherapy

Acute toxicity includes nausea and vomiting, alopecia and bone marrow depression. Neutropenic sepsis is a potential hazard of any such treatment. Peripheral neuropathy can develop from the use of vincristine or, less commonly, vinblastine.

Adriamycin has specific dose-related cardiotoxic effects and bleomycin can cause lung damage at high doses. Neither of these effects will be expected in standard treatment schedules but might become a potential hazard in patients requiring retreatment. Bleomycin also results in characteristic changes to the nails and skin.

The anthracycline-containing schedules such as ABVD have the advantage of preserving fertility, whereas after MOPP-type regimens most patients are sterile, men being more sensitive than women.

Second malignancies

There is increasing concern regarding the incidence of second malignancies in patients who are cured of their Hodgkin's lymphoma. There is an ongoing risk with time from treatment, which appears to be rising to over 15 per cent in patients who have survived for 20 years or more. In the early years occasional leukaemias or non-Hodgkin's lymphomas are diagnosed but the major problem appears to be an increasing risk of solid tumours, which develop towards the end of the first decade after treatment with an ongoing incidence thereafter. The greatest concern is the incidence of breast cancer in young women where a relative risk (RR) for breast cancer of between 2 and 4 in women between the ages of 25 and 35 when irradiated has been reported and an RR of over 20 for those under the age of 20. In smokers there is also a dramatic increase in lung cancer related to both radiation and chemotherapy exposure where the relative risk of developing lung cancer is again over 20.

More recently an increase in deaths from cardiac disease related to both chemotherapy and radiotherapy exposure has also been reported in these cohorts of patients.

Prognosis

Overall the prognosis for patients diagnosed with Hodgkin's lymphoma is good. Virtually all patients presenting with early localized disease will be cured and with intensive chemotherapy over 80 per cent of those with advanced disease (stages 3B or 4) can also expect cure.

Seven important prognostic factors have been identified, which now comprise the International Prognostic Index. These are:

- age >45 years
- male
- stage IV disease
- haemoglobin <10.5 g/dL
- total white cell count >16 × 10⁹/L
- lymphocyte count <0.6 × 10⁹/L
- serum albumin <40 g/L.

Future prospects

Increasingly the emphasis in Hodgkin's lymphoma now is to maintain the very high cure rates obtained while reducing morbidity. This can be achieved by individualizing treatment according to stage and risk factors. New, less toxic chemotherapy schedules could be appropriate for low-risk patients whilst the more intensive weekly drug schedules combined with involved field radiotherapy might be needed for those with high-risk disease. The use of PET scans early in chemotherapy could be valuable in identifying patients in whom treatment can be minimized and conversely intensified where early response is unsatisfactory. Modern radiotherapy techniques enable smaller volumes to be treated and lower doses will reduce the probability of late effects.

NON-HODGKIN'S LYMPHOMA (NHL)

Epidemiology

Each year in the UK there are around 10 000 cases of NHL, 5300 cases in men and 4800 cases in women, making it the sixth commonest form of cancer, accounting for a total of 4500 deaths per annum.

It occurs equally in men and women and the incidence increases with age, being relatively unusual under the age of 50 with 70 per cent of cases diagnosed over the age of 60 years. As with Hodgkin's lymphoma there is a marked low incidence in the Japanese and the US black population.

Aetiology

No single aetiological agent has been identified to account for the common forms of lymphoma found in the UK.

Infective agents

- EBV is associated with Burkitt's lymphoma found predominantly in Africa.
- Human T-cell lymphotrophic virus type 1 (HTLV1) is associated with T-cell lymphoma found in the Caribbean and Japan.
- HIV infection is also associated with an excess of lymphomas, which is probably a feature of the immunosuppressed status

rather than a direct causation by virus. The RR for a high-grade lymphoma in HIV infection is 400.

- *Helicobacter* is closely associated with gastric mucosal associated lymphoid tissue-type lymphomas (MALTomas) and eradication of *Helicobacter* has been accompanied by regression of gastric lymphoma in a high proportion of cases.

Altered immune status

In addition to HIV, NHL is also increased in other disease states associated with a depressed immune system including rheumatoid arthritis, coeliac disease and hypogammaglobulinaemia, and following iatrogenic immune suppression after renal transplantation. There are also associations with autoimmune disease such as Hashimoto's thyroiditis with thyroid lymphoma and Sjögren's disease with salivary gland lymphoma.

Irradiation

This could also be a factor in the development of NHL and increased incidences have been seen following exposure in Hiroshima and Nagasaki, and after low-dose therapeutic irradiation to the spine for ankylosing spondylitis.

Pathology

NHL describes a spectrum of neoplastic conditions as a result of which many complex and confusing classifications have arisen. The majority of NHL arise from the B lymphocyte but there is a well-recognized group which are T-cell derived neoplasms. Rare forms of histiocytic neoplasm also occur.

Macroscopically, NHL will occur as a mass of neoplastic lymphoid tissue, which can reach a considerable size. Ulceration, necrosis and haemorrhage are unusual. It can arise in recognized lymph node chains but, unlike Hodgkin's lymphoma, extranodal lymphoma is relatively common with up to 50 per cent involving sites such as Waldeyer's ring, the gastrointestinal tract, skin and bone.

Microscopically, the appearances are complex and interpretation can be difficult. In broad terms lymphomas can be low grade or high grade. Features of low-grade lymphoma are the preservation of follicular architecture and cellular composition of well-differentiated small lymphocytes. In contrast, high-grade lymphomas are characterized by diffuse infiltration of the node or extranodal site with large undifferentiated lymphoid cells. The current international classification for NHL is the WHO-REAL (Revised European American Lymphoma classification) shown in outline below, which attempts to define disease entities rather than a pure morphological categorization. It also introduces some new definitions such as mantle zone lymphoma and the MALTomas:

B-cell neoplasms

I – Precursor B-cell neoplasm
 – Precursor B-lymphoblastic leukaemia/lymphoma
II – Peripheral B-cell neoplasms
1. Small lymphocytic lymphoma/chronic lymphocytic lymphoma
2. Lymphoplasmacytic lymphoma
3. Mantle cell lymphoma
4. Follicular lymphoma
5. Splenic marginal zone lymphoma
6. Hairy cell leukaemia
7. Plasma cell myeloma
8. Diffuse large B-cell lymphoma
9. Burkitt's lymphoma

T-cell neoplasms

I – Precursor T-cell neoplasm
 – Precursor T lymphoblastic lymphoma/leukaemia
II – Peripheral T-cell and NK-cell neoplasms
1. T-cell CLL/prolymphocytic leukaemia
2. Large granular lymphocytic leukaemia
3. Mycosis fungoides/Sezary syndrome
4. Peripheral T-cell lymphomas, unspecified
5. Angioimmunoblastic T-cell lymphoma
6. Angiocentric lymphoma
7. Intestinal T-cell lymphoma
8. Adult T-cell lymphoma/leukaemia
9. Anaplastic large cell lymphoma

The histological diagnosis of lymphoma is now supported by a range of specific monoclonal antibody stains. Distinction from a poorly differentiated small cell carcinoma is made using the leukocyte common antigen (LCA). Distinction of one subtype of lymphocyte from another has become a complex

---

Indolent (low-grade): 40% having a long natural history but rarely if ever cured

■ Follicular lymphoma with any of the following cell types:
 – small cleaved cells
 – mixed small and large cleaved cells
■ Well-differentiated diffuse small cell lymphocytic lymphoma

Aggressive (intermediate/high-grade): 50% having a shorter natural history with a fatal course unless treated with combination chemotherapy with which long-term cure is possible

■ Follicular lymphoma containing predominantly large cells (Grade 3)
 – Diffuse lymphoma containing any of the following cell types:
 – small cleaved cells
 – mixed small and large cells
 – predominantly large cells
■ Immunoblastic
■ Peripheral T-cell lymphoma

Rarer types: requiring different management

■ Lymphoblastic; aggressive requiring leukaemia-type treatment

■ Small non-cleaved cell as in Burkitt's lymphoma: poorly responsive to standard chemotherapy requiring more intensive schedules
■ Mycosis fungoides: skin lymphoma having long natural history
■ MALTomas, arising in mucosal surfaces, usually low grade. In stomach respond to anti-*Helicobacter* therapy

science. Monoclonal antibody stains to identify surface markers can differentiate B cells from T cells from histiocytes, and a large library of stains has now been built up to enable subtyping of a suspected lymphoma.

Despite this relatively complex classification, in practice most lymphomas can be divided into low-grade indolent lymphomas or more aggressive intermediate/high-grade types, which will define their natural history, management and prognosis as shown on the previous page.

Natural history

Indolent low-grade lymphoma can remain asymptomatic for many years and, in the elderly, have little impact upon their life expectancy.

A high-grade immunoblastic or lymphoblastic lymphoma is an aggressive often rapidly fatal condition.

Extranodal lymphoma can have a relatively benign course as in a low-grade skin lymphoma, existing as purplish nodules requiring little other than gentle local treatment from time to time. In contrast it can follow an aggressive course as in a high-grade lymphoma of the bowel or central nervous system.

In general, NHL, unlike Hodgkin's lymphoma, does not have a clear pattern of contiguous spread from one area to the next. Dissemination is often wide and unpredictable following a pattern closer to that of a carcinoma with relatively frequent hepatic and lung involvement.

Symptoms

NHL usually presents with a painless lump in a lymph node area, most commonly the neck but also the axilla or groin. There can be backache owing to enlarged para-aortic nodes or upper abdominal pain from hepatosplenomegaly.

'B' symptoms as described for Hodgkin's lymphoma are also an important feature, namely weight loss, fever and night sweats.

Other symptoms relate to the site of origin of an extranodal lymphoma. NHL arising in Waldeyer's ring therefore will cause local symptoms similar to those of a carcinoma in these regions, with local pain or discomfort, and epistaxis or nasal discharge where the nasopharynx is involved. Gastrointestinal lymphoma usually presents with an acute abdominal event owing to haemorrhage, perforation or obstruction. CNS lymphoma can cause symptoms of raised intracranial pressure with headache, vomiting and fits. Focal neurological features can cause bulbar palsy, diplopia, limb weakness and altered sensation. Skin lymphoma usually presents as asymptomatic lumps but mycosis fungoides has a characteristic pretumour phase often lasting many years with chronic skin change, which can be itchy and resemble dermatitis in its clinical picture.

Signs

Enlarged lymph nodes will be palpable, typically painless, firm, 'rubbery' nodes clinically indistinguishable from those of Hodgkin's lymphoma but different from the hard craggy nodes of carcinoma. At extranodal sites lymphoma often has a characteristic purplish appearance, stretching overlying surfaces and ulcerating only rarely. Hepatosplenomegaly is a common finding in both nodal and extranodal lymphoma.

Investigations

Blood count

A full blood count can show signs of mild anaemia or pancytopenia if there is bone marrow involvement. A high white cell count composed predominantly of lymphocytes can also be found and is a relatively poor prognostic sign.

ESR

The ESR will be raised; an ESR >40 mm/h is a further poor prognostic feature.

Biochemistry

The serum lactate dehydrogenase (LDH) is a marker of disease activity.

Routine biochemistry can show signs of hepatic infiltration. Renal failure is an occasional

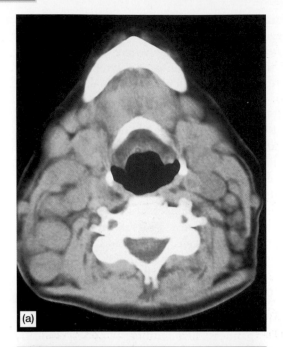

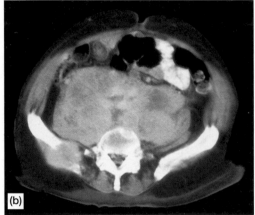

Figure 16.4 CT scans showing (a) extensive cervical lymphadenopathy and (b) para-aortic lymphadenopathy in non-Hodgkin's lymphoma.

complication of massive para-aortic node enlargement causing ureteric obstruction. Immunoparesis can be present and paraproteinaemia can occur. Hypercalcaemia is associated with HTLV-associated lymphomas.

Radiography

The chest X-ray might show mediastinal or hilar lymphadenopathy; more rarely infiltration of the lung parenchyma, pleural nodules or a pleural effusion will be found.

CT scan

Imaging of the abdominal and pelvic lymph nodes is best performed using a CT scan, which has now superseded the use of bipedal lymphangiography. Figure 16.4 demonstrates extensive lymphadenopathy in the neck and para-aortic region on CT scan.

PET CT

PET can give additional information showing evidence of active disease in normal sized lymph nodes resulting in upstaging in relation to CT stage, an example of which is shown in Figure 16.5. It can also be useful in assessing response, a negative PET scan at completion of treatment having a high predictive power for long relapse-free survival.

Bone marrow examination

Bone marrow examination will be required in all cases to assess the possibility of marrow infiltration.

Other imaging

Other imaging might be indicated depending on the site of origin. For bowel lymphoma a full barium series is performed since multiple foci of disease are well recognized. A CT scan of the brain will be performed for CNS lymphoma, which can be further supplemented by an MRI scan to image potential spinal disease.

Cerebrospinal fluid (CSF) examination

CSF examination for lymphoma cells will be required for central nervous system (CNS) lymphoma and can also be considered for other types considered to have a high risk of CNS involvement, in particular diffuse large cell and lymphoblastic lymphomas and those affecting the testis, tonsil or nasal sinuses.

Differential diagnosis

The main differential diagnosis rests between NHL and Hodgkin's lymphoma. Epithelial

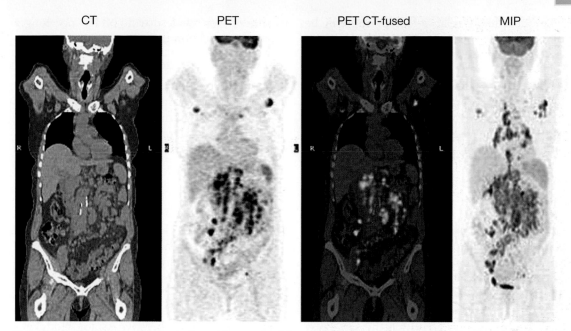

Figure 16.5 PET CT scan demonstrating widespread uptake of FDG in non-Hodgkin's lymphoma in nodes in both axillae, mediastinum, retroperitoneum and pelvis, with uptake also in the spleen. Maximum intensity projection (MIP) image reveals the total body uptake. (Courtesy of Dr RJ Chambers)

tumours could be considered where NHL arises in extranodal sites. It might be difficult to distinguish clinically an indolent diffuse small lymphocytic lymphoma with extensive bone marrow involvement from chronic lymphocytic leukaemia, and lymphoblastic lymphoma from acute lymphoblastic leukaemia.

Staging

The Ann Arbor staging system is used for NHL as for Hodgkin's lymphoma (see above) with the further addition of a suffix 'E' where the lymphoma has arisen in an extranodal site. For example, an NHL arising in the tonsil with involved nodes in the neck would be stage 2 by virtue of the presence of two or more sites all on the same side of the diaphragm and be designated stage 2E, having arisen in an extranodal site.

Treatment

Treatment is based on histological grade and stage.

Indolent low-grade NHL

(Common types are follicular and diffuse small cell lymphoma in WHO-REAL classification.)

This is a condition that is rarely curable but usually has a long clinical course. Localized low-grade NHL (stage 1A) is treated using local radiotherapy. The involved area only is treated, using low doses of 20–30 Gy in 2–3 weeks.

In the management of more advanced stage disease there is no proven advantage to immediate treatment in the asymptomatic patient who does not have bulky disease or potential organ failure. Such patients will be kept under surveillance until symptoms arise or they develop bulk disease, compromised bone marrow function, or other major organs are perceived at threat, e.g. early hydronephrosis from enlarging nodes.

The first-line chemotherapy of choice for this group of lymphomas is RCVP comprising rituximab, cyclophosphamide, vincristine and prednisolone. In elderly patients an alternative is to use single-agent oral chemotherapy, of which the most popular is chlorambucil or cyclophosphamide: 70–80 per cent of patients will enter remission with such treatment.

The subsequent relapse-free period can be prolonged with maintenance rituximab given every 3 months for 2 years.

Relapse

Low-grade lymphoma that is not localized is never cured, although survival for many years is to be expected. When relapse does occur further chemotherapy will be given; second-line treatment can include fludarabine often in combination with Adriamycin or mitozantrone and dexamethasone (FAD or FMD), which appear more active than the single drugs alone. Retreatment with an alkylating agent such as chlorambucil or cyclophosphamide is often successful and local sites causing symptoms can be irradiated. Patients who fail to respond to successive courses of chlorambucil can be treated with fludarabine or alternatively combination chemotherapy such as CHOP in the same way that a high-grade lymphoma will be treated (see below). Ritoximab (see above) will also achieve responses in chemotherapy-resistant disease.

There is some evidence now that patients achieving a second remission after relapse can benefit from proceeding to more intensive chemotherapy using either high-dose schedules such as BEAM (BCNU, etoposide, cytosine arabinoside, melphalan) with a stem-cell autograft or a low-dose allograft (see below).

Transformation

Richter's syndrome refers to the transformation from a low-grade to a high-grade lymphoma, which can occur in up to 15 per cent of patients presenting initially with low-grade lymphoma. For this reason re-biopsy of recurrent disease, particularly where there has been a period free from detectable disease or a change in growth rate is observed, should be considered before treatment.

Palliation

Steroids alone in moderate doses (40–60 mg of prednisolone) can have a valuable antitumour effect as well as conferring general effects such as improvement in appetite and general wellbeing.

Single-agent etoposide or vincristine can be used for progressive advanced disease at relapse. Hemi-body irradiation is a valuable palliative treatment for widespread NHL no longer responsive to chemotherapy.

Aggressive high-grade lymphoma

(Common type is a diffuse large cell lymphoma in WHO-REAL classification.)

This is a much more dangerous condition than low-grade lymphoma and in general requires more intensive therapy.

Nodal lymphoma

Localized high-grade NHL (stage 1A and 2A) is best treated with a short course of chemotherapy (typically three courses of RCHOP (rituximab, cyclophosphamide, Adriamycin, vincristine, prednisolone) followed by local irradiation to the involved sites delivering a dose of 30 Gy in 3 weeks.

Advanced disease (stage 1B, 2, 3 or 4) is treated with chemotherapy. As for Hodgkin's lymphoma, consideration should be given to sperm banking for young males and all patients should be well hydrated and started on allopurinol to prevent tumour lysis syndrome (see Chapter 22).

Specific chemotherapy

Usually, combination chemotherapy is given of which the most widely used is RCHOP, rituximab, cyclophosphamide, Adriamycin, vincristine, and prednisolone. The first four drugs are given intravenously on day 1 of a 21-day cycle with oral steroids on the first 5 days. Allergic reactions to the monoclonal antibody rituximab can be seen on initial exposure and so the infusion is given slowly for the first cycle, speeding up on subsequent cycles if no reaction is seen. A total of six to eight courses is usually given, the standard dictum being to deliver two courses of chemotherapy beyond complete clinical remission. Rapid responses can be seen after only one cycle of treatment, as illustrated in Figure 16.6.

Alternative schedules give weekly drugs over a 12-week course. These cycles are in general associated with greater toxicity, in particular neutropenia with the risk of sepsis and mucositis, and to date no advantage over standard chemotherapy in terms of patient survival has been shown.

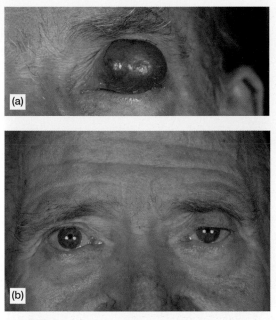

Figure 16.6 Conjunctival lymphoma (a) before and (b) after one cycle of CHOP chemotherapy.

Combined modality treatment

Sites of original bulky disease are often irradiated on the basis that these are frequently the sites of initial relapse. There is no good evidence that this practice significantly improves survival, particularly in those patients who achieve a complete response to chemotherapy, but a reduced rate of local relapse in the irradiated area is seen.

High-dose chemotherapy

Intensive chemotherapy using drug schedules such as BEAM (carmustine, etoposide, cytosine arabinoside, melphalan), which result in ablation of the bone marrow, are playing an increasing role in the management of NHL. The procedure of peripheral blood progenitor cell (PBPC) collection from the blood subsequently using the stem cells to reseed the marrow after treatment has become a routine procedure enabling high-dose marrow ablative chemotherapy schedules to be given safely in patients up to the age of 65 years; beyond this there is an increasing morbidity and mortality, which must be carefully considered.

PBPCs are obtained by using bone marrow stimulation with cyclophosphamide and colony-stimulating factors such as G-CSF. This increases the number of PBPCs in the peripheral circulation, which are then 'harvested' during plasmaphoresis. These cells are stored in liquid nitrogen until needed for reinfusion after an ablative dose of chemotherapy (or radiotherapy).

The role of high-dose chemotherapy in advanced high-grade NHL is principally in relapse or disease refractory to initial chemotherapy. In recurrent disease, challenge with conventional dose chemotherapy is essential to select those with chemosensitive disease. In this group further treatment with high-dose chemotherapy will result in prolonged remission in over 60 per cent. There is, however, no value of proceeding to such treatment in those patients having relapsed disease unresponsive to initial chemotherapy.

Lymphoblastic lymphoma

This form of high-grade lymphoma has a particularly aggressive course and resembles acute lymphoblastic leukaemia in many of its features, for example a propensity to spread to the CNS. Results from standard lymphoma chemotherapy as described above are poor and most of these patients will be treated in protocols similar to those for acute lymphoblastic leukaemia (ALL), including CNS prophylaxis.

Burkitt's lymphoma

This is a distinct high-grade lymphoma defined histologically as a diffuse small non-cleaved cell lymphoma. It is common in certain parts of Africa where an association with EBV infection is apparent, but is a rare lymphoma in Europe and the US. Results from standard lymphoma treatment are poor and current schedules use more intensive chemotherapy including CNS prophylaxis.

Extranodal lymphoma

In general these lymphomas are intermediate grade and will be treated in the same way as lymphomas arising in nodes as described above. There are, however, certain features of management particular to specific sites.

Waldeyer's ring lymphomas

These usually arise in the tonsils or nasopharynx and will be treated in the same way as nodal lymphomas, localized disease receiving three cycles of RCHOP followed by involved field radiotherapy, and more advanced disease receiving six to eight cycles of RCHOP. When radiotherapy is used the volume traditionally includes the whole of Waldeyer's ring.

Gastrointestinal tract lymphomas

These often present as a surgical emergency with obstruction or perforation when patients proceed to laparotomy at which bowel resection is performed. The diagnosis of NHL having been made, these patients will be treated with chemotherapy. A well-recognized hazard of initial chemotherapy in these patients is that of intestinal perforation as the lymphoma in the bowel wall regresses, and careful observation as an inpatient is usually recommended for the first course of treatment. Irradiation is difficult in these patients as it is a problem to demarcate clearly the affected area using standard localization techniques, and the bowel tolerates irradiation poorly.

A distinct pathological entity is the MALToma found particularly in the stomach and small bowel. Initial management of MALTomas in the stomach should be a course of anti-*Helicobacter* therapy using omeprazole and antibiotics such as ampicillin or tetracycline with metronidazole. Responses are seen in over 90 per cent of patients but close gastroscopic surveillance is required to detect those patients who relapse and then require standard lymphoma chemotherapy.

Skin lymphomas

These are often low grade (lymphoma cutis) and require only gentle local treatment from time to time, but more extensive high-grade lymphoma can develop, as shown in Figure 16.7. Mycosis fungoides is a characteristic T-cell skin lymphoma, which has a long pretumour phase before developing into the characteristic skin infiltration, which can be widespread. It responds poorly to chemotherapy. Less severe forms can respond to PUVA (psoralens and

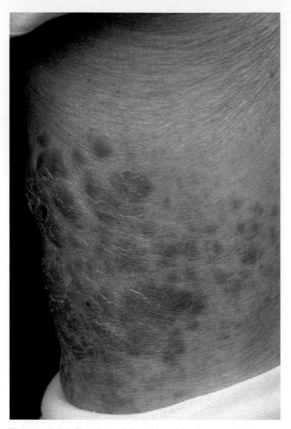

Figure 16.7 Infiltration of the skin with characteristic features of primary skin lymphoma.

ultraviolet A exposure) and for others local irradiation is required. In widespread disease the entire body can be affected when irradiation of the whole body with electrons will be required.

CNS lymphoma

This has a poor prognosis. It has a propensity to seed throughout the CNS via CSF circulation. Management will include high-dose methotrexate chemotherapy and radiotherapy despite which most patients will still relapse after only a relatively short time. Two distinct populations have now emerged: those with sporadic primary CNS lymphoma and those where it is associated with HIV infection. The prognosis for the latter is particularly poor. In patients who do survive after radiotherapy there are concerns with regard to long-term psychometric function.

CASE HISTORY: NON-HODGKIN'S LYMPHOMA

A 53-year-old man presents to his GP having had a sore throat for the past few weeks with discomfort on swallowing. On examination he is found to have enlargement of the left tonsil and a 2 cm lymph node palpable in the left side of the neck. He is referred urgently to an ENT surgeon who performs an excision biopsy of the tonsil. Histology of the tonsil shows diffuse large cell non-Hodgkin's lymphoma. He is referred to the oncologist who undertakes various staging investigations. A CT scan shows no evidence of further lymphadenopathy other than that detectable clinically in the neck. His bone marrow is normal and other blood tests including a full blood count, ESR, biochemical profile, immunoglobulins and serum lactate dehydrogenase are all normal. He is recommended to receive a short course of chemotherapy to be followed by radiotherapy.

Chemotherapy is started with a cycle of combination treatment using rituximab, cyclophosphamide, Adriamycin, vincristine and prednisolone (R-CHOP). He is warned about the possibility of infertility but has decided that he does not wish to store sperm having completed his family many years ago. An echocardiogram is also performed to check cardiac function before he receives anthracyclines, and this is also normal with a left ventricular ejection fraction of 65 per cent. Following his first cycle of R-CHOP chemotherapy he has some transient nausea but otherwise no significant side-effects. Three weeks later he receives a second cycle of R-CHOP chemotherapy. By this time he has noted marked thinning of his hair but otherwise remains well and reports that the lump previously palpable in his neck has already disappeared. A third course of R-CHOP chemotherapy is repeated after 3 more weeks.

Two weeks later he attends the radiotherapy planning clinic where a cast for a head shell is made. His head is placed in the correct position for the treatment and a close-fitting plastic shell is made. A CT scan for radiotherapy planning is then taken with him in position wearing the shell. These are used by the oncologist to define the areas to be treated and from this a plan of the radiation beams is defined by the radiation physicists. A week later he attends for the beam positions to be checked, X-ray images to be taken of the beams to check their accuracy, and marks made on the shell for them to be lined up against during his subsequent treatment. A week later he attends for his first of 15 daily radiotherapy treatments. During each treatment he is placed in position wearing the shell and the X-ray beams from the linear accelerator are set up by the light beam against the marks on the shell. He is treated by a total of three beams, two lateral beams covering the Waldeyer's ring area and a beam from the front covering the lower neck below this. Each beam exposure takes about a minute and the whole process around 10 minutes. He feels perfectly well during the procedure other than some minor discomfort on being kept still in the shell. By the end of the first week he notices some slight discomfort on swallowing again and as he continues treatment in the second week he becomes increasingly uncomfortable with pain on swallowing particularly hot foods. He also notices that the skin where the X-ray beams enters his face and neck has become red and starts to feel tight and uncomfortable, as if he had been exposed to excess sun. He is given dietary advice and later aspirin mucillage to take before food. He continues treatment on a daily basis through the third week. At completion of treatment he has marked skin reddening and some early peeling of the skin over the neck. Swallowing is very uncomfortable and he is warned to expect this to continue for a few days before a slow improvement develops. Two weeks later the skin is feeling itchy and peeling but he is otherwise comfortable. His throat has improved considerably and he is starting to return to a normal diet without the need for regular medication.

Three months after treatment his symptoms have resolved completely and the follow-up CT scan shows no evidence of detectable lymph node enlargement or other abnormalities. Examination of his oropharynx shows no abnormalities either. He is told that he is in complete remission.

He is seen regularly in the outpatient clinic. Five years later he remains well with no signs of recurrence of his lymphoma.

Primary lymphoma of bone

This can, if still localized to the bone of origin, be cured by local radiotherapy alone but will usually be treated with a combined schedule of RCHOP chemotherapy followed by radiotherapy. Conventionally the entire bone is included in the radiation field.

Tumour-related complications

Given the great heterogeneity of NHL, a vast range of clinical complications can arise, most of which have been covered in the above text.

Mass effects can be caused by malignant nodes or lymphomatous tissue compromising normal function so that, for example, mediastinal disease could cause SVC obstruction or dysphagia, abdominal disease could cause renal failure owing to ureteric obstruction, and pelvic disease could cause oedema of the lower limbs.

Gastrointestinal lymphoma can cause bowel haemorrhage, obstruction or perforation.

CNS lymphoma can cause focal neurological damage or obstructive hydrocephalus.

Treatment-related complications

Radiotherapy

This can cause late toxicity related to site, e.g. irradiating Waldeyer's ring can cause dry mouth, taste loss and dental problems. Abdominal and pelvic irradiation might result in postradiation bowel and bladder changes.

Chemotherapy

During treatment bone marrow depression, with the risks of neutropenic sepsis, occurs together with nausea, vomiting, alopecia and mucositis.

Rapid tumour regression can result in complications, in particular perforation at the site of gastrointestinal lymphoma, estimated to occur in around 5 per cent of patients with lymphoma in this site, and tumour lysis syndrome (see Chapter 22).

In the longer term, Adriamycin can cause dose-related cardiotoxicity, and bleomycin is associated with dose-related pneumonitis and lung fibrosis together with peripheral skin changes.

Infertility can result, particularly in males, after combination chemotherapy, although pregnancy is seen in women even after high-dose chemotherapy.

Second malignancy in patients with NHL is becoming more apparent as the results of treatment improve and more patients survive to develop a new malignancy. It is estimated that the risk of developing acute myeloblastic leukaemia in the first 5 years following treatment is between 6 and 8 per cent and as with Hodgkin's lymphoma appears most marked in patients treated with both chemotherapy and radiotherapy. There is a less clear association with the development of solid tumours (i.e. cancers or sarcomas) as yet, but since it is known that this risk increases with time over 20 or 30 years it is likely to emerge as cohorts of cured patients are followed for this length of time.

Prognosis

There are four major independent prognostic features in non-Hodgkin's lymphoma:

- age
- performance status
- stage (3 or 4 worse than 1 or 2)
- serum lactate dehydrogenase.

These have been validated and are referred to as the International Prognostic Index (IPI).

The overall prognosis for indolent low-grade lymphoma is better than that for intermediate or high-grade lymphomas, with median survivals of 8–10 years reported from most centres.

Early localized disease will be associated with high cure rates, over 90 per cent for indolent lymphoma and 85 per cent for aggressive forms following radiotherapy preceded in the latter by short-course chemotherapy

Extranodal lymphoma, even when localized, tends to have a worse prognosis than nodal lymphoma; Waldeyer's ring and skin do better than gastrointestinal tract, which does better than CNS.

More advanced aggressive high-grade NHL will respond to chemotherapy in most patients with complete regression of disease in 70–80 per cent; however, long-term survival figures tend to fall below 50 per cent at 5 years from treatment.

Future prospects

The main areas of development in the management of NHL are concerned with individualizing treatment according to risk factors and lymphoma subtype. PET is under investigation as an early predictive test of response to identify those patients who could benefit from early intensive therapy. Radiolabelled monoclonal antibodies against the CD20 surface marker for B cells such as ibritumomab are highly active and will undoubtedly find an important role in future treatment schedules.

Rare tumours

Nodular lymphocyte-predominant Hodgkin's lymphoma (NLPHL)

NLPHL accounts for around 5 per cent of Hodgkin's lymphomas and is a distinct entity characterized histologically by cells that are negative for the cell markers CD15 and CD30 but positive for CD20.

Clinically it typically presents with localized lymphadenopathy and has an indolent course. Optimal management varies between nothing more than observation after excision biopsy to involved site radiotherapy. In more advanced disease management is analogous to that of an indolent B-cell NHL.

Malignant histiocytosis

This is a rare form of lymphoma characterized by systemic symptoms of fever, weight loss, generalized lymphadenopathy, hepatosplenomegaly and pancytopenia. Histiocytic lymphoma is typically associated with coeliac disease, when it presents as a multicentric bowel lymphoma. It may respond to lymphoma-type chemotherapy but the prognosis is generally much worse than for other forms of lymphoma.

Castleman's disease

This is probably not a neoplasm but a hamartomatous condition of lymphoid tissue. It can present in a similar fashion to lymphoma and histological differentiation can be difficult. It is uncertain whether active treatment other than simple excision of affected nodes is of value, although there are reports of successful regression after irradiation.

Waldenström's macroglobulinaemia

This is lymphoplasmacytic lymphoma typically producing an IgM paraprotein and as such needs to be distinguished from myeloma. This is usually clear from the clinical findings, which are those of a lymphoma with lymph node and splenic involvement. Bone marrow examination shows infiltration with lymphoma rather than plasma cells. Haemolytic anemia owing to cold agglutinins is a further rare feature. Management and prognosis are similar to those of other low-grade non Hodgkin's lymphomas.

FURTHER READING

Armitage J, Cavalli F, Zucca E, Longo DL. *Text Atlas of Lymphomas*. Revised Edition. Martin Dunitz, London, 2002

Diehl V, Thomas RK, Re D. Part II: Hodgkin's lymphoma: diagnosis and treatment. *Lancet Oncology* 2004;**5**:19–26

Evans SL, Hancock BW. Non-Hodgkin lymphoma. *Lancet* 2003;**362**:139–46

Hennessy BT, O'Hanrahan EO, Daly PA. Non-Hodgkin lymphoma: an update. *Lancet Oncology* 2004;**5**:341–53

Thomas RK, Re D, Wolf J, Diehl V. Part I: Hodgkin's lymphoma: molecular biology of Hodgkin and Reed–Sternberg cells. *Lancet Oncology* 2004;**5**:11–18

Yung L, Linch DC. Hodgkin's lymphoma. *Lancet* 2003;**361**:943–51

SELF-ASSESSMENT QUESTIONS

1. Which of the following is true of Hodgkin's lymphoma?
   a. It arises from immunoblasts
   b. It is most common in middle age
   c. It is associated with previous infection with EB virus
   d. It is common in Japan and the Caribbean
   e. There is an increased risk in identical and non-identical twins

2. Which of the following is true of the pathology of Hodgkin's lymphoma?
   a. The cells stain with T-cell surface markers
   b. The presence of large binucleate cells is characteristic
   c. Extranodal sites are frequently involved
   d. Splenic involvement is rare
   e. The lymphocyte-depleted subgroup has the best prognosis

3. Which three of the following are typical in Hodgkin's lymphoma?
   a. Alcohol-related pain
   b. Hypercalcaemia
   c. Eosinophilia
   d. Raised levels of alpha-fetoprotein (AFP)
   e. Anaemia
   f. Lymphocytosis
   g. Hypercalcaemia

4. Which of the following is *not* a routine staging investigation in Hodgkin's lymphoma?
   a. CT scan of chest, abdomen and pelvis
   b. ESR
   c. Full blood count
   d. Bone marrow examination
   e. Liver function tests

5. In the treatment of Hodgkin's lymphoma which of the following is true?
   a. The common chemotherapy includes high-dose steroids
   b. Radiotherapy alone is preferred for stage I and II disease
   c. Rituximab is added to combination chemotherapy
   d. Tumour lysis is common
   e. Late complications include secondary breast cancer

6. Which three of the following are important adverse prognostic factors in Hodgkin's lymphoma?
   a. Age <45 years
   b. Male sex
   c. Haemoglobin <10.5 g/dL
   d. Serum albumin <40 g/dL
   e. B symptoms
   f. Lymphocytosis
   g. Mediastinal mass

7. Which of the following is true of non-Hodgkin's lymphoma?
   a. It is less common than Hodgkin's lymphoma
   b. It is most common in childhood
   c. In the stomach, may be associated with *Helicobacter* infection
   d. Is related to HTLV-I infection in China
   e. Is characterized by a translocation from chromosome 9 to 22

8. Which of the following is regarded as an indolent (low-grade) lymphoma?
   a. Burkitt's lymphoma
   b. Follicular lymphoma
   c. Mantle cell lymphoma
   d. Peripheral T cell lymphoma
   e. HTLV-associated T-cell lymphoma

9. Which three facts about the treatment of non-Hodgkin's lymphoma are true?
   a. The standard chemotherapy for aggressive disease is ABVD
   b. Rituximab improves results with chemotherapy for T-cell lymphomas

SELF-ASSESSMENT QUESTIONS

c. Localized indolent lymphoma may be cured by radiotherapy alone

d. MALToma of the stomach is best treated by surgical resection

e. Stage IV follicular lymphoma may need no active treatment

f. Mycosis fungoides is treated initially with amphotericin

g. Lymphoblastic lymphoma is treated with acute leukaemia therapy

10. Which three of the following are adverse prognostic factors in aggressive types of non-Hodgkin's lymphoma?

a. Age

b. Performance status

c. Weight loss

d. Haemoglobin

e. Lymphocyte count

f. Serum albumin

g. Serum lactate dehydrogenase

17 HAEMATOLOGICAL MALIGNANCY

■ Leukaemia   288   ■ Further reading   306
■ Multiple myeloma   299   ■ Self-assessment questions   308

LEUKAEMIA

Neoplastic conditions of the haemopoietic and lymphoid systems are closely related. Subclassifications of leukaemias and lymphomas tend to be complex but clinical management is usually based on a more simple and pragmatic division of leukaemias into acute or chronic, lymphoid or myeloid. There are around 7000 cases of leukaemia registered per year in the UK and these account for over 4000 deaths each year.

Acute leukaemia is subclassified by its cell of origin into two broad groups: lymphoblastic and myeloblastic. Chronic leukaemias are malignancies of cells that have differentiated beyond the blast stage. They are subdivided into chronic granulocytic leukaemia and chronic lymphocytic leukaemia. Despite their names, they do not necessarily have a more protracted natural history, and the prognosis for chronic leukaemia is overall no better than for acute leukaemia.

Acute lymphoblastic leukaemia (ALL)

Epidemiology

Each year in the UK there are 700 cases of ALL leading to a total of 260 deaths per annum. ALL is less common than acute myeloid leukaemia, affecting males and females in equal proportions. It is predominantly a malignancy affecting children with over 40 per cent occurring in the 2–5-year-old age group when it predominates in boys.

Aetiology

Down's syndrome is associated with a higher incidence as are other less common genetic syndromes including Bloom's syndrome and ataxia telangiectasia.

Environmental agents, e.g. viruses, might be implicated. Clustering of cases in certain areas of the UK has been described. There is an increased incidence in affluent and industrialized areas but no specific environmental agent has been identified.

Chromosomal translocations have been identified: around 25 per cent of B-cell ALL cases have a t(12;21)(p13;q22) translocation and more than 50 per cent of T-cell ALL cases have mutations involving the *NOTCH1* gene involved in the regulation of normal T-cell development and which can potentiate the overexpression of the oncogene *c-myc*. The most frequent translocation in adults is t(9;22), the Philadelphia chromosome, which is also found in chronic myeloid leukaemia.

TABLE 17.1 Staining characteristics of acute lymphoblastic leukaemia compared with acute myeloid leukaemia

Type	PAS	TdT	Sudan black
ALL	+	+	−
AML	−	−	+

Key: PAS, periodic acid Schiff; TdT, terminal deoxyribonucleotidyl transferase.

Radiation exposure might be implicated, although postradiation leukaemia is more commonly myeloblastic.

Pathology

Lymphoblastic leukaemia is characterized by the presence of large immature lymphoblasts throughout the reticuloendothelial system. These cells are distinguished from other cells such as myeloblasts by their staining, as shown in Table 17.1.

ALL is also subclassified according to the type of lymphoid cell that has become neoplastic, and by the cell morphology, as shown in Table 17.2.

In addition to de novo ALL, up to 15 per cent of cases represent transformation into an acute phase from chronic granulocytic leukaemia (CGL). These are characterized by possessing the Philadelphia chromosome (see below). Other chromosomal changes that may be identified and relate to a worse outcome are translocations affecting chromosome 4, t(4;11), deletions of chromosome 7 and trisomy 8.

Natural history

Progressive infiltration of the bone marrow and subsequent bone marrow failure ensues. It may also affect other sites, in particular the CNS, where diffuse meningeal infiltration can be seen, and the testes in males.

Symptoms

Patients present with bone marrow failure, which results in:

- malaise, lethargy, effort dyspnoea or angina owing to progressive anaemia
- infection owing to leukopenia
- bleeding in the form of epistaxis, haematuria or haemoptysis owing to thrombocytopenia.

Bone pains can also be present. There are also general symptoms of malignancy including fever, sweats and weight loss.

Signs

These can include

- peripheral lymphadenopathy
- splenomegaly
- palpable liver
- purpura, particularly on the lower limbs, and also other signs of recent haemorrhage from the nose or oral cavity
- signs of infection, with fever and oropharyngeal or chest signs.

TABLE 17.2 Subclassification of acute lymphoblastic leukaemia

Morphological	
L1	Small uniform blast cells with high nuclear/cytoplasmic ratio
L2	Larger blast cells lower nuclear/cytoplasmic ratio
L3	Vacuolated blasts, basophilic cytoplasm

Surface Ig	Rosette formation		Proportion (%)
B cell	+	−	2
T cell	−	+	1
Common	+	+	75
Null	−	−	8

Differential diagnosis

Other types of acute leukaemia or high-grade non-Hodgkin's lymphoma should be considered, as should other causes of pancytopenia, including aplastic anaemia. Infection with Epstein–Barr virus can give a similar picture, with abnormal blast cells seen in the peripheral blood.

Investigations

Blood count

A full blood count will show pancytopenia. The blood film will reveal the presence of lymphoblasts.

ESR

The ESR will be raised.

Liver function

Liver function tests might be abnormal.

Radiography

Chest X-ray or CT scan can show evidence of leukaemic infiltration or more commonly infection. A mediastinal mass of lymph nodes might be seen.

Bone marrow examination

A bone marrow aspirate and trephine is required to confirm the diagnosis with an excess (>5 per cent) of abnormal lymphoblasts. Specific stains will then be applied to subtype the cells into common, T, B or null ALL.

Staging

There is no formal staging system for the leukaemias. However, the important features that determine prognosis are:

- subtype, common ALL having a good prognosis
- total white blood cell count, a total count of more than 20 000 being associated with a poor prognosis.

Other favourable features are female sex, young age and the absence of a mediastinal mass.

Treatment

The treatment of acute leukaemias can be considered in three phases: induction, consolidation and maintenance. Alongside this, intensive supportive treatment might be necessary with blood products and antibiotics. In the UK most centres will treat patients within the national UKALL protocols through which modifications to treatment schedules have been tested in prospective randomized studies.

Induction

Induction consists of vincristine and prednisolone with the addition of a third drug such as Adriamycin, daunorubicin or L-asparaginase; high-risk cases may receive a four-drug combination based on these agents and including cyclophosphamide. Imatinib mesylate will be indicated in those patients with the t(9;22) translocation. Remission rates of >95 per cent in children and 80–90 per cent in adults are achieved. Induction therapy will usually continue over a period of 8 weeks.

Consolidation (intensification)

This will be necessary once remission is achieved, i.e. when abnormal leukaemic cells are no longer detectable in the peripheral blood and bone marrow, to ensure eradication of any relatively resistant cells surviving the induction phase. Various drug schedules are in use including further exposure to the initial induction agents and high-dose methotrexate. Prophylactic treatment to the CNS will be included since this site accounts for 30–40 per cent of all relapses including intrathecal injections of methotrexate. The use of low-dose cranial irradiation (18 Gy) is also included in some protocols but omitted in others because of concerns over late toxicity to brain function.

Maintenance

Chemotherapy will continue beyond the intensification phase for a total of 2–3 years using methotrexate and mercaptopurine with the dose adjusted to bone marrow tolerance through regular blood count monitoring.

Bone marrow transplantation

High-dose chemotherapy with allogeneic (donor) stem cell or bone marrow transplantation is considered for poor-risk patients who achieve initial remission. This is particularly the case for adults who have a much worse prognosis from ALL than children, especially those with Philadelphia chromosome present on the leukaemic cells. Bone marrow transplantation is also indicated for children who relapse with bone marrow disease after initial chemotherapy.

Bone marrow transplantation is an intensive treatment which involves exposure of the patient to very high doses of chemotherapy, usually cyclophosphamide or melphalan, and whole body irradiation. This has the effect of completely ablating the bone marrow, which then has to be replaced. This may be from a matched donor (allograft) or from the patient's marrow previously collected and stored while in remission (autograft). The patient's marrow can be treated with monoclonal antibody techniques in an attempt to purge it further of residual leukaemic cells.

Intensive support is required for the period from marrow ablation to the re-establishment of the grafted marrow, which might be 3–4 weeks. During this time blood and platelet transfusions are required. Antibiotic prophylaxis is given with aggressive treatment of any febrile episode using high-dose broad-spectrum antibiotics for bacterial, viral and fungal infections. Despite this, even in experienced units, a mortality rate of around 5 per cent is expected from the procedure, usually owing to neutropenic infection or pneumonitis. Mortality is in general related to age, and bone marrow transplantation is a hazardous undertaking in patients over the age of 50 years.

A further complication of allograft bone marrow transplantation is that of graft-versus-host disease in which the graft marrow reacts against the host tissues. This may manifest itself in a number of ways, most commonly through hepatic dysfunction, gastrointestinal disturbance and skin rashes. Various attempts have been made to reduce this event by treating the donor marrow to remove T lymphocytes, which are the principal cell type involved and by the use of immunosuppressive agents such as methotrexate or azathioprine.

Relapse treatment

When ALL has failed to respond to first-line chemotherapy or has relapsed following initial treatment, the usual pattern of relapse is with bone marrow disease. CNS relapse occurs in up to 10 per cent of cases despite CNS prophylaxis and will require treatment with local irradiation and intrathecal therapy. Testicular relapse is also well recognized representing a further site where chemotherapy has poor penetration. It is treated with local irradiation.

Salvage chemotherapy takes the form of using standard induction chemotherapy as above with alternative drugs added such as cytosine arabinoside. For those with a matched donor available then bone marrow transplantation is indicated.

Tumour-related complications

Pancytopenia with consequent anaemia, leukopenia predisposing to infection and thrombocytopenia-related haemorrhage can occur.

Treatment-related complications

- Tumour lysis syndrome is a rare complication arising as a result of the breakdown of large numbers of lymphoid cells when chemotherapy is initiated. This is discussed in full in Chapter 22.
- Bone marrow suppression with the particular risk of neutropenic sepsis is also seen.
- Bone marrow transplantation carries the added risks of graft-versus-host disease and prolonged immunosuppression.
- Total body irradiation during marrow transplantation can cause pneumonitis.
- CNS prophylaxis in young children could have effects on later intellectual development. Attempts are constantly being made to minimize this effect by reducing the dose and overall use of CNS irradiation.
- Testicular irradiation will result in sterility but not impotence.

Prognosis

The prognosis for childhood ALL is age-related. In babies <12 months the cure rate is 44 per cent, increasing in children aged 1–9 years to 88 per cent; in adolescents aged 10–15 years it is 73 per cent and for adults it falls to 69 per cent. Philadelphia-positive ALL has a worse outcome than other types of ALL.

Acute myeloid/ myeloblastic leukaemia (AML)

Epidemiology

Each year in the UK there are 2300 cases of AML leading to a total of 2100 deaths per annum. AML has an incidence of around 4 in 100 000 in the UK affecting males and females in approximately equal proportions. It is most common in young children under the age of 4 years but is less common in children than ALL, accounting for 20 per cent of childhood leukaemias. In adults it is typically seen in the over-40 age group with a median age of 60 years.

Aetiology

- *Radiation exposure*: increased incidence of AML appeared in populations exposed after the nuclear explosions in Hiroshima and Nagasaki. After therapeutic or diagnostic use of radiation it is a rare but recognized event.
- *Chemotherapy agents*: these include, in particular, alkylating agents such as chlorambucil and procarbazine when AML is usually preceded by a period of myelodysplasia. Topoisomerase II inhibitors of which etoposide is the most common example are also associated with an increased incidence of secondary AML, typically not preceded by myelodysplasia and associated with a specific gene rearrangement affecting 11q23.
- *Environmental agents*: benzene exposure has been associated with the development of AML.
- *Genetic predisposition*: an increase in Down's syndrome, trisomy 8 and syn-

TABLE 17.3 Subtypes of acute myeloid leukaemia

AML subtype	Cell type
MO	Undifferentiated myeloblastic
M1	Undifferentiated myeloblastic without maturation
M2	Differentiated myeloblastic
M3	Promyelocytic
M4	Myelomonocytic
M5	Monoblastic
M6	Erythroleukaemia
M7	Megakaryoblastic

dromes associated with defects in DNA repair including Bloom's syndrome, ataxia taelangiectasia and Fanconi's anaemia is seen.

The vast majority of cases of AML (over 90 per cent) have no clear association with environmental agents and appear to arise de novo.

Pathology

AML encompasses a much broader pathological spectrum of disease than ALL. The characteristics of the myeloblast are positive staining with Sudan black and peroxidase stains. Eight subtypes based on morphological and cytochemical differences are now recognized; their features are outlined in Table 17.3. The common forms are M1 and M2.

Clinically, all these forms of AML behave in a similar fashion. Around half of all patients with AML will have chromosomal abnormalities. Recognized changes include trisomy of chromosome 8, deletions affecting chromosome 5 or 7 and abnormalities of chromosome 11, all of which are poor prognostic features.

Natural history

There is progressive infiltration of the bone marrow with subsequent bone marrow failure. Testicular and CNS involvement is relatively rare. CNS involvement is most common in monoblastic AML. Extramedullary involvement is more common than with ALL, with infiltration of liver and spleen in over 50 per cent and characteristic skin and gum infiltration in myelomonocytic and monoblastic leukaemias.

Symptoms

Symptoms include bone marrow failure causing fatigue, recurrent infections and haemorrhage. There is also associated fever, sweats and weight loss. Scattered bone pains may also occur.

Signs

These may include:

- signs of anaemia, bruising, purpura and recurrent infection
- hepatosplenomegaly
- lymphadenopathy (less common than in ALL)
- gum hypertrophy with associated gum bleeding, particularly in myelomonocytic and monoblastic forms of AML.

Differential diagnosis

Other forms of acute leukaemia and non-Hodgkin's lymphoma together with aplastic anaemia and myelofibrosis should be considered.

Investigations

Blood count

A full blood count will show pancytopenia with the presence of primitive blast cells on examination of the blood film.

Biochemistry

Routine biochemistry may show abnormalities in liver function owing to infiltration.

Radiography

Chest X-ray could show signs of infection or, more rarely, leukaemic infiltration.

Coagulation studies

There can be coagulation abnormalities, particularly with promyelocytic leukaemia associated with disseminated intravascular coagulation.

Bone marrow examination

The diagnosis will be confirmed on examination of the bone marrow and the subtype of AML determined by specific stains.

Treatment

Induction

This consists of chemotherapy in the form of daunorubicin and cytosine arabinoside. Some schedules have included a third drug such as thioguanine (DAT) or etoposide but the added value is uncertain. Complete regression can be achieved in up to 85 per cent of patients on first exposure to these agents. It is highly dependent on age, the complete response rate in patients over 55 years falling to only 45 per cent.

Consolidation

Consolidation therapy in AML may be in the form of further chemotherapy for patients with good risk disease, and autograft transplant or allogeneic transplant for those with un-favourable features.

Chemotherapy will include further cycles of cytosine arabinoside; high-dose schedules have been advocated to achieve higher CNS drug levels. Patients with CNS disease will also require cranial irradiation and intrathecal methotrexate but prophylactic CNS treatment is not generally recommended in contrast to that in ALL.

Better long-term results have been associated with the use of more intensive treatment in the consolidation phase and this will be considered for patients under 55 years, particularly those with unfavourable presenting features.

Maintenance

Maintenance therapy has not been shown to have great value in AML and chemotherapy is not usually continued beyond 6 months after achieving initial remission.

Relapse treatment

Relapse carries a poor prognosis; re-induction chemotherapy using cytosine arabinoside-based schedules followed by allogeneic transplantation for those under 55 years with an HLA-matched donor gives the best chance of salvage; autologous transplant can be considered for older patients up to 65 years.

Tumour-related complications

These include in particular the effects of pancytopenia including anaemia, susceptibility to infection and haemorrhage.

Treatment-related complications

Tumour lysis can occur with induction chemotherapy, and prophylaxis with fluids, allopurinol or rasburicase should be given. Chemotherapy is also associated with further bone marrow depression and in particular the risk of neutropenic sepsis. Bone marrow transplant has its own specific risks of infection, graft-versus-host disease and radiation-induced pneumonitis.

Prognosis

The prognosis for AML is not as good as for ALL but has improved considerably in recent years with the use of bone marrow transplantation. Overall around 40 per cent of all patients are cured of AML. Cure rates of around 50 per cent are to be expected in those undergoing transplantation in first remission and 25 per cent for those who are transplanted in second remission. Poor prognostic features at presentation include a high white cell count >100 × 10^9/L and disseminated intravascular coagulation associated with M3. The outlook is worse for older patients (>40 years) who have a lower rate of initial remission and are less able to tolerate intensive chemotherapy regimens or bone marrow transplantation. Other features associated with a poor prognosis are AML secondary to previous treatment, previous myelodysplasia and tumours expressing CD34 or bcl-2.

Rare tumours

Promyelocytic leukaemia (M3) is characterized by the t(15;17) translocation. It is particularly sensitive to anthracyclines and to all-trans-retinoic acid (ATRA), which can alone induce remissions. Standard induction therapy will therefore include ATRA with cytosine arabinoside and daunorubicin. ATRA is also included in maintenance treatment with mercaptopurine for 2 years after induction. Cure rates of over 80 per cent with these schedules are achieved.

Chloroma or isolated granulocytic sarcoma is a localized tumour of myeloblasts. Around two-thirds will progress to widespread AML; localized treatment with surgery or radiotherapy is not appropriate and these tumours should be treated as for AML.

Screening and future prospects

Patients at risk of treatment-related AML, typically survivors from intensive chemotherapy treatment for germ cell tumours or lymphoma, are screened with regular examination of the peripheral blood.

Chronic granulocytic leukaemia (CGL)

Each year in the UK there are 550 cases of CGL leading to a total of 250 deaths per annum.

CGL increases in incidence with age; it is rarely diagnosed below the age of 30 and the median age is 60 years. Its annual incidence in the UK is around 0.8 in 100 000 and it affects men and women equally.

Aetiology

There are no recognized environmental agents although an increased risk in those populations exposed to excess radiation has been documented.

Pathology

CGL represents neoplastic proliferation of granulocyte precursors and is characterized by an excess of metamyelocytes and myelocytes in the peripheral blood. Promyelocytes and myeloblasts can also be present and often there is an excess of basophils and eosinophils.

Philadelphia chromosome is present in around 80 per cent of patients, formed by a translocation from chromosome 9 to chromosome 22 or less frequently another chromosome. Additional chromosomal abnormalities frequently develop in the acute phase of CGL (the blast crisis).

The translocated fragment from chromosome 9 is a proto-oncogene, *ABL*, which translocates to the break point cluster (BCR) region of chromosome 22. This results in a chimeric fusion gene *BCR-ABL* which encodes for a protein having tyrosine kinase activity. This is outside the tight control mechanisms that govern the normal expression of *ABL*. The downstream events from this are related to both proliferation and apoptosis of haemopoietic progenitor cells leading to a massive accumulation of myeloid cells.

Natural history

An initial indolent period gives way to a fulminating blast crisis indistinguishable from an acute leukaemia but in general is less responsive to treatment.

Blast crisis is usually myeloblastic in type although lymphoblastic crises may occur. Occasionally the blast crisis might be the first clinical manifestation of the disease when it can be distinguished from a de novo acute leukaemia by the presence of Philadelphia chromosome.

Symptoms

CGL can present with:

- symptoms of anaemia or thrombocytopenia owing to bone marrow failure
- abdominal distension and discomfort from splenic enlargement which may be massive
- bone pain
- general features of an active leukaemic process such as fevers and weight loss and also itching.
- very high white count resulting in hyperviscosity of the blood causing confusion and headaches
- priapism.

Signs

These may include:

- clinical signs of anaemia and purpura
- massive splenomegaly (Fig. 17.1)
- hepatomegaly
- lymphadenopathy – usually not prominent.

Differential diagnosis

Myelofibrosis can also present with a large spleen and pancytopenia. In the acute phase differentiation between de novo acute leukaemia and blast crisis of CGL can be diffi-

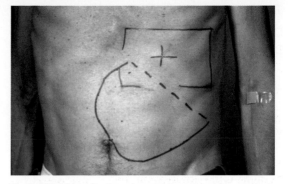

Figure 17.1 Massive hepatomegaly outlined in a patient with chronic granulocytic leukaemia.

cult unless the preceding history is known, but can be resolved by the finding of Philadelphia chromosome.

Investigations

Blood count

The peripheral blood usually has a characteristic picture with a very high white blood cell count of between 100 and 1000×10^9/L of which the majority will be metamyelocytes with other granulocyte precursors. This is usually associated with a mild thrombocytopenia and anaemia. Basophilia is also a characteristic finding.

Bone marrow examination

This will show a hypercellular picture with an excess of granulocyte precursors. Areas of myelosclerosis can also be seen. Philadelphia chromosome can be demonstrated in myeloid, erythroid and megakaryocytic cell lines.

Ultrasound

Abdominal ultrasound is performed to confirm the extent of hepatomegaly and splenomegaly.

Other investigations

Other characteristic abnormalities are a low leukocyte alkaline phosphatase and raised serum B12 and B12 binding proteins. Blast crisis is characterized by the appearance of more primitive blast cells and on bone marrow these will comprise over 50 per cent of the myeloid population.

Treatment

Chronic phase

Initial treatment is aimed at reducing the peripheral blood white cell count to under $15 \times 10^9/L$ and to alleviate symptoms of splenomegaly.

Chemotherapy using imatinib mesylate, a specific inhibitor of the *BCR-ABL* tyrosine kinase is now the treatment of choice. It is given orally as a single daily dose and with this after 12 months over 80 per cent of newly diagnosed patients will be in cytogenetic remission. However, more detailed polymerase chain reaction (PCR) analysis will still demonstrate residual leukaemic cells and on this basis it is recommended that younger patients who have an HLA-matched donor undergo elective allogeneic transplantation as the only recognized curative treatment. The small number of non-responders would also go down this route.

Older patients and those with no donor can be considered for autologous transplant procedures.

The traditional treatments for CGL – busulphan, hydroxyurea and alpha-interferon – are now only used in those with advanced disease refractory to imatinib and unfit for intensive chemotherapy.

Splenic irradiation is useful in the palliation of local symptoms from a large spleen and the effects of hypersplenism in disease refractory to chemotherapy.

Leukophoresis will achieve rapid reduction of very high white cell counts. The patient's blood is passed through a cell separator, being returned through a continuous flow into a second intravenous cannula. This results on average in a 35 per cent reduction in white cell count with each procedure, and also has the advantage of providing large numbers of redundant granulocytes, which can be used for therapeutic transfusion in other patients. However, no effect on the natural history of the CGL process is achieved by regular leukophoresis and it is therefore generally used only when hyperviscosity is a predominant feature.

Acute phase

The treatment of the blast crisis is essentially that of the acute leukaemia into which the CGL transforms. In around 70 per cent this will be an AML, around 5 per cent may have a mixed picture and the remaining 25 per cent will manifest ALL. As with de novo acute leukaemia, an ALL blast crisis has a better prognosis with around 40 per cent of patients reverting to a chronic phase with simple induction therapy such as vincristine and prednisolone. Bone marrow transplantation could be of value in those patients achieving remission from their acute phase.

Tumour-related complications

There might be bone marrow failure resulting in anaemia, reduced resistance to infection and a bleeding tendency from thrombocytopenia. This can be exacerbated by the effects of gross splenomegaly, causing the phenomenon of hypersplenism with pooling of blood within the large spleen. Massive splenomegaly can also cause local pain and might impair gastric emptying. Local areas of infarction can occur within the spleen, causing acute pain.

Large numbers of white cells in the circulation can cause hyperviscosity with headache, confusion, visual disturbance and priapism.

Treatment-related complications

Imatinib results in bone marrow depression and close monitoring of the peripheral blood count is required; titrating the dose is necessary in the first few weeks of administration. Tumour lysis is seen on rare occasions and prophylactic cover with fluids and allopurinol is important. Other side-effects from imatinib include nausea, muscle cramps, and fluid retention causing periorbital and peripheral oedema.

Splenic irradiation or surgical splenectomy can be hazardous because of thrombocytopenia and a subsequent predisposition to infection, particularly pneumococcal pneumonia.

Prognosis

The 5-year survival after allogeneic transplant is between 60 and 80 per cent; however, the median survival of all patients with CGL is around 4 years with death usually occurring in the acute blast crisis. Prognostic indices use age, platelet count, splenomegaly and peripheral blast counts to define good, intermediate and poor risk groups with survivals ranging from 60 months to 30 months. The full impact of imatinib has yet to be clearly defined and it is likely that these survival figures will show an upward trend as a result.

Future prospects

The role of low-dose allogeneic transplants, new agents targeting the *BCR-ABL* complex and vaccine therapy are currently areas of investigation.

Chronic lymphocytic leukaemia (CLL)

Each year in the UK there are 2400 cases of CLL leading to a total of 1100 deaths per annum. CLL represents the end of the leukaemic spectrum where the classification merges with that of non-Hodgkin's lymphoma. CLL is a neoplastic proliferation of the same cell type as lymphocytic lymphoma, the differentiating feature being the extent of bone marrow infiltration.

Epidemiology

CLL affects a somewhat older age group than CGL, with a median age of 70–75 years. Males and females are affected in approximately equal proportions.

Aetiology

The only specific aetiological agent relates to the use of herbicides in agricultural workers and an association with exposure to Agent Orange as used in the Vietnam war has been confirmed. No other environmental factors for the common form of CLL seen in Europe and North and South America have been recognized.

First-degree relatives are three times more likely than the general population to also develop CLL or another lymphoid malignancy.

Around half of all patients with CLL have demonstrable chromosomal abnormalities. The most common of these is a deletion on chromosome 13q seen in 55 per cent, trisomy of chromosome 12 in 18 per cent and a deletion on chromosome 11q in 16 per cent.

The rarer T-cell variant can be associated with HTLV-I infection, as found in Japan and the Caribbean.

Pathology

The cell of origin for CLL is in most cases a B lymphocyte, although in 5 per cent there might be markers of T-cell origin. The B-cell type will demonstrate surface immunoglobulin, which may be either kappa or lambda, and the surface antigens CD5, CD19, CD20 and CD23. The characteristic finding in the peripheral blood is of large numbers of mature lymphocytes with a total lymphocyte count of $>5 \times 10^9/L$ being required to confirm the diagnosis. This is associated with bone marrow infiltration by immature lymphocytes, which should account for more than 30 per cent of the total marrow. Three patterns of marrow involvement have been described: interstitial, nodular or diffuse. As with non-Hodgkin's lymphomas diffuse appearance is associated with a worse prognosis than the more focal forms.

Natural history

The natural history spans many years. Ultimately death occurs usually owing to bone marrow failure or to transformation into a high-grade lymphoma.

Symptoms

CLL can be asymptomatic for some time. When symptoms do appear they include:

- painless lymphadenopathy
- anaemia
- recurrent infections
- fever, sweats and weight loss.

Signs

These include:

- peripheral lymphadenopathy
- splenomegaly
- hepatomegaly – usually only mild.

Investigations

Blood count

A full blood count will reveal anaemia, thrombocytopenia and a high total white cell count, which on examination of the blood film consists of predominantly small, round, lymphocytes.

Bone marrow examination

This will confirm the diagnosis with the finding of excess lymphoid cells, at least 30 per cent of which will be immature forms.

Biopsy

Lymph node biopsy can be performed and will show infiltration of involved nodes with well-differentiated lymphocytes, usually in a diffuse pattern.

Other tests

Hypogammaglobulinaemia is a common association. Haemolytic anaemia might be associated with CLL with elevated conjugated bilirubin and a positive Coomb's test. In HTLV-associated CLL, hypercalcaemia and hyponatraemia are characteristic features.

Differential diagnosis

Non-Hodgkin's lymphoma should be considered, particularly the diffuse small cell types.

Staging

There are two staging systems in use, the Rai and the Binet sytems, both of which are similar and classify patients into good, intermediate and poor risk (Table 17.4).

TABLE 17.4 Rai Classification for chronic lymphocytic leukaemia

Stage	Features	Risk
0	Lymphocytosis in blood and marrow	Good
I	Lymphocytosis and enlarged nodes	Good
II	Lymphocytosis and large spleen/liver	Intermediate
III	Lymphocytosis and anaemia	Poor
IV	Lymphocytosis and thrombocytopenia	Poor

Treatment

Because CLL has a long indolent course and most patients present with no clinical signs or symptoms but simply an abnormal blood count, treatment is considered only when patients are symptomatic or when there are signs of bone marrow failure in the presence of very high peripheral white cell counts. No benefit to earlier treatment in the asymptomatic patient has been demonstrated.

When treatment is required there is usually a good response to simple oral chemotherapy using chlorambucil, cyclophosphamide or fludarabine with no advantages in long-term outcome apparent for any particular approach to date. Steroids can also be used and are of value when the disease becomes refractory to alkylating agents, but there is no evidence that adding them to chemotherapy in the early management of the disease is of value. Other combinations have also included anthracyclines, vincristine or vinblastine, but again no significant advantage over single-agent therapy has emerged. CLL comprises CD20 positive cells and is therefore responsive to rituximab. The addition of rituximab to chemotherapy undoubtedly improves response rates but the long-term implication of this in terms of overall survival remains uncertain. In refractory disease alentuzumab is also considered, as it has profound antilymphocyte activity.

Low-dose irradiation will result in rapid shrinkage of enlarged node masses or splenomegaly. Doses as low as 20 or 30 Gy over 2–3 weeks are usually sufficient and associated with little or no morbidity.

Currently stem cell autograft and bone marrow transplantation has no established role in CLL.

Tumour-related complications

The associated hypogammaglobulinaemia results in a high incidence of infections.

There can be chronic anaemia, which can have a haemolytic component requiring regular transfusions. Thrombocytopenia may also persist.

The rare HTLV-related CLL is sometimes associated with hypercalcaemia.

Treatment-related complications

Oral alkylating agents are usually relatively trouble free, provided careful attention is paid to the blood count and treatment stopped when there are signs of significant bone marrow depression.

With a large tumour burden there is always the possibility of provoking hyperuricaemia owing to cell lysis on initiation of chemotherapy. This should be prevented by administration of allopurinol and ensuring adequate fluid intake.

Prognosis

While remissions are usually readily achieved in CLL, cures are rare. Many patients will live with their disease for several years, the median survival being around 8 years.

The HTLV-associated T-cell form of CLL is a far more aggressive disease, however, and some patients succumb within a few months, although a more chronic form similar to sporadic CLL is also seen.

Rare forms of leukaemia

Prolymphocytic leukaemia

This is related to CLL, presenting in elderly men with splenomegaly and very high white cell counts. The cells are larger than the mature lymphocytes seen in CLL and the disease has a more aggressive course.

Hairy cell leukaemia

This is a chronic leukaemia occurring in the middle aged and is more frequent in men than women, sometimes classified as a variant of CLL, distinguished immunohistochemically by cells that are positive for CD19 and 25 but negative for CD5. It is rare, accounting for around 2 per cent of all cases of adult leukaemia. Typically it presents with massive splenomegaly and pancytopenia. The characteristic finding is of 'hairy cells' in the peripheral blood and bone marrow. These are B lymphocytes with cytoplasmic projections giving them a 'hairy' appearance under the microscope.

Hairy cell leukaemia usually has a long indolent course. It responds to treatment with interferon with which it may remain in remission for many years before it becomes resistant and bone marrow failure develops. The new purine analogue drugs pentostatin and cladribine are also highly active in this disease and can be used instead of interferon.

MULTIPLE MYELOMA

Epidemiology

Each year in the UK there are 3800 cases of multiple myeloma, 2100 cases in men and 1700 cases in women leading to a total of 2600 deaths per annum.

The incidence of multiple myeloma in the UK in men is around 55 per million; men and women are affected in equal proportions. There has been an apparent increase in incidence over the past 30 years from only 5 per million in 1960, which probably reflects improved diagnostic abilities rather than a true increase in the prevalence of the disease.

Aetiology

There are no recognized aetiological agents for multiple myeloma. An increased risk in those exposed to excess radiation after the atomic bomb and in radiologists prior to formal radiation protection has been seen. It has been suggested that the origin of the paraprotein production could be as a host antibody response to a foreign protein but no consistent antigen has been identified.

Pathology

Multiple myeloma is one of a spectrum of plasma cell neoplasms ranging from benign monoclonal gammopathy through solitary plasmacytoma to multiple myeloma. All these conditions are characterized by a neoplastic proliferation of B cells producing a characteristic paraprotein. Transformation within this group of conditions is well recognized, with around 20 per cent of benign monoclonal gammopathies and 60 per cent of apparent solitary plasmacytomas eventually developing multiple myeloma.

Cytogenetic abnormalities are found in around 50 per cent but no single characteristic change is recognized. The most common is found in the *14q32* gene locus but many others have also been reported.

Natural history

Three phases in the evolution of multiple myeloma have been described, not all of which will be seen in an individual patient:

- monoclonal gammopathy
- smouldering myeloma, which is usually asymptomatic with low levels of paraprotein and 10–20 per cent plasma cells in bone marrow
- typical myeloma, with symptoms, rising paraprotein levels and >20 per cent plasma cells in bone marrow.

Once established, myeloma affects the bone marrow, bones and kidneys. Bone invasion is facilitated by release of chemicals, which act as osteoclast-activating factors, including interleukins (in particular IL-1 and IL-6), tumour necrosis factor (TNF) and macrophage colony-stimulating factor (MCSF). Renal damage occurs from deposition of paraprotein and amyloid formation, hypercalcaemia and hyper-uricaemia.

Symptoms

Symptoms of multiple myeloma typically present in three ways:

- Bone marrow infiltration causes anaemia; thrombocytopenia is usually not prominent but more commonly there may be a bleeding disorder owing to the effects of macroglobulinaemia.
- Bone destruction results in local pain, pathological fracture or neurological complications such as nerve root or spinal cord compression – bone pain is present in two-thirds of patients presenting with myeloma.
- Metabolic and biochemical disturbance occurs, including:

- high levels of paraprotein causing hyperviscosity, resulting in confusion and headache;
- renal failure, which is present in around one-third of patients as defined by a raised blood urea and creatinine causing nausea, vomiting, malaise, fluid retention or itching, and
- hypercalcaemia, which is present in around one-third of patients who present with myeloma resulting in thirst, polyuria, dyspepsia, nausea, vomiting, constipation or confusion.

Signs

Clinical signs of myeloma can be few. Patients might be clinically anaemic and bone lesions present as locally tender or even swollen areas. There can be rib or spinal tenderness.

Patients presenting with pathological fracture will have obvious signs of swelling, tenderness and deformity.

Cord compression can present with weakness of the lower limbs, sphincter disturbance and neurological signs of an upper motor neurone lesion. In contrast cauda equina compression from disease in the lumbosacral spine will result in lower motor neurone weakness.

Hyperviscosity causes confusion. Papilloedema and retinal haemorrhage are also described.

Differential diagnosis

There are few conditions outside the spectrum of plasma cell neoplasms that will mimic myeloma; however, there are rare forms of non-Hodgkin's lymphoma that may produce high levels of paraprotein and cause initial confusion.

Waldenstrom's macroglobulinaemia will also present with a paraprotein but none of the other features of myeloma and must be distinguished from benign monoclonal gammopathy (see Chapter 16).

Other causes of bone metastases including primary tumours of the breast, lung, thyroid and prostate should be considered.

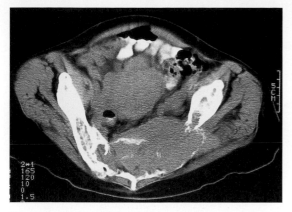

Figure 17.2 Solitary plasmacytoma arising in the ilium showing large soft tissue mass and bone destruction. This patient has an associated plasma paraprotein but no evidence of other sites of bone involvement and a normal bone marrow.

Patients who present with a solitary plasma cell lesion might have a true solitary plasmacytoma as shown in Figure 17.2, but 70 per cent will eventually manifest the characteristic features of widespread multiple myeloma.

Investigations

Blood count

A full blood count can show anaemia and the ESR will be raised. The blood film might have rouleaux formation.

Biochemistry

Biochemical tests will show a raised total protein and there might be hypercalcaemia, renal failure with raised urea and creatinine and hyperuricaemia.

Protein electrophoresis

This will demonstrate the characteristic M band containing the paraprotein, which can also be quantitatively measured. This will be an IgG in around 50 per cent of patients, IgA in 20 per cent, IgM in 10 per cent and light chain in only 10 per cent. Other rare types of paraprotein include IgD (2 per cent) and heavy chain fragments (1 per cent). In 1 per cent of patients there might be two different M proteins and in 1 per cent the paraprotein may be absent.

Serum β_2-microglobulin

The serum β_2-microglobulin is also raised in many patients and is an important marker of disease both for prognosis and for monitoring treatment.

Urine tests

Proteinuria could be present and, on electrophoresis of the urine, Bence–Jones protein might be detected.

Bone marrow examination

This will show infiltration with plasma cells; infiltration with more than 20 per cent plasma cells is diagnostic.

Radiography and scans

An X-ray skeletal survey might show lytic bone lesions, many of which are asymptomatic. Typical appearances are shown on the skull X-ray as in Figure 17.3. Because the bone metastases of myeloma are usually predominantly lytic with little osteoblastic reaction, they often do not show on isotope bone scan or might be seen as cold areas rather than hot spots. MRI will also demonstrate bone lesions well, as shown in Figure 17.3, and whole skeleton MRI is an alternative staging investigation where available (Fig. 17.4).

Other tests

Other investigations can be considered where indicated, including plasma viscosity, plasma volume, and rectal biopsy for amyloid.

Staging

A number of criteria for the diagnosis of myeloma have been defined:

- 1 – Presence of a monoclonal 'M' protein in serum or urine
- 2 – Bone lesions owing to a plasma cell infiltrate
- 3 – Marrow plasma cells accounting for >10 per cent of marrow infiltrate
- 4 – Associated features: anaemia, hypercalcaemia or renal failure.

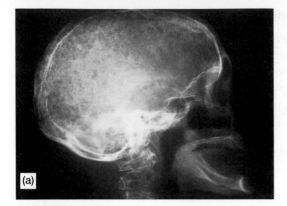

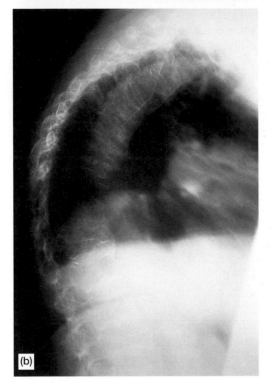

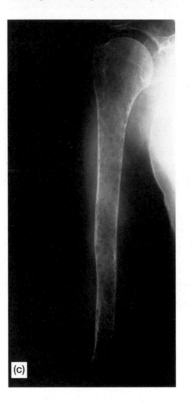

Figure 17.3 X-rays of (a) skull, (b) spine and (c) humerus, showing multiple lytic bone deposits of myeloma.

Diagnosis is confirmed on demonstration of any two of criteria 1–3.

Staging of myeloma is based on recognized prognostic factors, which include haemoglobin, blood urea, serum calcium, extent of bone lesions and level of paraprotein. The usual classification applied in the UK is the Durie–Salmon staging system:

■ Stage 1 – Hb >10 g/dL
  – calcium normal
  – normal bone skeletal survey (or solitary plasmacytoma)
  – low serum and urine paraprotein (serum IgG <6 g/dL; lgA <3 g/dL; urine <4 g/ 24 h).
■ Stage 2 – Neither stage 1 nor stage 3
■ Stage 3 – Hb <8.5 g/dL
  – calcium >12 mg/dL
  – multiple lytic bone lesions
  – high paraprotein levels (serum IgG >7 g/dL; lgA >5 g/dL; urine>12 g/24 h).

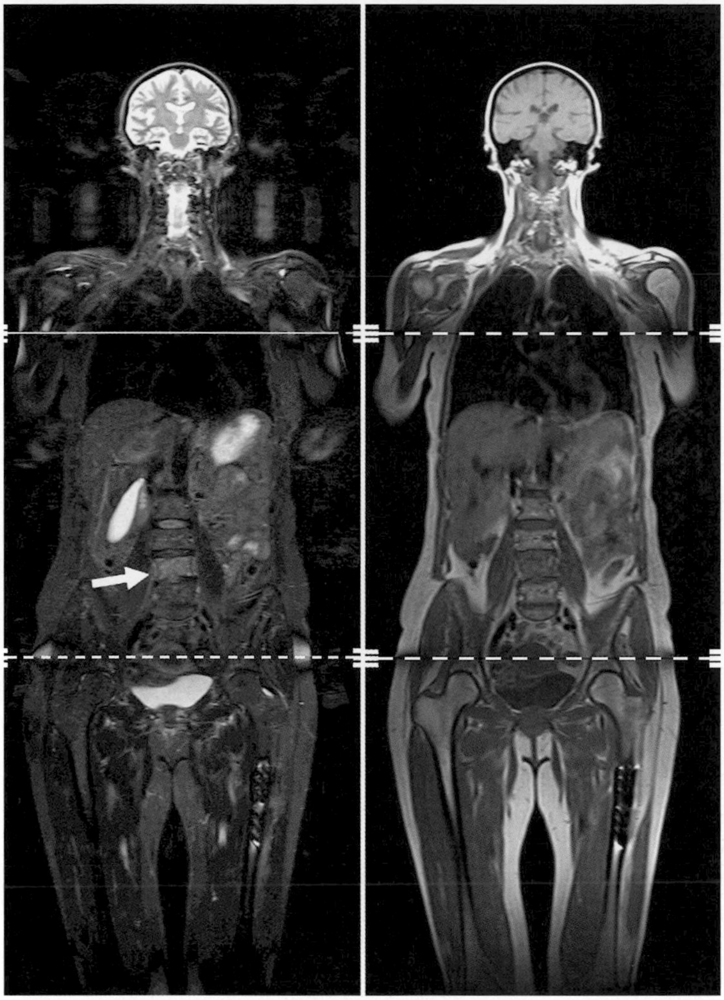

Figure 17.4 MRI scan of whole skeleton demonstrating lytic lesions of multiple myeloma in spine (arrowed) and surgical fixation of pathological fracture of the left femur. (Courtesy of Dr A Padhani)

There is a further subclassification into 'A' (normal renal function) or 'B' (raised serum creatinine).

It is proposed that the staging correlates with plasma cell mass, increasing from $<0.6 \times 10^{12}/m^2$ for stage 1 to $>1.2 \times 10^{12}/m^2$ for stage 3.

Serum β_2-microglobulin is a further important prognostic indicator.

Treatment

There is a small group of patients with indolent myeloma manifest by a few asymptomatic bone lesions or mild anaemia who require no specific treatment. They are managed by transfusion when appropriate and occasional monitoring of the serum paraprotein and β_2-microglobulin.

Solitary lesions (true plasmacytomas) are usually treated with local radiotherapy alone.

The remainder of patients will require treatment with chemotherapy and, where indicated, radiotherapy to sites of painful bone lesions.

Chemotherapy for myeloma

There are two main approaches to the drug treatment of myeloma.

- *Intravenous induction chemotherapy and autologous stem cell transplant*: offered to younger patients who are fit for the high-dose chemotherapy option; this will usually be those up to 65 years who have no other co-morbidities. Initial chemotherapy will comprise a combination of idarubicin and high-dose dexamethasone (Z-DEX) or cyclophosphamide, Adriamycin, vincristine and dexamethasone. Responding patients will then proceed to a stem-cell harvest and high-dose BEAM (BCNU, etoposide, cytosine arabinoside, methyl prednisolone) chemotherapy followed by stem-cell reinfusion.

- *Oral chemotherapy*: offered to older (>70 years) patients or those with other co-morbidities that would exclude them from a high-dose chemotherapy. The current schedule of choice is a combination of melphalan or cyclophosphamide, dexamethasone and thalidomide (MDT or CDT).

Supportive treatment

Alongside chemotherapy, management of the complications of myeloma will have a considerable impact on both the quality of life and the survival of the patient.

- Anaemia will require blood transfusion.
- Infections will require prompt treatment with appropriate antibiotics.
- Hypercalcaemia will require active hydration, diuresis and the use of bisphosphonates.
- Renal failure will require management of fluid balance and, in severe cases, dialysis, pending definitive chemotherapy, may be justified.
- Adjuvant bisphosphonate therapy (clodronate, pamidronate or zolendronate) has been shown to reduce the likelihood of complications such as pathological fracture owing to bone deposits and is given routinely.
- Pathological fracture will require internal fixation followed by local radiotherapy.
- Spinal canal compression will require steroids and urgent radiotherapy or surgical spinal stabilization.
- Active rehabilitation is also important as immobility is a further adverse prognostic factor.

Relapse treatment

Treatment on relapse will depend upon initial management. Further response induction may be attempted using one of the high-dose dexamethasone-based schedules (Z-DEX or CVAD) or further exposure to alkylating agent-based schedules with thalidomide. In young patients a further intensive chemotherapy option can be considered. Other new agents now available include:

- bortezomib (Velcade®), a new drug, which is a proteosome inhibitor and has high levels of activity against myeloma even after previous treatment
- lenolidamide, derived from thalidomide, which appears more active against myeloma
- bevacizumab, an antiangiogenic agent, which has activity against myeloma.

Tumour-related complications

These have been covered in the above discussion on supportive treatment in myeloma.

Treatment-related complications

Chemotherapy will cause bone marrow depression and the blood count must be carefully monitored with aggressive treatment of neutropenic infections. This is particularly the case when high-dose therapy is given where there will be a period of 2–3 weeks when the patient is pancytopenic.

Steroid infusions can cause Cushingoid symptoms and, particularly in the elderly, fluid retention, causing cardiac failure.

Prognosis

The median survival for patients with stage 1 disease is around 5 years falling to only 2 years for stage 3. Increasing age, poor renal function and a high β_2-microglobulin are associated with a poor prognosis with survival of less than 1 year.

Those with solitary plasmacytoma in a site other than bone, usually in the head and neck

MULTIPLE MYELOMA

A 68-year-old man presents to his GP with a 3-month history of increasing back pain. His GP elicits local tenderness in the thoracolumbar spine and sends him for an X-ray. This showed scattered lytic abnormalities in the vertebral bodies and it is commented that similar lesions are seen in adjacent ribs taken on the thoracic spine views. His GP proceeds to take blood for a full blood count, ESR, biochemical profile and paraproteins. A urine sample is tested at the local surgery and found to be positive for protein. A further sample is therefore sent to the pathology laboratory for detection of Bence–Jones proteins. In addition to this being positive he is found to have a paraprotein consisting of an immunoglobulin G with a level 48 g/L. His other tests show that he is mildly anaemic with a haemoglobin of 10.3 but his other blood count parameters are normal. His ESR is 97 mm/hour. His urea is marginally elevated at 7.5 with a serum creatinine of 160. Serum calcium and other biochemical parameters are normal. He is referred to the haemato-oncology clinic. Further investigations performed there include an X-ray skeletal survey that shows scattered bone lesions, and his bone marrow is reported as consisting of 35 per cent plasma cells. A formal diagnosis of multiple myeloma is confirmed.

He is started on treatment with oral chemotherapy using cyclophosphamide, dexamethasone and thalidomide. He finds this treatment is surprisingly easy to take but does note a lack of energy and drowsiness, which he is told may be due to side-effects from the thalidomide. He also attends every 3 weeks for intravenous pamidronate infusions.

His paraprotein level falls satisfactorily and after his third month of treatment it has reached 12 g/L. Over the next 2 months he continues with his treatment but no further change in the paraprotein level is seen and, his paraproteins having reached a plateau, chemotherapy is discontinued. He does, however, continue the 3-weekly pamidronate infusions.

He remains well for the next 8 months, seen occasionally in the clinic. A slow rise in his paraproteins is observed and, whilst out walking, he stumbles and develops severe pain in the right thigh; he is unable to weight bear and is brought to the accident and emergency department where an X-ray confirms a pathological fracture through a lytic area of myeloma in the femur. The orthopaedic team perform internal fixation with an intramedullary nail and he makes a good postoperative recovery, being mobile with sticks when he is discharged 2 weeks later. He is then referred to the radiotherapy department and a short 5-day course of radiotherapy is given to the femur covering the site of fracture.

He makes a good recovery but investigations in the haematology clinic reveal a further rise in the paraprotein to 46 g/L, a rising creatinine which has reached 230 and a fall in his haemoglobin to 8.2 g/dL. His myeloma is clearly progressing and he is offered further chemotherapy with idarubicin and dexamethasone. Once again after 6 months of treatment his paraprotein stabilizes at around 15 g/L, he maintains his haemoglobin steady at around 10 g/dL and his renal function is stable with only mild impairment.

A paraprotein level measured 6 months later again starts to show a slight rise and when seen 2 months later he is complaining of some new back pain. X-rays show that he still has quite extensive lytic abnormalities in the bone. When seen at the end of the first month of restarting treatment his back pain is becoming more and more troublesome and he is referred for local radiotherapy. He attends the radiotherapy department and receives a single treatment to the thoracolumbar spine treating the painful area. That night he has quite troublesome nausea despite the dose of steroids and ondansetron given to him at the time of radiotherapy treatment. This, however, settles over the next 24 hours when he takes regular metoclopramide tablets. He notices little change in the pain over the first few days but after 10 days there has been some gradual improvement and 2 weeks later he is left with a mild ache but otherwise untroubled by the previous pain.

When seen in the clinic, however, 2 weeks later it is noted that his paraprotein is continuing to rise. He is offered further chemotherapy with bortezomib. This involves coming to the hospital twice a week for 2 weeks out of 3 for an intravenous infusion. After the second cycle of bortezomib his paraprotein has fallen by 50 per cent; he is feeling tired and has developed some tingling in his fingers and toes, which he was told are recognized side-effects. He continues with two further cycles of bortezomib. It is noted that his platelet count has been steadily falling and it is decided to stop the bortezomib at that point. Within a few weeks of discontinuing the treatment his energy level have improved; he is left with some numbness in his finger ends and occasional tingling but is reassured that this is an expected side-effect and that a slow improvement can be expected.

He remains well again for a period of 8 months. He returns to the clinic complaining of general malaise and lack of energy. It is found that his haemoglobin has fallen to 8.6 and his white cell count is only 2.9 with a neutrophil count of 1.2. His platelet count is 112. His paraprotein level has risen once more to 42 g/L. He is given a 3-unit blood transfusion. The role of further chemotherapy is discussed with him and he is told that it is unlikely he will get a long response to further treatment but he is anxious to try further alternatives and is started on weekly injections of cyclophosphamide. After the first month his paraprotein level has risen to 56 g/L and his haemoglobin is once again falling. He is started on erythropoietin injections given subcutaneously three times a week, which improve his haemoglobin and maintain it at a level between 10.5 and 11 g/dL, which he finds tolerable and keeps him free from symptoms. His paraprotein, however, continues to rise inexorably and the weekly cyclophosphamide injections are discontinued. It is noted that his creatinine level has risen to 230. He starts complaining of increasing pain in the ribs with localized tenderness in several sites. He is started on diclofenac tablets with some improvement in his pain. The next week he stumbles whilst coming down stairs at home and has severe pain in the left hip following which he can no longer weight bear. An ambulance is called and he is admitted through casualty. X-rays show that he has a pathological fracture of the left femur through a large lytic lesion. Following admission he develops a temperature and a productive cough. His blood count shows that, whilst the erythropoietin has maintained his haemoglobin, his white cell count has fallen with a neutrophil count of 0.9. He is started on intravenous antibiotics. His chest infection, however, progresses with signs of widespread pneumonia. Three days later he has become semiconscious and confused with widespread signs of bronchopneumonia on his chest X-ray. His serum creatinine has risen to 380. The role of further antibiotics is discussed with his family who agree that in this circumstance it is unlikely to improve the situation and they are discontinued. He lapses into unconsciousness and dies peacefully over the next 24 hours.

region, have the best prognosis with progression to myeloma being unusual; plasmacytoma in bone will progress to myeloma in 55 per cent of patients with a further 10 per cent developing multiple lesions confined to the skeleton.

FURTHER READING

Chiorazzi N, Rai KR, Ferranini M. Chronic lymphocytic leukaemia. *New England Journal of Medicine* 2005;**352**:804–15

Dighiero G, Hamblin TJ. Chronic lymphocytic leukaemia. *Lancet* 2008;**371**:1017–29

Estey E, Dohner H. Acute myeloid leukaemia. *Lancet* 2006;**368**:1894–907

Hehlman R, Hochhaus A, Baccharani M *et al.* Chronic myeloid leukaemia. *Lancet* 2007;**370**:342–50

Kyle RA, Rajkumar SV. Multiple myeloma. *New England Journal of Medicine* 2004;**351**:1860–73

Pui C-H, Robison LL, Look AT. Acute lymphoblastic leukaemia. *Lancet* 2008;**371**:1030–43

SELF-ASSESSMENT QUESTIONS

1. Which of the following is true of acute lymphoblastic leukaemia (ALL)?
   a. It is most common in girls over 5 years
   b. It is increased in incidence in Down's syndrome
   c. The T-cell type may exhibit the t(12;21)(p13;q22) translocation
   d. Exhibits Philadephia chromosome when it develops in CLL
   e. Is characterized by cells which stain positive with Sudan Black

2. Which three of the following are common presenting features of ALL?
   a. Anaemia
   b. Gum hypertrophy
   c. Purpura
   d. Peripheral neuropathy
   e. Erythema nodosum
   f. Fevers
   g. Diarrhoea

3. Which of the following is true of the treatment of ALL?
   a. Induction treatment will include cranial irradiation
   b. Vincristine and prednisolone are used in induction
   c. Consolidation will be given with bone marrow transplant
   d. There is no role for maintenance treatment once remission is achieved
   e. Testicular irradiation will cause impotence

4. Which of the following is true of acute myeloid leukaemia (AML)?
   a. It accounts for 50 per cent of childhood leukaemias
   b. The common form is the M3 subtype
   c. Involvement of soft tissues is less common than in ALL
   d. Disseminated intravascular coagulation occurs in the M1 subtype
   e. The presence of *11q23* gene rearrangement is seen after etoposide

5. In the treatment of AML, which of the following is true?
   a. Induction is usually with vincristine, prednisolone and daunorubicin
   b. Consolidation includes bone marrow transplant for high-risk cases
   c. Intrathecal methotrexate is an important component of induction
   d. Response increases with age beyond 40 years
   e. AML secondary to myelodysplasia has a better prognosis than de novo

6. Which of the following is true of chronic granulocytic leukaemia (CGL)?
   a. The incidence increases with age
   b. Translocation from chromosome 9 to 22 is seen in 80 per cent
   c. Massive hepatomegaly is characteristic
   d. There may be preceding myelofibrosis
   e. The blood film will show an excess of neutrophils

7. Which three of the following are true of the treatment of CGL?
   a. Imatinib mesylate is an inhibitor of tyrosine kinase
   b. Patients with hyperviscosity may require leukophoresis
   c. Intrathecal methotrexate is used in induction
   d. Interferon is used to improve the response rates to chemotherapy
   e. Up to 15 per cent of patients will never require treatment
   f. Thrombocytosis is a poor prognostic feature
   g. Blast crisis should be treated as an acute leukaemia

8. Which of the following is characteristic of chronic lymphocytic leukaemia (CLL)?
   a. Gum hypertrophy
   b. Joint pains
   c. Massive splenomegaly
   d. Neutrophilia
   e. Painless lymphadenopathy

SELF-ASSESSMENT QUESTIONS

9. Which of the following is true in the treatment of CLL?
   a. Induction therapy is the same as for acute lymphoblastic leukaemia
   b. Many patients require no active treatment
   c. Imatinib mesylate has improved the outcome of this disease
   d. Leucophoresis may be required for hyperviscosity
   e. Consolidation is with maintenance rituximab

10. Which of the following is true of multiple myeloma?
    a. Hypercalcaemia is a diagnostic criterion
    b. Paraproteinaemia is present in all cases
    c. Bence–Jones protein is found in serum
    d. The marrow having >10 per cent plasma cells is a diagnostic criterion
    e. It is usually asymptomatic

11. Which three of the following apply to the treatment of myeloma?

    a. Thalidomide is a useful drug
    b. Pathological fracture is best treated with radiotherapy
    c. Transfusion is contraindicated owing to hyperviscosity
    d. Autologous bone marrow transplant is used in younger patients
    e. Bisphosphonates reduce the incidence of pathological fracture
    f. Rituximab improves the response to chemotherapy
    g. Bortizemab is a monoclonal antibody against plasma cell receptors

12. Which three of the following are poor prognostic factors in myeloma?
    a. Raised serum IL-6
    b. High β_2-microglobulin
    c. Extraskeletal plasmacytoma
    d. Serum creatinine >350 μmol/L
    e. Hyponatraemia
    f. Circulating plasma cells
    g. Haemoglobin <10 g/dL

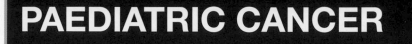

18 PAEDIATRIC CANCER

■ Leukaemia 310
■ Central nervous system tumours 310
■ Bone and soft tissue tumours 313
■ Lymphoma 315
■ Neuroblastoma 316

■ Nephroblastoma (Wilms' tumour) 318
■ Other tumours 321
■ Further reading 322
■ Self-assessment questions 323

Malignant tumours are rare in children, with an incidence of around 1 in 500 children per year in the UK accounting for just over 1500 cases per year. The greatest incidence is under the age of 5 years when around half of all paediatric cancers are diagnosed. Childhood cancer is the most common cause of death in the age groups up to 14 years. Leukaemias account for 32 per cent of cancer deaths in children and central nervous system (CNS) tumours for 30 per cent.

Tumours in children differ from those in adults with relatively more leukaemias and lymphomas and fewer solid epithelial cancers. The general distribution is shown in Table 18.1.

TABLE 18.1 Frequency and type of common paediatric cancers

Cancer	Incidence (%)
Leukaemia	30
CNS tumours	20
Bone and soft tissue	15
Lymphoma	10
Neuroblastoma	7
Nephroblastoma (Wilms')	7
Others	11

Overall, the outlook for paediatric malignancy is far better than for adults, with an overall cure rate approaching 75 per cent. Because of the high cure rate there is now increasing emphasis on the long-term effects of treatment, in particular the influence of chemotherapy and radiotherapy on growth and both physical and intellectual development.

LEUKAEMIA

Leukaemias in childhood are predominantly acute lymphoblastic or less frequently acute myeloblastic leukaemias. Chronic leukaemia, although recognized, is extremely rare. Details of these conditions have been covered in Chapter 17.

CENTRAL NERVOUS SYSTEM TUMOURS

Around 70 per cent of childhood CNS tumours are astrocytomas, predominantly low grade, the management of which has been covered in Chapter 12. Of the remainder, the most common are primitive neuroectodermal tumours (PNETs) of which in turn, medulloblastoma is the most common accounting for 15–20 per cent of the total.

Medulloblastoma

Epidemiology

Medulloblastomas are more common under 5 years than over 5 years and occur in twice as many boys as girls.

Aetiology

There are no recognized aetiological factors in the development of this tumour other than the small proportion, estimated around 2 per cent, which have an inherited component developing within the context of Gorlin's syndrome.

Pathology

Medulloblastoma is a PNET arising in the posterior fossa.

Medulloblastoma accounts for 85 per cent of PNETs; other sites are the pineal (pineal blastomas) and supratentorial regions.

Local growth can result in obstruction of the fourth ventricle or aqueduct causing secondary hydrocephalus. A characteristic feature of this tumour is its propensity to seed throughout the neuroaxis so that meningeal deposits are found at any site both within the skull and down the spinal cord.

Blood-borne metastases have been described, particularly in bone, but these are rare.

Microscopically, the cells are derived from precursors of neuronal tissue and have a characteristic appearance likened to short carrots, forming circles or rosettes.

Cytogenetically around 50 per cent have a deletion of the short arm of chromosome 17, and up to 18 per cent have an abnormality of the short arm of chromosome 9, which is also implicated in Gorlin's syndrome.

Symptoms

In children CNS tumours can have an insidious onset with irritability and failure to achieve appropriate milestones. Children or their parents might complain of specific difficulties with walking or headache. Spinal disease can cause nerve root pains and arm or leg weakness.

Signs

Posterior fossa tumours can cause specific signs of cerebellar dysfunction with incoordination, ataxic gait and scanning dysarthria. There might also be lower cranial nerve signs.

Spinal involvement will cause weakness of limbs and sensory changes, particularly the development of nerve root pains.

Hydrocephalus, causing raised intracranial pressure, can in the young child result in bulging of the fontanelle and increased head circumference.

Differential diagnosis

Other tumours of the posterior fossa should be considered of which the most common is a low-grade astrocytoma. Other rarer tumours include ependymoma and germ cell tumours. Unlike in adults, metastases in the posterior fossa are rare in children.

Investigations

Routine tests such as a full blood count and biochemical screen are usually unremarkable as is routine radiology including a skull X-ray.

CT scan

The tumour will be seen on CT scan, which should be enhanced with intravenous contrast. CT will also demonstrate any degree of hydrocephalus.

MRI

This is superior to CT in imaging the posterior fossa (Fig. 18.1). Some form of spinal imaging is essential to complete the staging process. In the past this has required a myelogram but this can now be replaced by MRI scan as demonstrated in Figure 18.2.

Staging

There is no TNM staging for medulloblastoma, although various other staging systems have been proposed. Essentially patients can be divided by certain prognostic factors into two groups:

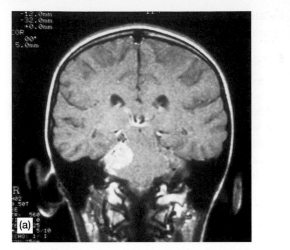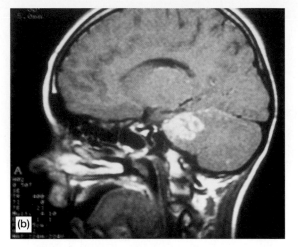

Figure 18.1 MRI showing medulloblastoma arising in posterior cranial fossa. (a) Coronal and (b) sagittal views.

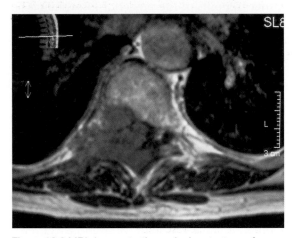

Figure 18.2 MRI demonstrating spinal metastases from medulloblastoma.

■ Good risk – age >3 years; posterior fossa tumour with no dissemination; total excision or <1.5 cm³ residual tumour postoperatively
■ Poor risk – defined by any one of the following criteria: age <3 years, primary site outside posterior fossa; metastatic disease; subtotal resection, i.e. >1.5 cm³ residual tumour.

Treatment

Initial treatment following the diagnosis of a posterior fossa tumour will be surgery. Surgery has three roles in the management of this tumour:

■ to confirm the histological diagnosis from resected tissue
■ to remove all visible tumour if technically possible
■ to relieve hydrocephalus if present by the insertion of a ventriculoperitoneal shunt.

Following surgery, postoperative radiotherapy will be given. This involves treatment of the whole craniospinal axis, i.e. the whole brain and spinal column down to the level of S2 where the thecal sac terminates.

There may also be some benefit from chemotherapy for poor-risk patients as defined above.

Tumour-related complications

Obstructive hydrocephalus may occur. There can be permanent neurological deficits, in particular incoordination and ataxia. Spinal disease can result in permanent limb weakness.

Treatment-related complications

Immediate postoperative complications include meningitis and transient loss of speech (cerebellar mutism). Ventriculoperitoneal shunts may become infected or blocked requiring surgical revision. Craniospinal irradiation can cause significant bone marrow depression, particularly in those patients receiving chemotherapy. Late effects of this treatment include impaired growth, particularly of the spine, resulting in a disproportionate reduction in sitting height compared with standing height. The ovaries are usually included in the sacral radiation field and, unless they are surgically placed outside the irradiated area (oophoropexy), sterility will occur.

Pituitary irradiation within the whole brain volume can result in varying degrees of hypopituitarism requiring appropriate replacement therapy. Late results of whole brain irradiation include long-term neurocognitive effects with a reduction in IQ scores greatest with younger age at the time of irradiation.

Despite these concerns, many patients achieve good results and function normally within society.

Prognosis

The overall long-term cure rate using the above treatment strategies is around 50 per cent.

Rare tumours

Ependymomas

These account for around 8 per cent of childhood brain tumours. When occurring in the posterior fossa, they behave in a very similar fashion to medulloblastomas and the principles of treatment are the same. Cure rates are also similar.

BONE AND SOFT TISSUE TUMOURS

The common bone tumours in children are osteosarcoma and Ewing's sarcoma, both of which are discussed in Chapter 15.

The common soft tissue tumour to occur in children is the embryonal rhabdomyosarcoma. This differs significantly from the alveolar form, which occurs particularly in adolescents, and pleomorphic forms of rhabdomyosarcoma found in adults.

Rhabdomyosarcoma (embryonal type)

Epidemiology

These tumours are usually seen in the first 5 years of life and two-thirds are seen under the age of 10 years. There is an overall incidence of 3 per million children under 15 years of age in the UK. They arise in any site, the most common being the head and neck region and the genitourinary tract.

Aetiology

There are no known aetiological factors.

Pathology

Approximately one-third arise in the head and neck region, one-third in the genitourinary tract and a quarter in the soft tissues of the trunk or extremities. The orbit is also a relatively frequent site, accounting for 10 per cent of the total.

Macroscopically, they appear as pink fleshy masses and proliferative forms are likened to bunches of grapes ('sarcoma botryoides').

Microscopically, they are embryonal cells rich in glycogen and within which myofibrils can be demonstrated. Immunohistochemistry will be positive for desmin, myoglobin, myo-D1 and muscle-specific actin. The embryonal subtype is distinct from the alveolar rhabdomyosarcoma of adults, although this type can be seen in older children and adolescents.

A specific chromosome deletion has been identified at chromosome 11p15 associated with embryonal type distinct from the other subtypes of rhabdomyosarcoma. Other associated genetic mutations include point mutations in the N-ras and K-ras oncogenes.

Natural history

The natural history of this form of rhabdomyosarcoma is for rapid local growth with infiltration along tissue planes and early blood-borne metastases. Around one in five patients will have bone marrow infiltration at presentation and 15–20 per cent will have evidence of distant metastases. Lymph node spread also occurs, particularly in those tumours arising in the genitourinary tract and limbs.

Symptoms

Presenting symptoms depend on site of origin. Many arise as rapidly enlarging but painless masses. Other local symptoms can be present including nasal obstruction and epistaxis from the nasopharynx, haematuria from the urinary tract, vaginal bleeding from the vagina or uterus. Orbital tumours can cause local discomfort and blurred or double vision.

Signs

Clinical signs will go along with the presenting symptoms. There might be an obvious mass visible. Vaginal tumours can present with a fleshy mass of 'botryoid' tumour at the introitus. Orbital tumours will cause proptosis and ophthalmoplegia.

Differential diagnosis

In childhood there are few other tumours likely to arise in similar sites to rhabdomyosarcoma. Other causes of presenting symptoms such as epistaxis or haematuria in the absence of an obvious mass should be sought.

Investigations

Routine tests such as full blood count and biochemistry may well be normal.

Radiography

Chest X-ray sometimes demonstrates lung metastases.

CT scan and MRI

CT scan or MRI of the affected site will be valuable in delineating the extent of local tumour most accurately.

Bone marrow examination

Bone marrow examination should be performed in view of the high incidence of marrow involvement and skeletal X-ray survey or isotope bone scan should also be performed.

Biopsy

A full examination of the affected site under anaesthetic with biopsy of the tumour is essential to confirm the diagnosis.

Lumbar puncture to examine CSF is indicated for parameningeal tumours to exclude meningeal disease.

Staging

TNM staging is used and is based on postsurgical status:

- ■ T1 – Tumour limited to site of origin with microscopic margins of excision clear
- ■ T2 – Tumour extending beyond site of origin but complete microscopic clearance of tumour
- ■ T3 – Tumour extending beyond site of origin with incomplete excision
- ■ N0 – Regional nodes negative
- ■ NI – Regional nodes involved
- ■ M0 – No metastases
- ■ M1 – Distant metastases.

In practice group staging as used by the Intergroup Rhabdomyosarcoma Studies (IRS) may be of more value:

- ■ Stage I: – Localized disease completely resected
- ■ Stage II: – Either localized disease with residual microscopic disease or node involvement completely resected (IIB) or node involvement with microscopic residual disease (IIC)
- ■ Stage III: – Incomplete resection or biopsy only
- ■ Stage IV: – Distant metastases at diagnosis.

Around 50 per cent of patients will be stage III at diagnosis and 20 per cent will present with metastases.

Treatment

Radical treatment

Chemotherapy

Chemotherapy is given to all cases; good risk patients, which includes stage I orbital and paratesticular tumours, can receive vincristine and actinomycin D alone. Others will have VAC (vincristine, actinomycin D and cyclophosphamide). In advanced disease additional agents can be used such as topotecan or irinotecan.

One or two courses are given followed by definitive surgery or radiotherapy and then chemotherapy is continued for a period of up to 1 year.

Surgery

This is the treatment of choice in the absence of advanced distant metastases. For urogenital, truncal and limb rhabdomyosarcoma, wide resection is usually performed.

Radiotherapy

This is used for inoperable tumours such as orbit and nasopharynx, delivering doses of around 50 Gy in 5 weeks.

Palliative treatment

For recurrent disseminated disease a course of palliative chemotherapy or radiotherapy could be valuable in minimizing symptoms. Second-line chemotherapy using drugs such as ifosfamide and etoposide might achieve good responses, although further relapse is usual. Local recurrence, particularly in patients with the botyroid type of tumour, should be treated actively as there is a high salvage rate in this group.

Tumour-related complications

These will depend on the site. Urogenital tumours can permanently affect renal, urinary and reproductive function, and orbital tumours can affect sight.

Treatment-related complications

Chemotherapy using VAC can cause nausea, vomiting and alopecia during the period of administration. In the longer term peripheral neuropathy from vincristine can persist.

Radical surgery sometimes has late sequelae depending on the type of procedure. There are obvious effects of cystectomy or hysterectomy for urogenital tumours.

Radical radiotherapy can have late sequelae also, in particular growth impairment in the treated area. In a young child, this can result in quite marked disfigurement if significant asymmetry develops, as may be the case following, for example, orbit irradiation.

Prognosis

The overall prognosis for embryonal rhabdomyosarcoma confined to the site of origin is good with cure rates of around 80 per cent. Once metastatic, the outlook is poor with less than 20 per cent surviving.

Age and site are important predictors of cure. The best prognoses are associated with tumours of the orbit, paratesticular region and vagina. Poor prognosis sites are parameningeal, prostate and perineum. Patients with metastatic disease aged <10 years have a significantly better outcome than older patients.

LYMPHOMA

Both Hodgkin's disease and non-Hodgkin's lymphoma occur in children. While they obey the general rules discussed in Chapter 16, there are certain features of paediatric lymphomas which should be considered.

Non-Hodgkin's lymphoma

NHL in children is usually a high-grade nodal disease with a particular propensity for diffuse lymphoblastic or undifferentiated tumours, and also T-cell lymphomas associated with a mediastinal mass. Low-grade NHL is rare in children.

Treatment usually involves combination chemotherapy and, for extensive high-grade disease, bone marrow transplant can be considered. Local radiotherapy can also be given in doses of 25–30 Gy.

Hodgkin's disease

Hodgkin's disease is relatively more common in boys than in girls, which is in contrast to a more even sex distribution in adults. Lymphocyte-predominant histology is relatively more common and the less favourable lymphocyte-depleted form uncommon.

Treatment is based on the same principles as in adult Hodgkin's disease but with even greater emphasis on minimizing late effects. For this reason chemotherapy is often preferred for relatively early disease, avoiding the local growth problems after radiotherapy. Schedules containing vincristine, procarbazine, prednisolone and Adriamycin (OPPA) and OEPA, which substitutes etoposide for procarbazine, combined with localized radiotherapy, have been highly successful. Where irradiation is used, lower doses of around 20–30 Gy are given compared with 30–35 Gy in adults.

NEUROBLASTOMA

Epidemiology

Neuroblastoma is a tumour of young children, 50 per cent occurring before the age of 2 years and 80 per cent under 5 years. It has an annual incidence of 8 per million in the UK and is slightly more common in boys than in girls. There is some geographical variation: it is rare in Africa compared with Europe and the US.

Aetiology

There is an association with von Recklinghausen's disease (multiple neurofibromatosis) and colonic aganglionosis, but most cases have no recognizable causal factor. There is some evidence that it arises as a congenital anomaly and cases in utero have been reported.

Specific chromosome abnormalities have been identified in neuroblastoma, including amplification of the *N-myc* oncogene, deletions affecting chromosome 1 and gain of the long arm of chromosome 17(17q).

Pathology

Two-thirds of neuroblastomas are intra-abdominal tumours, of which 60 per cent occur in the adrenal and 40 per cent at other sites related to the sympathetic chain. The remaining third are divided between the chest, pelvis and head and neck region. In a small number of these tumours, widespread metastatic disease may be present with no recognizable primary site.

Macroscopically, the tumour is usually encapsulated but soft and friable, containing areas of haemorrhage, necrosis, cystic degeneration and calcification.

Microscopically, there is a spectrum of appearances depending on the degree of differentiation. Typically it is composed of densely packed, small round cells which can form rosettes. In the more differentiated forms neurofibrils and ganglionic elements and granule-containing chromaffin cells can be seen.

Natural history

Local infiltration of surrounding tissues is seen.

Regional lymph nodes can be involved but the predominant pattern of metastases is by early blood-borne dissemination with around two-thirds of children having widespread disease at presentation, affecting in particular bone and liver. Lung metastases are relatively rare.

Spontaneous maturation and regression may occur. At post mortem there is a much higher incidence of asymptomatic tumours in patients dying from unrelated conditions than in the general population.

Symptoms

These will depend on the site and age at presentation.

Abdominal tumours, which are the most common, will present with abdominal discomfort and bowel or urinary obstruction.

In the head and neck a painless mass may be the first manifestation.

There also may be fever, anorexia, malaise and weight loss.

Metastatic disease can cause the first symptoms, particularly bone pain from bone metastases.

Excessive catecholamine production from the tumour cells causes flushing, palpitations, diarrhoea and headache.

Rarely in utero it presents with pre-eclampsia in the mother.

Signs

These may include:

■   a palpable mass

- intrathoracic tumours, causing venous obstruction with dilated neck veins, plethora and oedema
- catecholamine secretion, causing hypertension.

There are rare neurological syndromes associated with neuroblastoma, in particular an acute cerebellar disturbance (opsomyoclonus) characterized by truncal ataxia and rapid random eye movements (so-called 'dancing feet', 'dancing eyes').

Differential diagnosis

A palpable mass must be distinguished from other types of tumour. In the abdomen this will include Wilms' tumour and in the neck a lymph node from lymphoma.

The differential diagnosis of a small round cell tumour in bone includes not only neuroblastoma but also rhabdomyosarcma, Ewing's sarcoma and lymphoma. A benign couterpart, ganglioneuroma, and the transitional tumour, ganglioneuroblastoma, might also have similar pathological appearances.

Investigations

Routine blood tests can be unremarkable but extensive bone metastases can cause pancytopenia and there could also be obstructive renal impairment.

Radiography

X-ray of the tumour can demonstrate speckled calcification within it.

CT scan or MRI

CT scan or MRI is needed for more accurate definition of the tumour.

Bone marrow examination

This examination is important because of the high incidence of bone metastases.

Urine tests

Twenty-four-hour urine collections will be made to measure catecholamines such as vanillylmandelic acid (VMA) and homovanillylmandelic acid (HVA), the ratio of the two having prognostic importance. Other peptides such as vasoactive intestinal peptide (VIP) might also be raised.

Biopsy of the accessible tumour confirms the diagnosis; ploidy and cytogenetics should be undertaken to give additional prognostic information.

Other tests

Because many of the tumours will contain cells synthesizing catecholamines from their precursors a labelled precursor called meta-iodobenzyl guanidine (mIBG) may be used as a tracer in scanning labelled with radioactive iodine. This also has therapeutic uses.

Serum levels of neurone-specific enolase (NSE), ferritin and ganglioside GD2 have prognostic value.

Staging

The International Staging System, which combines the older Audrey Evans and COG (Childrens' Cancer Group) classification, is used based on postoperative status:

- Stage 1 – Confined to the site of origin with complete macroscopic excision; lymph nodes negative
- Stage 2
  - Stage 2A – Unilateral tumour with incomplete gross excision; lymph nodes negative
  - Stage 2B – Unilateral tumour with incomplete gross excision; positive ipsilateral lymph nodes but contralateral nodes negative
- Stage 3 – Unresectable tumour extending beyond site of origin across midline with or without positive lymph node involvement; or unilateral tumour with contralateral positive lymph nodes or midline tumour with bilateral positive lymph nodes
- Stage 4 – Distant metastases
  - Stage 4S – Infants (<2 years) with local tumour not crossing midline but with liver, skin or bone marrow involvement (<10 per cent) but without bone metastases.

Treatment

Stages 1 and 2

Local treatment alone is given by radical surgical excision. Postoperative radiotherapy is given for older children (>1 year) or those with poor prognostic features on histology, in particular poorly differentiated tumours and those with aneuploidy or *N-myc* amplification. Neuroblastoma is very sensitive to irradiation and doses of only 20–30 Gy over 3–4 weeks are adequate.

Stages 3 and 4

Chemotherapy using a combination of cyclophosphamide and vincristine with the addition of Adriamycin, etoposide or cisplatin is given to those over 1 year of age. Resection of or radiotherapy to the primary tumour can be considered before or after cytoreduction with chemotherapy.

Intensive chemotherapy using high doses of drugs such as melphalan with or without autologous bone marrow transplant could be of value and has been shown to be superior to conventional dose consolidation chemotherapy for those with poor prognostic features.

Targeted radiation using iodine-131-labelled mIBG, which is actively concentrated in cells synthesizing catecholamines, is also used.

13-cis retinoic acid can be used in consolidation programmes for high-risk tumours.

Palliative treatment

Local radiotherapy for painful bone metastases or large tumour masses can be given.

Stage 4S disease

With little or no treatment spontaneous regression of tumour occurs. Vincristine or low-dose irradiation might be indicated for pressure symptoms from a large liver or other tumour mass.

Tumour-related complications

Mediastinal, renal or intestinal obstruction can occur, depending on primary site. Excess catecholamine secretion can cause hypertension and tachycardia with arrhythmias. Diarrhoea occurs if vasoactive intestinal peptide (VIP) is produced.

Treatment-related complications

Irradiation of the abdomen of a child can cause bowel or renal damage. It is important to design symmetrical fields of irradiation to minimize deformity from growth retardation.

Intensive chemotherapy regimens result in profound bone marrow suppression with the risks of neutropenic sepsis. Treatment-related mortality is 2–3 per cent with such intensive schedules.

Prognosis

The prognosis for localized neuroblastoma is good with virtually all patients with stage 1 disease and 80 per cent of those with stage 2 cured. Stage 4S also has a good outlook with cure rates approaching 80 per cent. In contrast older patients with metastatic disease have a very poor prognosis with long-term survival between 10 and 40 per cent. Important prognostic factors are hyperploidy conferring a good prognosis and diploidy or *N-myc* expression predicting a poor outcome.

Future developments

More dose-intensive chemotherapy regimens are being evaluated in those patients identified as having a poor prognosis on the basis of chromosomal changes. 13-cis retinoic acid has an increasing role in consolidation and remains under active evaluation in current trials. In experimental systems vaccines have been developed which are under evaluation together with monocloncal antibody therapy.

NEPHROBLASTOMA (WILMS' TUMOUR)

Epidemiology

Wilms' tumour (WT) is a tumour of young children with a peak incidence at 3 years and the majority occurring before the age of 5 years. The annual incidence is 1 in 20 000 children in the UK and there is equal distribution between boys and girls.

Aetiology

WT is familial in 1–2 per cent of cases and there is marked racial variation with an incidence of 2.5 per million in Chinese children to 10.9 per million in African American children.

There is an association with certain rare congenital abnormalities including Beckwith–Weidemann syndrome, hemi-hypertrophy, aniridia, Bloom's syndrome and other abnormalities of the urogenital tract. Trisomy 18 is another associated disorder and a deletion on the short arm of chromosome 11 (11p13) is seen in around one-third of cases of WT as well as certain other abnormalities of the genitourinary system such as hypospadias and cryptorchidism. The gene that causes aniridia is also located close to this position on chromosome 11. This has led to identification of the *WT1* gene associated with WT; this encodes a transcription factor critical for normal kidney develoment. Other deletions in WT are seen on chromosomes 16 and 1p.

Genetic linkage studies have identified two loci on chromosomes 17 and 19, *FWT1* and *FWT2*. Loss of heterozygosity at either of these sites conveys a relatively poor prognosis.

Pathology

The tumour arises in the kidney and 5 per cent are bilateral. It can be lobular and is surrounded by a pseudocapsule as it compresses surrounding tissue. There might be areas of haemorrhage, necrosis and cyst formation.

Microscopically, there is often considerable variety within the tumour with areas of primitive mesenchymal cells, which can show differentiation into fat, muscle or cartilage within which are areas of recognizable embryonal glomerular and renal tubular elements.

Certain microscopic features are of prognostic importance. Anaplastic areas are associated with a worse prognosis, particularly if there are

diffuse rather than focal areas of anaplastic change. Previously subtypes labelled sarcomatous and clear cell are now thought to be distinct entities rather than variants of WT and also have a poor prognosis.

Natural history

Local invasion from the renal parenchyma into the renal pelvis and renal vein will occur. Lymph node involvement is relatively infrequent.

Blood-borne metastases are the usual means of spread beyond the kidney, the most common distant site being the lungs.

Symptoms

Abdominal pain is the most common presenting feature.

Haematuria occurs in about 20 per cent and a similar proportion can have unexplained fevers. Other systemic symptoms, however, are unusual.

Pulmonary metastases can cause cough, haemoptysis or dyspnoea.

Signs

The majority have a palpable abdominal mass at presentation which can be entirely asymptomatic. Hypertension can be present but is relatively unusual.

Differential diagnosis

Abdominal neuroblastoma can also present with a large abdominal mass but is usually associated with greater systemic upset and bone metastases rather than lung metastases.

Investigations

Blood tests

A full blood count might show anaemia and urea and electrolytes can be disturbed.

Urine tests

Urinalysis can show both blood and protein in the urine.

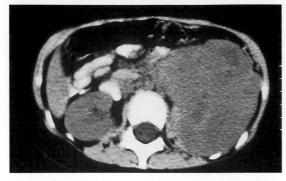

Figure 18.3 CT scan demonstrating large renal mass in nephroblastoma.

Radiography

Chest X-ray can demonstrate lung metastases, but CT is now preferred to give higher and more accurate resolution.

Other tests

The primary tumour will be seen on abdominal ultrasound; CT has replaced IVU as the diagnostic imaging of choice as shown in Figure 18.3.

Staging

The largest group investigating Wilms' tumour is the National Wilms' Tumour Study Group in the US and their staging system is commonly reported:

- Stage 1 – Tumour completely excised and retained within capsule
- Stage 2 – Tumour completely excised but extending beyond capsule
- Stage 3 – Tumour incompletely excised but no blood-borne metastases
- Stage 4 – Blood-borne distant metastases
- Stage 5 – Bilateral tumours.

Around 5 per cent will present with bilateral tumours and a second tumour develops in the contralateral kidney in up to 3 per cent.

Treatment

Surgery by laparotomy and radical resection of the tumour is performed, which will usually entail a nephro-ureterectomy and regional node dissection. An important feature of the operation should be mobilization and careful inspection of the contralateral kidney in view of the significant incidence of bilateral tumours.

Postoperative radiotherapy or chemotherapy are used as follows:

- Where histology shows no anaplastic elements:
  - Stage 1 and 2 disease is given a short course (usually over 18 weeks) of vincristine with actinomycin D
  - Stages 3 and 4 are given chemotherapy using vincristine, actinomycin D and Adriamycin with radiotherapy to the renal bed delivering 20–30 Gy in 3–4 weeks
- Where histology shows anaplastic tumour:
  - Stage 1 disease is given a short course of vincristine with actinomycin D
  - Stages 2, 3 and 4 are treated with more intensive chemotherapy using vincristine, Adriamycin, etoposide, and cyclophosphamide. In patients who respond satisfactorily, radiotherapy to the renal bed and metastatic sites can be given
  - Stage 5 disease is a special and more difficult case. Initial chemotherapy will be given to achieve tumour shrinkage and allow surgery with the intent of performing nephron-sparing surgery or partial nephrectomy. Postoperative treatment will then continue as above.

Palliative treatment

This can take the form of chemotherapy or local radiotherapy to symptomatic disease. High-dose chemotherapy with bone marrow rescue has been used but may be no better than alternative alternating chemotherapy regimens using ifosfamide, etoposide and carboplatin. Around 50 per cent of patients might be salvaged after recurrence. For chemotherapy-resistant lung disease low-dose whole lung irradiation can be given, delivering 10–12 Gy in 7 or 8 small fractions.

Tumour-related complications

Most survivors will have normal renal function, the incidence of renal failure being 1 per cent or less.

Treatment-related complications

Radiotherapy to the renal bed will include the lumbar vertebrae and there will therefore be growth retardation in this area. Because of this it is extremely important that the radiotherapist includes the entire width of the vertebral body to avoid a scoliotic deformity owing to differential growth across the vertebral body.

Immediate side-effects of chemotherapy include nausea, vomiting and alopecia. In the longer term vincristine can be associated with a peripheral neuropathy, actinomycin D with liver dysfunction and Adriamycin with dose-related cardiomyopathy.

Prognosis

Wilms' tumour is both radio- and chemosensitive and the prognosis for localized disease is therefore very good with 80–90 per cent of patients with stage 1 or 2 disease being cured. Even those presenting with distant metastases (stage 4) have a cure rate of up to 40 per cent.

Rare tumours

The rhabdoid tumour of kidney is highly malignant metastasizing widely to lungs and CNS in particular. Clear cell sarcoma of the kidney also disseminates widely and both have a far worse prognosis than WT.

OTHER TUMOURS

Langerhans' cell histiocytosis

This is a complex condition arising from a proliferation of histiocytes. Three distinct forms are recognized:

- Letterer–Siwe disease
- Hand–Schüller–Christian disease
- Eosinophilic granuloma.

Letterer–Siwe disease affects infants and is usually rapidly fatal owing to widespread infiltration of liver, spleen, skin and lymph nodes with proliferating histiocytes.

Hand–Schüller–Christian disease occurs at any age with a less fulminant course and is once again characterized by widespread infiltration of histiocytes which in this case is characterized by intracellular accumulation of lipid. Bones in particular are affected and patients survive for many years, although most ultimately succumb. It cn be treated using drug combinations such as VAC (vincristine, Adriamycin or actinomycin D and cyclophosphamide).

Eosinophilic granuloma is the least aggressive form of the disease and is usually localized, presenting as solitary lytic bone lesions. Deposits around the pituitary are a recognized cause of diabetes insipidus. They are characterized by accumulations of lipid-filled histiocytes, eosinophils and giant cells. They can regress spontaneously. If symptomatic they respond well to low doses of irradiation.

Retinoblastoma

This is a rare tumour present in around 1 in 20 000 live births in the UK and usually presents in the first 2 years of life. There are two distinct forms: 40 per cent are hereditary bilateral or multifocal tumours characterized by germ-line mutations in the retinoblastoma gene and the remainder are non-hereditary unifocal or unilateral tumours.

The retinoblastoma gene is located on chromosome 13q,14 and was one of the first tumour-suppressor genes to be identified.

Retinoblastoma presents with reduced vision, characteristic white pupils or strabismus. As the tumour occludes fluid drainage within the eye secondary glaucoma can develop. The diagnosis is confirmed on examination of both eyes under anaesthetic. An example is shown in Figure 18.4.

Small tumours can be treated by light coagulation using a xenon arc laser or cryotherapy. Larger tumours can be treated with neoadjuvant chemotherapy using carboplatin, vincristine and etoposide followed by radiotherapy, which can be delivered either by placing over the tumour cobalt discs or with external beam treatment where most of the eye has to be included. Enucleation is avoided but could be necessary if the optic nerve is invaded.

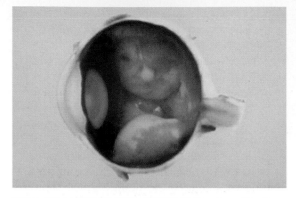

Figure 18.4 Lateral section of eyeball showing extensive primary retinoblastoma.

Most tumours are cured using this approach with preservation of vision.

Genetic counselling is an important feature of further management; the risk of retinoblastoma developing in children of a patient with the hereditary bilateral form of the tumour is 45 per cent; it is only 2.5 per cent for those with unilateral non-hereditary tumours.

Germ cell tumours

Teratomas present in the first 5 years. The majority are benign but 20 per cent or so will be malignant. The common sites are the ovary and the sacrococcygeal region but they are also found in the mediastinum, neck, nasopharynx, retroperitoneum or brain.

The management of these tumours is essentially that of germ cell tumours in the adult. Initial treatment will be surgical removal where possible followed by appropriate adjuvant chemotherapy using combinations such as BEP (bleomycin, etoposide and cisplatin). Local radiotherapy is considered where surgical excision is not feasible, as in the brain. Overall the prognosis, as in adult germ cell tumours, is good.

FURTHER READING

Voute P, Barrett A, Stevens MCG, Caron HN (eds). *Cancer in Children: clinical management*. Fifth Edition. Oxford University Press, Oxford, 2005

SELF-ASSESSMENT QUESTIONS

1. Which of the following is true of childhood cancer?
   a. Acute leukaemia causes one-third of childhood cancer deaths
   b. The peak incidence is in the 5–10-year age group
   c. The most common solid tumour is nephroblastoma
   d. It is more common in lower socioeconomic groups
   e. After trauma it is the second most common cause of death up to the age of 15 years

2. Which three of the following apply to medulloblastoma?
   a. It is a primitive neuroectodermal tumour (PNET)
   b. It occurs in the posterior fossa of the skull
   c. It is related to hypoxic birth injury
   d. It is most common over 5 years of age
   e. It disseminates to distant blood-borne sites at an early stage
   f. It can be cured by radical surgery
   g. Seeding along the craniospinal axis is characteristic

3. Which of the following is true of bone and soft tissue tumours in children?
   a. The most common bone tumour is chondrosarcoma
   b. Ewing's sarcoma is usually extraskeletal in children
   c. Osteosarcoma typically affects the limb girdles
   d. Embryonal rhabdomyosarcoma is the common form in children
   e. The prognosis is worse in children than adults

4. Which of the following is true of rhabdomyosarcoma in childhood?
   a. Initial surgery may be curative
   b. They typically arise in the limbs

   c. Urogenital tumours commonly seed to the CNS
   d. Chemotherapy containing vincristine will be given to all patients
   e. Over 50 per cent have metastases at presentation

5. Which three of the following are true of neuroblastoma?
   a. The majority are intra-abdominal
   b. Most present in the first 2 years of life
   c. It may be associated with the retinoblastoma gene
   d. Stage IVS usually requires no treatment
   e. Catecholamines are detectable in the urine
   f. CNS prophylaxis is required after induction treatment
   g. Lung metastases are relatively common

6. Which of the following is true of nephroblastoma?
   a. It arises from the suprarenal gland
   b. Lymph node metastases are common
   c. It is bilateral in 5 per cent of cases
   d. It is more common in trisomy 21
   e. The majority occur between 5 and 10 years of age

7. Which of the following is true of the treatment of nephroblastoma?
   a. Initial treatment is with chemotherapy
   b. Chemotherapy is followed by radiotherapy to the involved side
   c. Nephro-ureterectomy is the usual operation
   d. Chemotherapy is reserved for anaplastic tumours
   e. Radiotherapy should avoid as much of the vertebra as possible

8. Which three of the following are true of retinoblastoma?
   a. Hereditary forms account for 40 per cent
   b. Enucleation is the treatment of choice

SELF-ASSESSMENT QUESTIONS

c. Meningeal infiltration is common
d. Survival beyond 5 years is unusual
e. Lung metastases are common
f. The retinoblastoma gene is a tumour-suppressor gene
g. Genetic counselling is important in management

9. Which of the following is true of germ cell tumours in children?
   a. The testis is the common site in boys
   b. The majority are malignant teratomas
   c. They are common in the sacrococcygeal region
   d. Initial treatment will be with BEP chemotherapy
   e. Benign teratomas are best managed with local radiotherapy

10. Which of the following is true of Langerhans' cell histiocytosis?
    a. The most aggressive form is Hand–Schüller–Christian disease
    b. Letterer–Siwe disease may regress spontaneously
    c. They may transform into a histiocytic lymphoma
    d. Eosinophilic granuloma is usually a solitary lytic bone lesion
    e. More than one form may be present at initial diagnosis

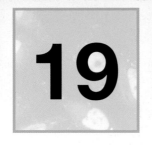

19 SKIN CANCER

■ Squamous and basal cell carcinoma   325
■ Melanoma   331
■ Metastases   338

■ Rare tumours   338
■ Further reading   339
■ Self-assessment questions   340

The skin is the largest organ in the body. Its large surface area and location make it particularly vulnerable to environmental carcinogens. Recent cultural, economic and environmental changes have resulted in many more people being exposed to high levels of ultraviolet radiation. As this is the main risk factor for developing skin cancer, many more cases can be expected in the decades to come.

SQUAMOUS AND BASAL CELL CARCINOMA

Epidemiology

Each year in the UK there are 72 000 cases of non-melanomatous skin cancer, 39 000 cases in men and 33 000 cases in women, accounting for 26 per cent of all cancer cases and leading to a total of 500 deaths per annum. Basal cell carcinoma (BCC) is twice as common as squamous cell carcinoma (SCC). The peak incidence is at 60–80 years and it is exceptional in the under-40s in whom a strong aetiological factor can usually be identified, e.g. Gorlin's syndrome, arsenic exposure. It is more common in white people living in a sunny climate, particularly South Africa and Australia, the incidence increasing as one moves closer to the equator. It is only rarely encountered in dark-skinned races.

Aetiology

Ultraviolet radiation is the most important cause accounting for the geographical and racial distribution of skin cancers. They are therefore most frequent on sun-exposed areas of the body. Previous radiotherapy can lead to skin cancer at the entry or exit site of the radiation. Radiation-induced cancers were a particular problem to the pioneering radiologists who used to calibrate their X-ray machines by exposing their hands to a dose sufficient to cause erythema of the skin.

Tar and soot are rich in aromatic hydrocarbons. SCC of the scrotum was described in nineteenth-century chimney sweeps where soot had become trapped in the rugose skin of the scrotum. Similarly, occupational exposure to tar and bitumen can lead to tumours on the exposed skin, and mineral oils were the cause of SCC described in yarn workers where they used to lubricate the spinning mules.

Arsenic is a potent cause of skin cancers and a history of exposure should be sought in patients with multiple BCCs and SCCs. It was once used as a 'tonic' and is found in some pesticides.

SCC has been described arising in chronic varicose (Marjolin's) ulcers, burn scars, cutaneous TB, sinuses from chronic osteomyelitis, and epidermolysis bullosa.

Gorlin's syndrome is a very rare, dominantly inherited syndrome predisposing to multiple BCCs and should be considered in all cases arising in those under 40 years of age. Palmar pits are characteristic but other features include bifid ribs, a calcified falx cerebris, frontal bossing of the skull and mandibular cysts. Xeroderma pigmentosum is even rarer, recessively inherited, and patients inevitably develop multiple BCCs and SCCs at a very young age.

Chronic immunosuppression by agents such as azathioprine and cyclosporin in organ transplant recipients is associated with an increased incidence of BCC and SCC.

Pathology

The tumours usually arise on sun-exposed skin such as the scalp, nose, ears, periorbital tissues and dorsum of hand. BCC is very rare in non-hair-bearing skin such as the palms and soles. They are frequently multiple, with changes of solar damage in surrounding skin such as keratoses. An invasive SCC can arise in an area of in situ carcinoma such as Bowen's disease. SCCs are usually well circumscribed, appearing as nodules, nodules with some central ulceration or ulcers with raised, everted, nodular edges (Fig. 19.1). A BCC can also appear predominantly nodular, ulcerating or mixed, and often have characteristic surface telangiectasia and a 'pearly' appearance (Fig. 19.2).

They vary greatly in rate of growth, some persisting unnoticed for many years, others growing rapidly over a period of several months. Large, neglected tumours (Figs. 19.3 and 19.4) are accompanied by local tissue destruction and secondary infection. Both BCCs and SCCs can occur concurrently in the same patient.

Microscopically, these tumours are locally invasive, often for some distance beyond their macroscopic margins. The cell of origin of a

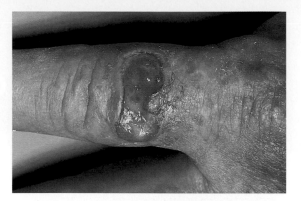

Figure 19.1 A typical ulcerating squamous carcinoma arising on the skin of a finger. Note the irregular, slightly everted edge.

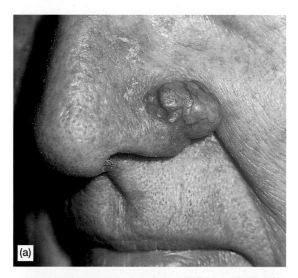

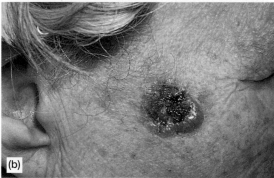

Figure 19.2 Basal cell carcinoma. (a) Nodular variant. (b) Ulcerating variant.

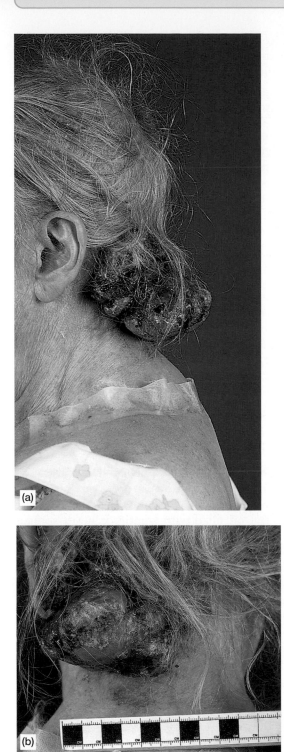

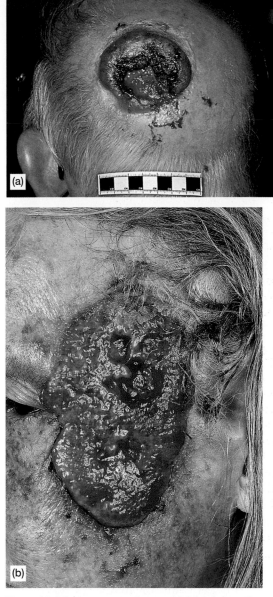

Figure 19.4 Squamous carcinoma. (a) Arising from the skin overlying the vertex of the skull. Such tumours may penetrate into the skull and involve the underlying brain. (b) Large plaque of tumour arising from temple.

Figure 19.3 Basal cell carcinoma. This lesion had been neglected for 20 years and covered by a headscarf. Surgical excision was curative. (a) Side view. (b) Rear view.

BCC is uncertain, but thought to be a basal cell of a hair follicle giving rise to small dark-staining cells. SCCs arise from keratinocytes, are well differentiated, demonstrate intercellular bridges on electron microscopy and produce

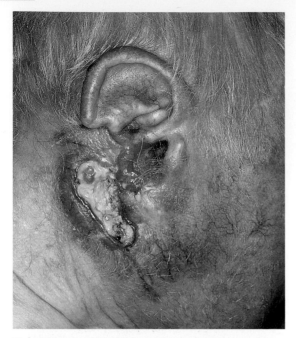

Figure 19.5 Nodal relapse of squamous carcinoma. This man had originally undergone surgery for a carcinoma arising from the pinna. There is now invasion and ulceration of skin overlying an enlarged lymph node.

keratin. Sometimes the appearances are those of a mixed 'basisquamous' tumour.

Natural history

Both types of tumour are characterized by relentless local infiltration of the surrounding skin and normal tissues lying deep to or adjacent to the skin leading to their eventual destruction. About 5 per cent of SCCs and less than 0.1 per cent of BCCs spread to the regional lymph nodes (Fig. 19.5).

Blood-borne spread is rare for SCCs and extremely rare for BCCs. Lung and bone are the most common sites of metastatic spread.

Symptoms

The patient can be asymptomatic, the lesion being noticed at a routine medical examination, or the patient might complain of a skin lesion which is causing concern or cosmetic defect.

Ulcerating lesions can bleed spontaneously if traumatized and irritation is a common complaint, although pain is exceptional.

Signs

Careful inspection under a bright light with a magnifying glass is recommended as it is the most accurate way of defining the macroscopic extent of the tumour, which may be much greater than naked eye inspection would suggest. Telangiectasia suggests a BCC. Otherwise, it is difficult to distinguish an SCC from a BCC by appearance alone. The tumour can be tethered or fixed to underlying tissues depending on the depth of invasion. There can be much destruction of the surrounding tissues and secondary infection of the tumour. Regional lymph nodes should be examined in all cases.

Differential diagnosis

This includes:

- keratoacanthoma
- solar keratosis
- Bowen's disease.

Keratoacanthoma is a benign lesion. It is confused with an SCC and can grow very rapidly to form a large conical lesion with a characteristic central pit filled with keratin. It never spreads beyond the skin and usually resolves spontaneously within several weeks/months. Solar keratosis is a benign lesion seen in sun-damaged skin. It is usually a hyperkeratotic plaque with no evidence of nodularity, ulceration or invasion of the adjacent tissues.

Investigations

It is essential to obtain a tissue diagnosis in all cases prior to treatment.

Skin scraping cytology

This is the least traumatic means of obtaining a sample for analysis. A scalpel is used to scratch the surface of the tumour until the skin begins to bleed lightly, and the debris smeared onto a microscope slide. In conjunction with interpretation by a skilled cytopathologist, it is a sensitive test and can give a result within hours, but equivocal or obviously inconsistent results mean that a biopsy is necessary.

Incision biopsy

A wedge of tissue is removed, with care taken to include representative tumour and surrounding normal skin. This is usually performed when the lesion is too extensive to be treated with surgery.

Excision biopsy

This is best for small lesions that can be easily excised as it provides an accurate histological diagnosis and can be curative if microscopically complete.

Fine needle aspiration (FNA) of any enlarged regional lymph nodes

Although unusual, enlarged lymph nodes should be sampled by FNA to confirm malignancy.

Radiological investigations

Plain radiographs or a limited CT scan are indicated for very large, deeply invasive tumours to delineate their margins when treatment is being planned.

Staging

There is no formal staging system in routine clinical use.

Treatment

Both surgery and radiotherapy achieve local control in about 95 per cent of cases. The choice is dependent on the anatomical site, size of lesion, convenience and previous treatment.

Surgery

This is the treatment of choice for:

- very large tumours involving bone (radiotherapy would have a reduced local control and risk of osteonecrosis)
- scalp lesions (where radiotherapy would produce an area of permanent alopecia)

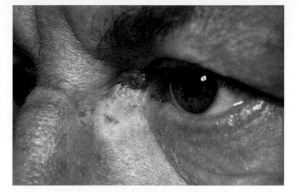

Figure 19.6 Recurrent basal cell carcinoma. This lesion has arisen at the edge of a previous radiation field. Such recurrences are best treated surgically.

- tumours arising in regions that do not tolerate radiotherapy well, e.g. skin overlying lower third of tibia in the elderly
- tumours of the upper eyelid where radiotherapy scarring could cause repeated trauma to the cornea
- local recurrences after radiotherapy (Fig. 19.6) or arising in previously irradiated skin
- young patients in whom the late cutaneous effects of radiotherapy will have longer to become manifest.

Excision is usually performed under local anaesthetic, although large lesions requiring a skin graft or flap reconstruction can be removed under general anaesthetic. Facial lesions are best dealt with by a plastic surgeon to optimize the cosmetic result. Complete macroscopic and microscopic excision will be curative for SCC and BCC and so a margin of macroscopically normal skin of up to 10 mm (depending on size of tumour, cytological type and how well circumscribed it is) should be taken away en bloc.

Surgery is the treatment of choice for cases with involved regional lymph nodes when a block dissection is indicated. Overall local control rates of 95 per cent or more are to be expected after excision alone. Patients with involved resection margins should be considered for re-excision or referred for radiotherapy as these patients will be at high risk of local recurrence.

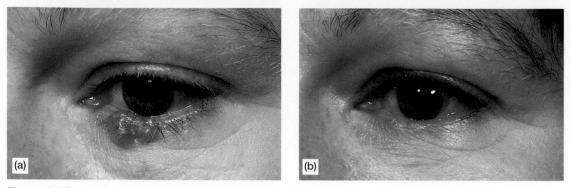

Figure 19.7 Basal cell carcinoma arising from the lower eyelid in a young woman (a) before treatment and (b) after radiotherapy. Note the permanent loss of eyelashes along the lower eyelid.

Radiotherapy

Radiotherapy is equivalent to surgery in terms of local control and is better for:

- tumours at sites where surgery would lead to an inferior cosmetic result, e.g. nasolabial fold
- tumours at sites where surgery would lead to an inferior functional result, e.g. lower eyelid (Fig. 19.7).

Superficial X-rays or electrons are used to limit irradiation of subcutaneous tissues. Treatment can be given as a large single fraction or a course of daily treatment over 2–6 weeks. A custom-shaped lead cut-out is used to shape the beam to allow irradiation of a small annulus of apparently normal surrounding skin (Fig. 19.8). The former is preferred for patients with small tumours who would find travelling difficult owing to age or infirmity, but this approach gives an inferior cosmetic outcome.

Chemotherapy

Topical 5-fluorouracil can cause complete regression of Bowen's disease (squamous carcinoma in situ) and small, flat BCCs/SCCs, but has to be applied regularly, is inconvenient and requires careful follow-up. It is not routinely used.

Cryotherapy

Thorough and sustained freezing with liquid nitrogen is very effective for small superficial tumours. It is usually administered by a dermatologist, who will have the greatest expertise.

Curettage

Suitable for small (≤1 cm), well-circumscribed and superficial tumours. However, there is a higher risk of local recurrence as the margins are more likely not to be free of tumour.

Tumour-related complications

Local tissue destruction will cause loss of function, disfigurement and predispose to secondary infection and bleeding. Secondary infection will lead to discharge and discomfort and can predispose to delayed healing after surgery or radiotherapy.

Treatment-related complications

After radiotherapy an acute skin reaction is inevitable, characterized by erythema, hyperpigmentation, itching, dry desquamation and in some cases moist desquamation. This begins after 10–14 days of treatment and resolves within 2–4 weeks of completing radiotherapy. Occasionally, healing of a large area of skin can take many months. Chronic radionecrosis is a rare complication and could require skin grafting (Fig. 19.9).

Prognosis

It is exceptional for a patient to die from non-melanoma skin cancer. Local control should be expected in over 95 per cent, with most recurrences being successfully salvaged by further local treatment.

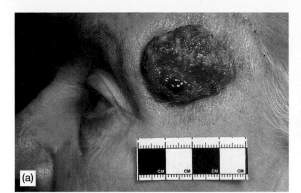

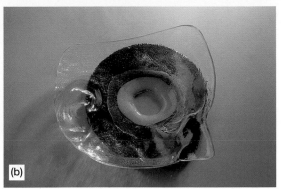

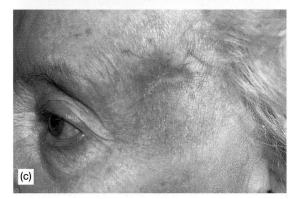

Figure 19.8 (a) A large squamous carcinoma. (b) Lead cut-out incorporated into a thermoplastic immobilization mask for the patient to wear during radiotherapy. (c) 12 weeks after radiotherapy.

Screening/prevention

The risks of ultraviolet radiation need to be appreciated, particularly by children and young adults. Avoidance of the sun during the midday period and use of sunblocks is recommended in sunny climates. Patients with a past history of skin cancer are at risk of developing others subsequently and benefit from surveillance and/or instructions regarding the early signs of a new tumour.

MELANOMA

This is a rarer but more serious form of skin cancer arising from the melanocytes of the skin. It is completely curable if detected and treated at an early stage.

Epidemiology

Each year in the UK there are 9000 cases of melanoma, 4000 cases in men and 5000 cases in women, accounting for 3.1 per cent of all cancer

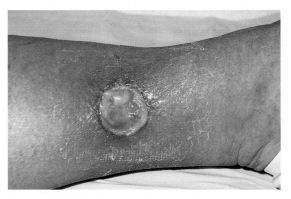

Figure 19.9 Necrosis after radiotherapy for a basal cell carcinoma arising from the skin of the lower calf region.

cases and leading to a total of 1900 deaths per annum. There has been a 50 per cent increase in incidence over the last decade. It is one of the few cancers that has a significant impact on young adults, 22 per cent arising in the under-40s. The geographical and racial distribution is similar to that of non-melanomatous skin

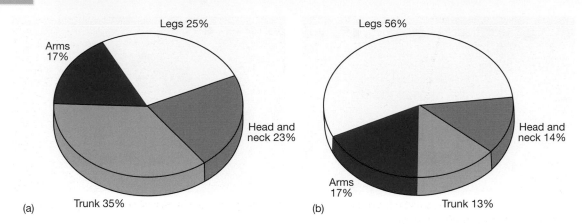

Figure 19.10 Site distribution of malignant melanoma in (a) males and (b) females.

cancer. Malignant melanoma does occasionally arise in dark-skinned people but is 10 times less common than in white people living a similar lifestyle. Severe sunburn (and therefore skin type) and childhood UV exposure are high-risk factors.

Aetiology

Ultraviolet radiation is the main causative factor, sun exposure being very important in determining risk, particularly if this happened during childhood. Additional risk factors include blond or red hair colour, and intense episodic sun exposure, particularly in those who tan poorly and burn easily. The vast majority of naevi confer no additional risk of melanoma, although individuals with large numbers (>100) are at increased risk. Dysplastic naevi can be congenital and are usually large lesions with irregular pigment and an irregular edge. Affected individuals should be watched very closely.

Pathology

The site distribution in men and women differs and is shown in Figure 19.10. Mucosal melanoma is rare and described in the upper aerodigestive tract, anus and vagina. Melanoma of the choroid of the eye is also described as the pigment cells are homologous with those of the skin. A melanoma is typically brown/black in

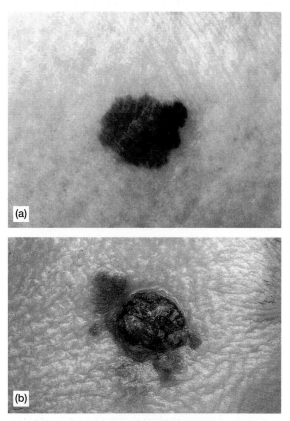

Figure 19.11 Malignant melanoma. Note the irregular edge, uneven pigmentation in both examples. (a) Superficial spreading melanoma. (b) Nodular melanoma.

colour owing to increased melanin production by the melanocytes, frequently with irregularity of pigment at its edge or centrally (Fig. 19.11).

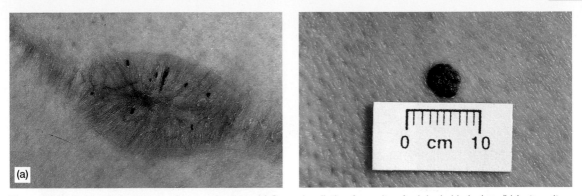

Figure 19.12 In-transit metastases from melanoma. (a) Spread radiating from site of original skin lesion. (b) In-transit metastasis in skin some 20 cm away.

Amelanotic tumours are seen in about 5 per cent of cases. They can be nodular or flat and seen to be spreading along the superficial layers of the skin. Fifty per cent are superficial spreading melanomas and have a more favourable prognosis than nodular types, which have an early vertical growth phase. In advanced cases there can be associated ulceration or satellite lesions on the adjacent skin. Like hypernephroma of the kidney and neuroblastoma of the adrenal, spontaneous regression in both primary and metastatic tumours is recorded, although this is seen in less than 5 per cent.

Microscopically, the tumour is composed of melanocytes that invade along the superficial layers of the skin and penetrate the basement membrane into the deeper layers of the dermis. The cells characteristically stain for S100, reflecting their origin from neural crest cells. A lymphocytic infiltrate is common, reflecting a host cellular immune response.

Natural history

Melanoma can remain at a superficial spreading phase for many months before it grows into the papillary dermis, reticular dermis and subcutaneous fat. Nodular melanomas tend to spread into the dermis at an early stage, which accounts for their poorer prognosis. Regional lymph nodes can be involved when the melanoma invades the deeper layers of the skin. Permeation of the dermal lymphatics sometimes leads to satellite nodules adjacent to the main bulk of disease (Fig. 19.12). Melanoma is a tumour that disseminates to any tissue in the body. Lung, bone (Fig. 19.13), brain and skin metastases are the most common and it is one of the few extra-abdominal tumours to spread to the bowel and its mesentery. Primary melanoma of the choroid of the eye has a propensity to spread to the liver.

Symptoms

Presentation is usually with a pigmented skin lesion. Changes in a preceding naevus or appearance of a new pigmented lesion frequently go unnoticed, particularly if on the back. Itchiness or bleeding are sinister symptoms.

Signs

The lesion will usually be on a sun-exposed area. The degree and pattern of pigmentation is variable but is characteristically irregular, particularly at the edge of the lesion, and is ideally assessed with a magnifying glass. Ulceration is an ominous sign. Regional lymph nodes should be palpated for enlargement, which may be due either to tumour infiltration or in reaction to the tumour/secondary infection. There can be signs of distant metastases such as hepatomegaly, pleural effusion/collapse/consolidation, or focal neurological signs. Patients with a heavy burden of metastases might have a slate grey complexion owing to increased circulating

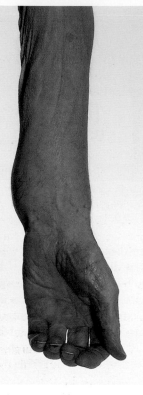

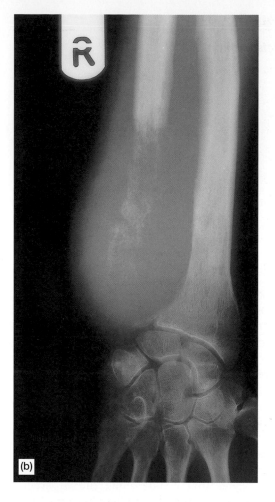

Figure 19.13 Bone metastasis from melanoma. (a) View of affected limb. (b) There is significant bone destruction at a site that is less frequently affected by other solid tumours.

melanin released by the tumour cells. Skin metastases have a typical blue/black colour (Fig. 19.14).

Differential diagnosis

A number of benign pigmented skin lesions could be confused with melanoma, including benign naevi, seborrhoeic warts, dermatofibromata and pigmented BCC/SCC.

Lentigo maligna (Hutchinson's melanotic freckle) deserves special mention. It typically occurs in the elderly on the face as a large, slow-growing, superficial, pigmented and irregular lesion, which represents a melanoma in situ, and it might become invasive.

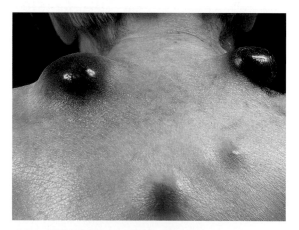

Figure 19.14 Multiple cutaneous metastases from malignant melanoma. Note the characteristic pigmentation of the lesions reflecting their origin.

Investigations

Excision biopsy

This is preferable to incision biopsy as it will provide a large specimen for detailed histological analysis and remove the lesion in toto. It is mandatory for any atypical pigmented lesion. Only a small macroscopic margin of normal skin is taken.

Fine needle aspiration (FNA) of any enlarged regional lymph nodes

This should differentiate between reactive and metastatic enlargement.

Exclusion of metastatic disease

A chest X-ray is performed in all cases to exclude lung metastases. A CT scan of chest, liver and regional lymph nodes is indicated in those at high risk of metastatic disease, e.g. deeply invasive (4 mm or deeper) lesions, lymph-node positive cases.

Staging

Clark's levels measure the depth in relation to histological landmarks:

- Level I – Confined to the lamina propria
- Level II – Reaches the papillary dermis
- Level III – Reaches the papillary/reticular dermis
- Level IV – Reaches the reticular dermis
- Level V – Reaches subcutaneous fat.

The Breslow thickness measures absolute depth in millimetres and is the distance of the deepest malignant cell from the stratum granulosum. Categories include thickness of:

- <0.75 mm
- 0.76–1.50 mm
- 1.51–4.0 mm
- >4.0 mm.

The TNM staging incorporates both Clark's level and Breslow thickness.

Treatment

Surgery

This is usually curative for localized lesions, a wide excision down to subcutaneous fat being necessary including a margin of macroscopically normal skin the size of which is dependent on the depth (if known). A centimetre of clearance for every millimetre of depth (clinical estimate or from result of previous excision biopsy) up to a maximum of 2 cm is adequate and an immediate re-excision is necessary if the margins are not clear microscopically. A skin graft or vascularized skin flap might be needed to close the defect if too large to heal by itself. In the case of subungual melanoma, amputation of the digit is performed.

The role of elective regional lymph node dissection has always been controversial. To some extent, this debate has become less important with the development of sentinel lymph node mapping (see Chapter 4 on Surgical Oncology Chapter 8 on Breast Cancer). This technique has proved very valuable in the surgical management of melanoma. Firstly, surgical clearance of all locoregional disease offers the only chance of cure, and sentinel lymph node removal can be applied to all cases, ensuring that only selected patients undergo a full lymph node dissection with its greater morbidity whilst the opportunities for surgical cure are maximized.

Second, for truncal melanomas, the regional lymph node zone might not be obvious because of the highly variable pattern of lymph drainage – sentinel lymph node mapping overcomes this issue by guiding the surgeon to the appropriate zone. All patients relapsing in the regional nodes after successful local treatment and with no evidence of distant metastases should have a lymph node dissection.

Surgery also has a role in the management of distant metastatic relapses. If limited to one anatomical site, resection should be considered. This will occasionally result in successful salvage and long-term remission.

Radiotherapy

Melanomas are considered relatively radioresistant tumours. The treatment technique is similar to that used for other skin tumours, and there is evidence that a few large doses are more effective than a prolonged course. In the rare case of melanoma of the choroid, very high doses of radiation administered using radioactive plaques sewn to the eye are curative in a high proportion. Otherwise, radiotherapy has little role as a curative treatment, being used when the patient refuses surgery or the tumour is inoperable, e.g. some mucosal melanomas. Low doses of radiation are valuable in palliating pain from skeletal metastases and focal, symptomatic metastases elsewhere.

Chemotherapy

Melanoma is not a chemosensitive tumour and is therefore incurable once distant metastasis has occurred. Adjuvant chemotherapy for high-risk patients does not have any proven benefit. The most active agents for metastatic disease are DTIC, BCNU/CCNU, cisplatin/carboplatin, vindesine and Taxol. Objective responses of 20–30 per cent can be expected. In recent years, the oral drug temozolomide has been shown to yield objective response rates of 20–25 per cent.

Biological therapy

The recognition of spontaneous regression in melanoma and rich lymphocytic infiltrate seen in and around the lesions suggests that host immunity might play a role in the rate of growth of these tumours. Lymphokines are chemical messengers produced by T lymphocytes, which stimulate lymphocyte proliferation and in turn the body's capacity for immunosurveillance and lymphocyte cytotoxicity.

There is evidence from initial randomized trials that adjuvant α-interferon given for approximately 1 year after surgery for melanomas 1.5 mm or greater in depth could improve the 5-year recurrence-free survival from 40–50 per cent to 60–70 per cent. As yet, a significant survival prolongation is yet to emerge from these studies. A similar improvement in disease-free survival has been shown for higher risk patients treated with high-dose α-interferon (10 MU × 3 weekly).

In metastatic disease, α-interferon, given subcutaneously at a dose of 3 MU three to five times weekly, produces objective responses of about 20 per cent. Similar response rates in metastatic disease have been observed to the lymphokine interleukin 2 (IL-2). Both drugs are expensive and have both physcial and neuropsychiatric toxicity, which may prove worse than the symptoms they are being used to palliate (see below). Recipients of such treatment should therefore be selected carefully.

Other strategies under development and investigation include administration of gangliosides and the development of tumour-specific vaccines.

Hormone therapy

There are reports of objective responses to the antioestrogen tamoxifen when given for metastatic disease. Tamoxifen also acts as a modifier of the chemotherapy agent DTIC and has therefore more often been used in combination with chemotherapy. In some trials, this did enhance the overall response rate. This is the subject of ongoing trials rather than routine practice.

Tumour-related complications

Secondary infection is an uncommon complication, predisposing to local discomfort, discharge and bleeding. Uncontrolled nodal disease may lead to lymphatic obstruction and lymphoedema of a limb.

Treatment-related complications

α-Interferon and IL-2 invariably have substantial systemic toxicity. The symptoms resemble influenza and include headache, malaise, fever, rigors, myalgia, lethargy, muscular weakness, depression, confusion, hypotension, renal failure and hypothyroidism.

Prognosis

Poor prognostic factors correlate with the risk of developing distant metastases and include:

- deep Clarke's level
- large Breslow thickness (5-year survivals for lesions <1.5 mm, 1.5–3.5 mm and >3.5 mm

are approximately 90, 70 and 40 per cent respectively)

- ulceration
- mucosal melanoma versus cutaneous (detected earlier)
- nodular melanoma versus superficial spreading (longer horizontal growth phase)
- male sex
- age >50 years.

Overall 5-year survival is 50–60 per cent for men, and 70–80 per cent for women.

Screening/prevention

As far as melanoma is concerned, early detection during the horizontal growth phase is essential. Education of community physicians and other healthcare professionals is important in facilitating this. People should be encouraged to visit their general practitioner or specialist dermatology clinic for an opinion if a pigmented lesion:

- increases in size
- changes shape or colour, particularly if pigmentation becomes irregular
- develops an inflammation at its edge
- itches
- bleeds or crusts.

Regular photographs of dysplastic naevi will aid early diagnosis of malignant change and screening of other family members should be undertaken if they have similar lesions.

Four out of five melanomas are preventable. Health education is again vital to inform people to:

- avoid visible sunburn, e.g. avoiding midday sun by seeking shade, use of sunscreen creams and clothing to protect skin
- take measures to protect skin of children
- take care to avoid excessive UV exposure in Northern Europe and not just when overseas
- take extra care if involved in outdoor occupations and/or leisure pursuits.

CASE HISTORY

CASE HISTORY: MELANOMA

A 34-year-old woman with a fair complexion presents to her GP with a mole on her right calf. This had been present for at least 10 years but over the last 6 months had enlarged in diameter, become more nodular, irregularly pigmented and itchy. She is referred to a fast-track dermatology clinic set up for such lesions.

Clinical examination reveals a pigmented lesion 1 cm in diameter suspicious for a melanoma. A detailed survey of the rest of the skin shows 20 to 30 benign naevi randomly distributed over the trunk and upper limbs. There is no popliteal, inguinal or femoral lymphadenopathy. There is no hepatomegaly. There are no other signs of disseminated malignancy.

Excision biopsy confirms a nodular melanoma with strong S100 immunostaining, 12 mm in diameter with a Breslow thickness of 4 mm. The margins of excision are clear but by <1 mm at the superior and a lateral margin.

She therefore undergoes a further wide excision and split skin graft to attain skin closure. Histology reveals a few residual nests of melanoma cells but the margins of excision are confirmed to be clear by 5 mm or more at all points. Baseline staging CT scan of the thorax and abdomen shows no evidence of visceral disease.

In view of the depth of the melanoma, she receives 12 months of adjuvant α-interferon. Four years after diagnosis, she notices a lump in the right groin. Fine needle aspiration confirms melanoma cells. Further CT scan shows no evidence of metastatic disease and no iliac lymphadenopathy. She therefore undergoes a radical groin lymph node dissection yielding three involved nodes.

Despite occasional swelling of the right lower leg, she remains well 8 years after diagnosis and we hope that she is cured of melanoma. She and her GP keep the other naevi under regular surveillence and she always avoids excessive sun exposure.

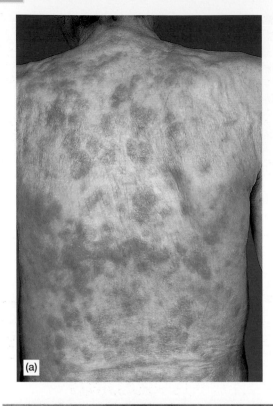

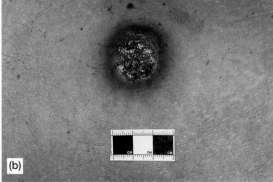

Figure 19.15 Cutaneous metastases from breast cancer. (a) Generalized rash. The skin infiltration was intensely irritating. (b) Solitary lesion. Note the dark areas corresponding to diathermy used to treat bleeding.

There is some evidence in at-risk populations that use of a powerful sunscreen can reduce the incidence of solar keratoses, the precursor lesion for cutaneous squamous carcinoma. Chemo-prevention programmes using isotretinoin or β-carotene have to date been ineffective.

METASTASES

The skin is frequently the site of distant metastases in patients with advanced cancer, particularly from breast and lung primaries (Fig. 19.15), usually presenting as one or more well-circumscribed subcutaneous nodules. They can be asymptomatic, cause irritation or fungate. If the diagnosis is in doubt, incision/excision biopsy or fine needle aspiration provide the definitive diagnosis. Symptomatic lesions can be treated by any of the usual local/systemic cancer therapies to which the primary tumour is sensitive.

RARE TUMOURS

Mycosis fungoides

This is a cutaneous T-cell lymphoma with a peak incidence at 30–50 years. The eruption has a predilection for body creases, buttocks and face and is initially non-specific, resembling chronic eczema or psoriasis. This stage can last for several years before progression to plaques that are well demarcated, erythematous, sometimes itchy lesions. The plaque stage progresses to the tumour stage consisting of erythematous nodules arising in the plaques or in normal skin. Erythroderma is described when the whole skin is affected, and Sézary syndrome when abnormal lymphocytes are seen in the peripheral blood (see Chapter 16). Treatment options include phototherapy with UV light, steroids, radiotherapy either locally or to the whole skin, topical or systemic chemotherapy, retinoids and interferon. The clinical course is protracted and many will die of unrelated causes.

Non-Hodgkin's lymphoma

B-cell non-Hodgkin's lymphoma may also affect the skin (Fig. 19.16).

Kaposi's sarcoma

This arises from vascular endothelial cells (see Chapter 20 for a detailed description).

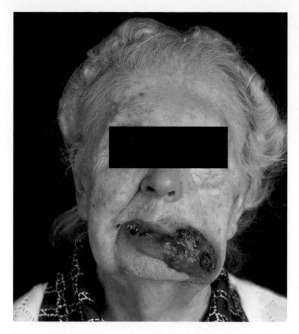

Figure 19.16 Cutaneous non-Hodgkin's lymphoma. There was no clinical or radiological evidence of disease elsewhere.

Merkel cell carcinoma

The mean age at diagnosis is 65–70 years and it presents as a solitary lesion, most frequent on head and neck in sun-damaged skin. It arises from neuroendocrine cells and is locally aggressive, spreading to regional lymph nodes and to distant sites. Even with combined wide local excision and postoperative radiotherapy, over one-third will recur locally and about half will eventually die from their disease.

Hidradenocarcinoma

This is a carcinoma arising from the sweat glands.

Sarcoma

These arise from the soft tissues of the skin and include leiomyosarcoma, liposarcoma, malignant fibrous histiocytoma, and angiosarcoma.

FURTHER READING

Nouri K. *Skin Cancer.* McGraw-Hill, New York, 2007
Rajpar S, Marsden J. *ABC of Skin Cancer.* Blackwell, Oxford, 2008
Schwartz RA. *Skin Cancer.* Blackwell, Oxford, 2008

SELF-ASSESSMENT QUESTIONS

1. Which one of the following is true about skin cancer?
   a. Only seen in the elderly
   b. Never occurs in dark-skinned races
   c. It is the commonest form of malignant disease
   d. Only caused by exposure to ultraviolet radiation
   e. With better public awareness the incidence is decreasing

2. Which three of the following are recognized causes of skin cancer?
   a. Immunosuppression
   b. Strychnine
   c. Chronic skin ulceration
   d. Gorlin's syndrome
   e. Phosphorus
   f. Microwaves
   g. Sarcoidosis

3. Which three of the following statements apply to basal cell carcinoma of the skin?
   a. Most commonly seen on legs
   b. Less common than squamous carcinoma
   c. Usually slow growing
   d. Only metastasize after many years
   e. Lymph node spread is common
   f. Highly sensitive to radiotherapy
   g. Can be treated by cryotherapy

4. Which three of the following statements apply to squamous cell carcinoma of the skin?
   a. More common than malignant melanoma
   b. Usually well differentiated
   c. Rarely arise on hair-bearing skin
   d. 10 per cent will have evidence of lymph node spread
   e. Much higher rate of cure compared with non-cutaneous squamous carcinoma
   f. Produce melanin
   g. May metastasize to the lungs

5. Which three of the following statements apply to malignant melanoma?
   a. Usually pigmented
   b. More common than squamous carcinoma
   c. Spreads to regional lymph nodes
   d. Higher mortality rate than other forms of skin cancer
   e. Can be treated by cryotherapy
   f. Highly sensitive to radiotherapy
   g. Highly sensitive to chemotherapy

6. Which three of the following are typical signs of melanoma?
   a. Hyperkeratosis
   b. Irregular pigmentation
   c. Spontaneous regression of a mole
   d. Itching
   e. Sun damage in surrounding skin
   f. Bleeding
   g. Secondary infection

7. Which one of the following is not a prognostic factor for melanoma?
   a. Mucosal origin
   b. Intensity of pigmentation
   c. Depth of invasion
   d. Thickness of lesion
   e. Ulceration

8. Which three of the following statements apply to Merkel cell carcinoma?
   a. Signet ring cells are characteristic
   b. More frequent in head and neck area
   c. Affects older age group than melanoma
   d. Higher risk of local recurrence than other forms of skin cancer
   e. Usually pigmented
   f. Treated with cryotherapy
   g. More common than melanoma

20 AIDS-RELATED CANCER

■ Management problems   341
■ Kaposi's sarcoma (KS)   342
■ Primary cerebral lymphoma   343
■ Non-Hodgkin's lymphoma   344
■ Hodgkin's disease (HD)   345
■ Other tumours   345
■ Further reading   345
■ Self-assessment questions   346

The acquired immune deficiency syndrome (AIDS) is a major health issue throughout the world, and its incidence relentlessly continues to increase. The advent of highly active anti-retroviral therapy (HAART) in recent years has to some extent reduced the magnitude of malignant disease in this special patient group. The types of tumours encountered are particularly rare in the rest of the population and present at a relatively advanced stage in patients who do not tolerate treatment well. Malignant disease can also be the first manifestation of infection with the human immunodeficiency virus (HIV), and should be considered in those presenting with Kaposi's sarcoma, high-grade B-cell non-Hodgkin's lymphoma and primary cerebral lymphoma. In such patients, risk factors for AIDS should be sought:

■ male homosexual sexual contact
■ sexual contact with an infected heterosexual partner
■ HIV-positive parent
■ intravenous drug abuse
■ blood/blood product transfusion in AIDS endemic area.

If appropriate, HIV positivity should be confirmed by a blood test after appropriate counselling.

MANAGEMENT PROBLEMS

Coping with the diagnosis

The patient has already been diagnosed as having an incurable illness with a poor prognosis, which compounds any psychological difficulties in coping with the diagnosis of either condition alone.

Poor prognosis from the tumour and AIDS

The prognosis from the underlying tumour will usually be very poor owing to the tumour presenting at an advanced stage and growing rapidly in an environment of a suppressed cellular immune system. The combination of HIV infection and malignancy will make the risk of opportunistic infection extremely high and indeed many may die from infection rather than their tumours. Much of the oncological management of such patients is therefore directed towards the prevention, early identification and treatment of opportunistic infections. However, the advent of HAART in recent years has improved life expectancy to an extent where the tumour poses a much more significant threat than AIDS itself.

Poor performance status

Patients with AIDS can have a poor performance status, which influences the treatment that they will tolerate, particularly as many present with advanced disease requiring aggressive chemotherapy.

Risk of infection to healthcare professionals

All healthcare workers who could potentially come into contact with bodily secretions should be aware of the patient's illness. Surgeons should double glove, consider wearing eyeshields during surgery, take care of any specimens obtained and notify the pathology laboratory of the risk of infection using appropriate biohazard labels. Radiographers should avoid routine use of skin tattoos, and take care with immobilization devices, e.g. bite blocks. Care should also be taken with needles and cannulae during and after administration of chemotherapy and when venepuncture is performed, and the laboratory notified of any blood specimens sent for analysis.

Predisposition to myelosuppression

Some of the drugs used in the combination chemotherapy for HIV can cause bone marrow suppression and therefore exacerbate the myelosuppressive effect of radiotherapy, chemotherapy and biological agents. This can in turn limit the intensity of anticancer treatment that is given. Patients with CD4 counts of 200 or less are at particular risk in the context of their oncological management.

KAPOSI'S SARCOMA (KS)

This is the most common AIDS-related malignancy but also occurs sporadically in Eastern Europeans, Africans and renal transplant patients on long-term immunosuppressants. In recent years, with the emergence of combination antiviral therapy for AIDS, its prevalence in the HIV-positive population has declined. It has not been reported in HIV-positive patients who contracted the disease through intravenous drug abuse. Recent research has suggested that it is caused by infection with human herpes virus type 8. The tumour is derived from the vascular endothelial cells of the skin. There are usually multiple skin lesions, particularly on the lower limbs (Fig. 20.1). Extracutaneous disease is common, particularly in the oral cavity and gastrointestinal tract (Fig. 20.2). The lesions have a characteristic purplish hue reflecting their vascular nature, appear as macules, plaques or nodules, and may ulcerate or bleed. They can spread to the regional lymph nodes or distant sites such as liver and lungs. Biopsy will confirm the diagnosis. KS may lead directly to death when there is extensive gastrointestinal involvement leading to haemorrhage. Otherwise, most will die of other AIDS-related complications. Indications for active management of KS lesions include:

- pain
- ulceration
- bleeding
- oedema
- disfigurement and stigma felt by patient
- mass effects, e.g. upper airways obstruction.

KS is a radiosensitive tumour and, although it is difficult to assess response owing to residual pigmentation, there is usually a visible regression in terms of flattening of the lesion and relief of symptoms, with 60–70 per cent attaining a complete response. A single fraction of radiotherapy is suitable for cutaneous sites. Candida superinfection of mucosal surfaces and enhanced radiation mucositis are problems when the oral cavity is irradiated.

Immunotherapy has also been used as a therapeutic strategy in KS owing to the following observations:

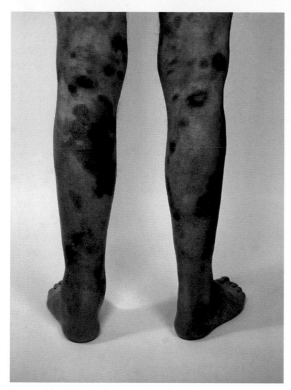

Figure 20.1 The multiple nodules and plaques of cutaneous Kaposi's sarcoma.

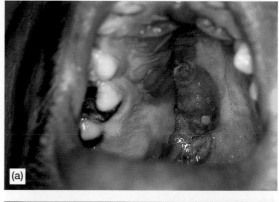

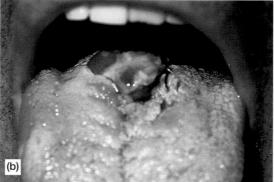

Figure 20.2 Kaposi's sarcoma. (a) Ulcerating plaques of tumour arising on the palate of a male homosexual. (b) Nodular tumour arising on posterior tongue.

- regression of KS in renal transplant patients with a decrease in their immunosuppression
- antitumour, antiviral effects of some biological modifiers
- recognized spontaneous regression of KS (4 per cent) in the more immunocompetent patients.

Up to 40 per cent respond to high-dose interferon with occasional complete responses. Objective responses have also been seen with chemotherapy. The drugs used are chosen to minimize the risk of myelosuppression and systemic toxicity. Bleomycin and vincristine are effective with response rates of 20–25 per cent, and usually well-tolerated by patients. In recent years, liposomal doxorubicin has been shown to be active and well tolerated in HIV-positive patients with objective response rates of 50–60 per cent. Taxol has a comparable activity to liposomal doxorubicin.

PRIMARY CEREBRAL LYMPHOMA

This is an extremely rare primary extranodal site of lymphoma in the general population but relatively more common in HIV-positive patients, representing approximately 20 per cent of non-Hodgkin's lymphomas (NHL) in HIV-positive patients. It tends to arise in those with more severe HIV immunosuppression than those who develop NHL, with lower basal CD4 counts, and is therefore rarely the defining HIV presentation. It usually arises in the cerebral hemispheres and can be multifocal (Fig. 20.3).

It presents with non-specific symptoms such as headache, somnolence and epilepsy, which may mimic atypical CNS infections such as toxoplasmosis, cerebral tuberculosis or progressive multifocal leukoencephalopathy. Histologically

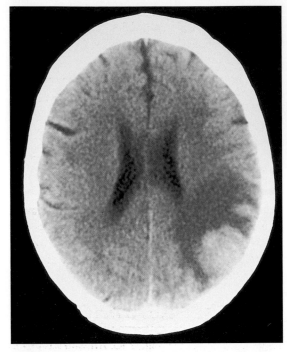

Figure 20.3 CT image of the brain in a patient with primary cerebral lymphoma. Note the two separate areas of contrast enhancement suggesting multifocality, and the surrounding cerebral oedema.

it is an aggressive high-grade B-cell NHL associated with evidence of infection with the Epstein–Barr virus (EBV) in all cases, in contrast with 40 per cent in AIDS-related NHL. It infiltrates the brain widely in the hemisphere of origin and can cross to the contralateral hemisphere. MRI is the best diagnostic imaging investigation and low toxoplasma IgG levels help to exclude an infective cause. Lumbar puncture can yield positive cytology or a positive test for EBV DNA. A brief trial of toxoplasma chemotherapy can be diagnostically useful in equivocal cases prior to undertaking craniotomy and biopsy. Standard lymphoma staging will exclude extracranial NHL. Aside from progressive cerebral dysfunction, CSF dissemination through the subarachnoid space will lead to nerve root deposits in the spine. The tumour is not particularly sensitive to either radiotherapy or chemotherapy. The preferred treatment is whole brain irradiation, with chemotherapy for those of good performance status. Intrathecal

methotrexate and cytosine arabinoside can be used for proven spinal metastases. Primary cerebral lymphoma has an extremely poor prognosis in patients with AIDS, with median survival times of around 3 months.

NON-HODGKIN'S LYMPHOMA

NHL is relatively uncommon in the general population, but a significant proportion of HIV-positive patients will develop it within the natural history of their AIDS illness. Indeed, in 30 per cent of those developing NHL it will be the presenting feature of a hitherto undiagnosed HIV seropositivity. Unlike KS, which has a higher prevalence amongst male homosexuals, NHL is seen in all HIV-positive subgroups. The diagnosis of NHL might be made before or at the time of discovery of positive HIV serology. These are usually high-grade, aggressive, large cell or immunoblastic B-cell lymphomas, frequently resembling Burkitt's lymphoma. Forty per cent are EBV-associated. Most patients present with stage 4 disease (Fig. 20.4), often with extranodal features at unusual sites e.g. heart, anus. 'B' symptoms such as fever can mask or be confused with an opportunistic infection. Treatment is with combination chemotherapy such as CHOP, but tolerance of such treatment can be a problem owing to bone marrow suppression and poor performance status of some patients. Increasing immunosuppression from

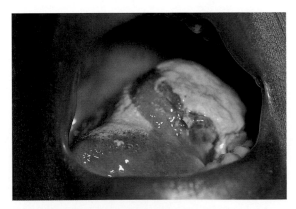

Figure 20.4 Non-Hodgkin's lymphoma of the tongue in a 27-year-old Ugandan woman.

chemotherapy exposes the patient to an even greater risk of atypical infections. Concurrent use of optimal HAART reduces this risk. Those with bone marrow involvement, evidence of EBV in the tumour or CSF positive for EBV using the polymerase chain reaction should have CNS prophylaxis with intrathecal chemotherapy. Rituximab does not have a proven role in these patients. Despite a good initial response to treatment, this is often short lived and the prognosis remains very poor.

The human herpes virus type 8 (HHV 8), implicated in the causation of KS, can also cause a variant of non-Hodgkin's lymphoma in these patients known as 'primary effusion lymphoma'. This presents with a 'liquid phase', affecting serous membranes without the usual formation of lymphoid masses. HHV 8 also causes multicentric Castleman's disease.

HODGKIN'S DISEASE (HD)

HD is 10 times less frequent than NHL in this group. As with NHL in this patient group, it is more likely to present with stage 4 or extranodal disease. It is usually mixed cellularity or lymphocyte depleted in type. Mediastinal involvement is less frequent than with HD in HIV-negative cases and stage for stage the prognosis is worse for HIV-positive cases with median survival of around 18 months.

OTHER TUMOURS

Possible associations have been described for:

- carcinoma of the tongue
- carcinoma of the anus
- squamous carcinoma of the conjunctiva
- testicular tumours
- hepatocellular carcinoma.

Many of these tumours are thought to have a viral aetiology (e.g. human papilloma virus and carcinoma of the anus and conjunctiva), which might account for their prevalence in this immunosuppressed population.

FURTHER READING

Feigal EG, Levine AM, Biggar RJ. *AIDS-Related Cancers and Their Treatment*. Dekker, New York, 2000
http://www.cancer.gov/cancertopics/pdq/treatment/
AIDS-related-lymphoma/healthprofessional/
http://www.cancer.gov/cancertopics/pdq/treatment/
kaposis/healthprofessional/
http://www.cancer.gov/cancertopics/pdq/treatment/
primary-CNS-lymphoma/healthprofessional/

SELF-ASSESSMENT QUESTIONS

1. Which three of the following are tumours associated with AIDS?
   a. Glioblastoma multiforme
   b. Uterine sarcoma
   c. Non-Hodgkin's lymphoma
   d. Small cell carcinoma of the prostate
   e. Primary cerebral lymphoma
   f. Squamous carcinoma of the conjunctivae
   g. Carcinoma of the pancreas

2. Which one of the following is characteristic of Kaposi's sarcoma?
   a. Does not involve lymph nodes
   b. Pigmentation
   c. Purplish colour
   d. Secondary infection
   e. Itching

3. Which three of the following are typical of primary cerebral lymphoma?

   a. Often multifocal
   b. Does not occur in absence of HIV infection
   c. May be confused with intracerebral infections
   d. Usually associated with extracerebral non-Hodgkin's lymphoma
   e. Arises in those with the greatest degree of immune suppression
   f. Very sensitive to chemotherapy

4. Which three of the following are typical of HIV-associated non-Hodgkin's lymphoma?
   a. Usually T cell
   b. Usually high grade
   c. Associated with EBV infection
   d. Relatively insensitive to chemotherapy
   e. Presents at an advanced stage
   f. High rate of cure

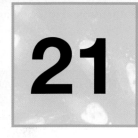

21 CARCINOMA OF UNKNOWN PRIMARY

■ Differential diagnosis   347
■ Investigations   348
■ Management   350

■ Prognosis   351
■ Further reading   352
■ Self-assessment questions   353

Some patients are diagnosed as having disseminated cancer but with no evidence of the site of origin, many presenting with their disease as an incidental finding, e.g. enlarged cervical lymph node(s), bone metastases or pulmonary metastases on chest X-ray. Their management is a difficult problem, the oncologist having to determine whether the patient has a curable tumour such as a teratoma or lymphoma, one that can benefit from systemic therapy (e.g. a hormone-responsive cancer such as from the breast or prostate), or one where treatment would not be justified.

A detailed history should be taken. Questions should be aimed at eliciting symptoms of the underlying primary neoplasm, judging its time course and rate of progression, as well as gauging the performance status of the patient. The presence of 'B' symptoms could suggest an underlying lymphoma. The possibility (albeit rare) of choriocarcinoma should be considered in a young woman with a recent history of pregnancy. The development of breast tenderness in a young male can suggest an underlying trophoblastic germ cell tumour.

A detailed physical examination should include the skin, oral cavity, thyroid, breasts, peripheral lymph node groups (cervical chains, Waldeyer's ring, supraclavicular fossae, axillae and groins), spleen, rectum including prostate and testes in males, and pelvic examination in females. If the patient has presented with lymphadenopathy, the region that drains to those nodes should be examined particularly thoroughly. For example, inguinal lymphadenopathy should prompt a thorough survey of both lower limbs, perianal region and anal canal, penis and scrotum in males, vulva and vagina in females. Some women will present with adenocarcinoma in one or more axillary lymph nodes and this should trigger breast-specific imaging to exclude an occult ipsilateral breast primary.

DIFFERENTIAL DIAGNOSIS

The most likely primary sites vary with histology (Table 21.1). The common solid tumours (lung, breast, colorectal, prostate, pancreas) should be considered. Anaplastic tumours are mainly poorly differentiated carcinomas, the rest being undifferentiated teratomas, lymphoma, melanoma (particularly amelanotic variant), sarcomas and neuroendocrine tumours.

TABLE 21.1 Most likely sites of primary carcinomas according to histology

Histological type	Most likely sites of primary
Adenocarcinoma	Lung
	GI tract (stomach, colon, pancreas)
	Breast
	Prostate
	Ovary
	Kidney
Squamous carcinoma	Lung
	Head and neck
Small cell carcinoma	Lung

INVESTIGATIONS

Patients with distant metastases should not undergo exhaustive investigation in the relentless search for a primary that is ultimately unlikely to be curable and where local treatment of the primary will not be justified. For those with distant metastases, localization of the primary tumour site is unlikely to affect materially the diagnosis or immediate management. However, histological typing of the tumour will influence assessment of prognosis and the type of systemic therapy chosen.

Biopsy

A balance has to be struck between the need to confirm the histological diagnosis, how it will affect ultimate management, and what is reasonable for the patient to undergo. The general principle is to obtain a sizeable piece of tissue from a representative part of the tumour that is not necrotic. This should ensure adequate tissue for immunocytochemistry so that an accurate histological analysis is possible. If several sites of bulk disease are accessible, the safest and least traumatic route of access should be followed. The simplest option is fine needle aspiration of a palpable lump with immediate cytological examination. However, this does not always yield adequate material for an accurate pathological diagnosis particularly for conditions such as lymphoma. A needle biopsy, open biopsy or

excision biopsy is therefore preferred in most circumstances. The lesion for biopsy might need to be localized using CT (Fig. 21.1) or ultrasound depending on its anatomical location and accessibility.

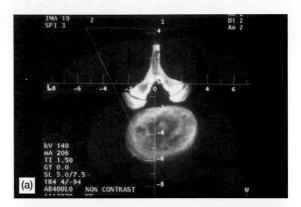

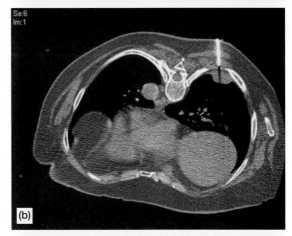

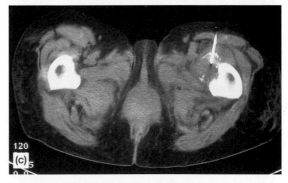

Figure 21.1 CT-guided percutaneous biopsy for a tissue diagnosis. (a) Vertebra. A safe trajectory has been selected to sample a lytic area. (b) Pleural mass. (c) Inguinal lymph node.

Immunocytochemistry

Some tissues have staining characteristics depending on their embryological origin and constituent cells:

- α-fetoprotein (AFP) – teratomas, hepatomas
- β-human chorionic gonadotrophin (HCG) – teratomas, choriocarcinomas
- prostate-specific antigen (PSA) – carcinomas of the prostate
- carcinoembryonic antigen (CEA) and CK20 – gastrointestinal cancers
- TTF–1 – lung cancer
- CA125 – carcinomas of the ovary
- oestrogen/progesterone receptors and/or CA15-3 – carcinoma of the breast
- CA199 – carcinoma of the pancreas
- CD45, CD20 – lymphoma
- cytokeratin 7 (CK7) – carcinomas
- desmin – leiomyosarcomas, rhabdomyosarcomas
- myoglobin – rhabdomyosarcomas
- vimentin – sarcomas
- neurone-specific enolase (NSE) – neuroblastomas, primitive neuroectodermal tumours (PNETs)
- calcitonin – medullary carcinomas of the thyroid
- thyroglobulin – follicular carcinomas of the thyroid
- α_1-antitrypsin – hepatomas
- S100 – melanomas, small cell lung cancers
- chromogranin – carcinoids
- CD117 (c-kit) – gastrointestinal stromal tumours (GISTs).

Cytogenetic studies

These are of value in tumours arising in children and adolescents as many tumours have characteristic chromosomal abnormalities, e.g. translocations in Ewing's sarcoma (t11;22), rhabdomyosarcoma (t2;13), non-Hodgkin's lymphoma (NHL) (t8;14). Extragonadal germ cell tumours can have abnormalities of chromosome 12. These are of less value in adult solid tumours.

Recent advances in genomic studies have led to the development of a test whereby fixed tissue is analysed using gene microarrays and matched against a tissue bank of different tumours to cross reference it and thereby identify a likely site of origin (CupPrint® test). This is commercially available but expensive.

Polymerase chain reaction (PCR)

PCR detection of Epstein–Barr virus genome can suggest an occult nasopharyngeal primary or NHL.

Radiological investigations

CT scan of the thorax, abdomen and pelvis not only allows a detailed radiological survey of a number of possible sites of origin of metastases that are clinically impalpable (e.g. pancreas, ovaries), but also allows full staging, which is of prognostic value and of use in planning treatment. An isotope bone scan is useful to assess the skeleton for staging purposes. Bilateral mammography should be considered in women with adenocarcinoma of unknown primary to exclude an occult breast primary that would be amenable to aggressive locoregional therapy or hormone manipulation. A transrectal ultrasound should be considered if the prostate feels suspicious or the PSA elevated, and if clinically indicated, will facilitate a needle core biopsy of the prostate under direct vision. A transvaginal ultrasound is useful in evaluating the lower female genital tract. A whole body PET survey sometimes discloses the location of an occult primary cancer amidst the known metastatic disease (Fig. 21.2).

Blood tests

Serum tumour marker assays can be useful for giving a clue as to the likely origin of the metastases and therefore allow a more focused approach to investigations. A normal PSA test makes carcinoma of the prostate unlikely. A very high CEA can suggest a gastrointestinal primary. CA15-3 and CA125 should be measured in women presenting with adenocarcinoma of unknown primary to exclude carcinoma of the breast and ovary respectively. Young adults presenting with undifferentiated cancers should have blood taken for AFP and HCG to exclude a trophoblastic germ cell tumour. In an urgent situation, a urinary pregnancy test is a crude way of checking for excess HCG levels in a male.

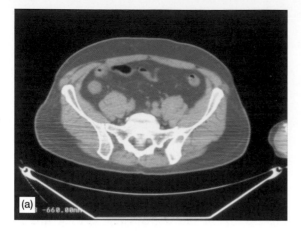

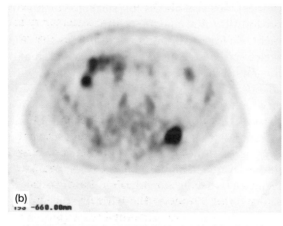

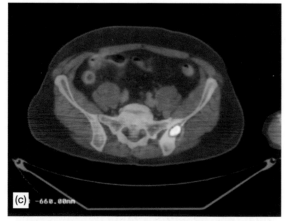

Figure 21.2 Whole body PET survey. The patient presented with bone metastases. (a) CT study. (b) Corresponding PET image. There are several areas of focal uptake. (c) Fusion PET/CT image. This confirms uptake in the pelvic bone posteriorly. Importantly, it suggests a hypermetabolic, rounded density within the right side of the pelvis, which turned out to be a primary colon cancer.

Other investigations

Patients presenting with squamous carcinoma in lymph nodes draining the head and neck region must be referred to an ENT surgeon for an endoscopy of the upper aerodigestive tract (especially nasopharynx, tonsils, posterior third of tongue, supraglottic larynx and pyriform fossa) as the patient could still have a curable occult primary cancer.

MANAGEMENT

The problem is usually one of systemic disease at the outset and so it is logical to consider some form of systemic therapy. The patient should be managed according to their age, general condition, site and stage of disease and symptomatology. In cases of widespread distant metastases in a patient with a very poor performance status, local treatment directed towards symptom relief is likely to be most appropriate as the patient will be incurable and unlikely to gain from chemotherapy. Conversely, the patient should be treated with curative intent if there are distant metastases and the tumour is particularly chemosensitive (e.g. teratoma, lymphoma) or if there are regional lymph node metastases from a tumour that could be cured by aggressive locoregional therapy, e.g. in the head and neck or breast. For this reason, women presenting with isolated axillary lymphadenopathy containing adenocarcinoma and no other primary site should be assumed to have an occult carcinoma of the breast and treated accordingly. A young person presenting with a rapidly enlarging mediastinal mass or retroperitoneal mass and a biopsy showing poorly differentiated tumour cells and negative lymphocyte markers should be suspected as having a non-gonadal germ cell tumour, and treated accordingly with a cisplatin chemotherapy regime, even if serum AFP and HCG levels are not elevated.

Most patients fall between these two extreme ends of the spectrum, in which case systemic therapy can be employed to maximize the symptom-free interval with the expectation that this may in turn lead to a prolongation of survival. Hormonal therapy should be initiated in selected tumours, e.g. prostate cancer and breast cancer. Chemotherapy is frequently used in good performance status patients. For those where the primary tumour origin is found or suspected from biopsy, the regimens specific for that disease are most appropriate. For those where it is impractical to obtain a histological diagnosis, it is rational to select several drugs that cover the most common solid tumours, e.g. an anthracycline, an alkylating agent, 5FU and/or platinum derivative. Examples therefore include combinations such as:

- ECF – epirubicin, cisplatin, protracted infusion of 5FU (or oral capecitabine – ECX)
- CAP – cyclophosphamide, Adriamycin, cisplatin.

PROGNOSIS

The prognosis is poor, with a median survival of approximately 3–4 months in most studies with less than 25 per cent and 10 per cent of patients alive at 1 and 5 years, respectively. This can be due to a selection bias as such tumours will have a strong propensity to spread widely before the primary discloses its presence, and hence have an innately poorer prognosis. Male gender, increasing number of involved organ sites, adenocarcinoma histology, and hepatic involvement are all unfavourable prognostic factors. Only the few with lymphoma or a germ cell tumour stand a higher chance of cure.

Unfortunately, the site of the primary tumour might never be found during life. A post-mortem examination can be very instructive for the clinicians and relieve uncertainty for the next of kin, although even then the primary origin can prove elusive.

CASE HISTORY

CASE HISTORY: CARCINOMA OF UNKNOWN PRIMARY

A previously fit 51-year-old woman is well until she joins a gym. Following a quadriceps toning exercise, she develops persistent discomfort in the right thigh. This persists for 2 weeks despite use of a topical anti-inflammatory gel. She is climbing a flight of stairs when she hears a loud 'crack', and collapses with severe acute pain in the thigh. She is taken to the accident and emergency department where a plain radiograph confirms a transverse fracture of the femoral midshaft. There is some lysis of the cortex either side of the fracture suggesting a pre-existing condition, which had led to bone absorption. The diagnosis of a pathological fracture is made, the radiologist confirming that there is almost certainly a metastasis at this site. She is referred to an orthopaedic surgeon and undergoes an emergency open reduction and internal fixation. A specimen is sent for histology but this shows normal connective tissue and bone.

Postoperatively, she is referred to an oncologist. A full history fails to reveal any symptoms of an underlying malignant process and therefore does not give any clue as to the likely underlying cause. She has had a recent normal cervical smear and her first screening mammogram was unremarkable. A detailed physical examination reveals a hard, solitary 1.5 cm lymph node in the left supraclavicular fossa. There is no abnormality within the breasts or axillae and all other lymph node groups are normal. The thyroid is unremarkable and there is no mucosal abnormality within the oral cavity and oropharynx. The chest is clear and there is no hepatomegaly. Digital examination of the rectum and vaginal examination are normal. There are a few benign naevi but no obvious cutaneous manifestation of primary or secondary malignancy.

Full blood count is normal. Liver function tests show a moderate elevation of both γ-glutamyltransferase and alkaline phosphatase at 125 U/L and 340 U/L, respectively. The serum calcium corrected for the serum albumin is 3.2 mmol/L (normal range 2.1–2.6). Fine needle aspiration of the supraclavicular lymph node reveals adenocarcinoma cells, which are both CEA negative and oestrogen receptor negative. Bilateral mammography is normal. Chest X-ray is clear but CT scan shows low volume bilateral lung metastases and multiple liver metastases. Isotope bone scan confirms increased isotope uptake at the site of recent bone surgery and in the dorsal spine, lumbar spine and contralateral humerus. Plain radiographs are obtained of the latter, which confirm that this area is not at risk of imminent fracture and therefore does not require prophylactic internal fixation. The CA15-3, CA125, thyroglobulin and CEA tumour markers are all within the normal range. Taking account of the extent of metastatic disease, it is not felt appropriate to investigate the gastrointestinal tract for an occult primary.

In view of the presentation and asymptomatic hypercalcaemia, she is encouraged to maintain a high fluid intake and commenced on infusions of disodium pamidronate 90 mg 4 weekly. A short course of radiotherapy is delivered to the fracture site to consolidate the surgical fixation. Bearing in mind her good performance status and extent of disease, having discussed the option of best supportive care with chemotherapy kept in reserve for symptomatic progression, an indwelling venous catheter is inserted and she starts chemotherapy with continuously infused 5-FU and 3-weekly boluses of epirubicin and cisplatin. Restaging after three cycles shows stable disease but after six there is evidence of progression within the thorax and liver. Repeat physical examination at this point reveals an ill-defined 2 cm lump within the left breast. Core biopsy confirms adenocarcinoma cells with similar staining characteristics to those obtained from the original lymph node. The tumour is HER2 negative. Her chemotherapy is changed to taxotere and she attains a good partial response which is sustained for 4 months. At second relapse, she fails to respond to further chemotherapy and dies of her disease. The certified cause of death is metastatic breast cancer.

FURTHER READING

DeVita VT, Lawrence TS, Rosenberg SA. Chapter 56 – Cancer of Unknown Primary Site. In: *Principles and Practice of Oncology* Vol. 2 part 3. Lippincott Williams and Wilkins, Philadelphia, 2008

http://www.cancer.gov/cancertopics/pdq/treatment/ unknownprimary/health professional/

SELF-ASSESSMENT QUESTIONS

1. Which three of the following are true for carcinoma of unknown primary?
   a. It is an uncommon clinical scenario
   b. The primary cancer is found in most cases after investigation
   c. Biopsy is mandatory
   d. Treatment is withheld until the primary tumour is identified
   e. Tissue immunohistochemistry is useful
   f. Investigation is futile
   g. Most cases will lead to the death of the patient

2. Which three of the following are true associations?
   a. CK20 and bowel cancer
   b. TTF-1 and lung cancer
   c. CA15-3 and ovarian cancer
   d. S100 and melanoma
   e. CA125 and pancreatic cancer
   f. CD117 and lymphoma
   g. Calcitonin and lung cancer

22 ONCOLOGICAL EMERGENCIES

- Hypercalcaemia 354
- Spinal cord and cauda equina compression 355
- Superior vena cava obstruction 357
- Neutropenic sepsis 359
- Tumour lysis syndrome 360
- Further reading 360
- Self-assessment questions 361

There are few conditions in the management of malignant disease that are true emergencies. However, it is important to identify those patients in whom urgent treatment is required. The following conditions can be associated with rapid deterioration and even death, and should be considered emergency situations:

- hypercalcaemia
- spinal cord or cauda equina compression
- superior vena cava obstruction
- neutropenic sepsis
- tumour lysis syndrome.

HYPERCALCAEMIA

Malignant hypercalcaemia is the most common cause of a raised serum calcium in oncology patients. It is associated in particular with lung cancer, breast cancer, prostatic cancer and myeloma. It is generally found in patients with disseminated metastatic disease although this is not essential.

Aetiology

There is increasing evidence that hypercalcaemia associated with malignancy is due prin-cipally to the effects of chemical agents released by the tumour, which disturb the normal mechanisms of calcium balance. A number of these have now been identified that act as osteoclast-activating factors (OAFs) and include parathyroid hormone-like peptides, prostaglandins, interleukins and transforming growth factor β (TGFβ). They result in osteo-clast activation and mobilization of calcium from bones.

Symptoms

These include anorexia, nausea, vomiting, con-stipation, confusion, polyuria, thirst, polydipsia and bone pains.

Signs

There are usually no specific physical signs. The patient might appear drowsy and have signs of confusion or dehydration.

Differential diagnosis

Other causes of similar symptoms including polyuria, polydipsia and confusion that should be considered include diabetes mellitus, cerebral metastases, hepatic failure, renal failure and neutropenic sepsis.

Investigations

The diagnosis is confirmed on measuring the serum calcium. It is important to correct the total level for the serum albumin which is often low in patients with advanced malignant disease. The simple correction is to add to the serum calcium level 0.02 mmol/L for every g/dL of albumin below 40 g/dL, which is the conventional standardization level. For example, a reading of calcium at 2.3 mmol/L with an albumin of 30 gives a corrected serum albumin of 2.5 mmol/L. The normal range after correction is between 2.1 and 2.6 mmol/L but symptoms are not often seen until the level reaches 3.0 mmol/L or above.

Treatment

There are two components to the treatment of malignant hypercalcaemia:

- Correction of dehydration and establishing good urine flow. An intravenous infusion of normal saline giving 1 litre every 6 hours should be started. Careful attention to fluid balance is essential, particularly in the elderly who may easily become fluid overloaded. Frusemide can be added which, in addition to acting as a diuretic, also promotes urinary excretion of calcium. Thiazides should be avoided as they increase calcium reabsorption.
- Specific therapy to reduce calcium levels using intravenous bisphosphonate once good urine flow has been established. Pamidronate, clodronate, zolendronate or ibandronate are all effective.

Although rapid correction of serum calcium is often possible with the above approach, rebound hypercalcaemia is common unless regular bisphosphonate infusions are continued at 3–4-weekly intervals.

The ultimate prognosis for malignant hypercalcaemia is poor with most patients surviving for only a few months, succumbing to either refractory hypercalcaemia or the effects of widespread malignancy.

SPINAL CORD AND CAUDA EQUINA COMPRESSION

This condition arises most commonly as a result of extradural tumour, typically secondary to carcinoma of the lung, breast or prostate. It should be treated as an emergency because the outcome in terms of final neurological disability is determined by the speed of diagnosis and neurological function at the time of starting treatment.

Aetiology

Extradural metastases are usually a result of blood-borne dissemination. Less often paravertebral tumour or tumour within the vertebral body can infiltrate directly into the spinal canal.

Symptoms

Spinal cord compression presents with neurological symptoms of weakness and reduced or altered sensation below the site of cord damage. This is accompanied by constipation and hesitancy in micturition leading to urinary retention.

Cauda equina compression similarly presents with weakness and sphincter disturbance. The sensory disturbance can be of reduced or altered sensation but nerve root pain affecting the lumbosacral segments is also seen.

Signs

Spinal cord compression causes a spastic paraparesis or, if it affects the cervical spine, quadriparesis, with a cut-off of sensory changes corresponding to the anatomical level of the compression – a sensory level. In contrast, cauda equina compression will result in a flaccid paraparesis with loss of sensation in a dermatome pattern affecting the lumbosacral segments (the lower limbs and buttocks). Reflexes are increased with extensor plantars in cord compression whilst, with cauda equina compression, reflexes are reduced or lost with flexor plantar responses.

Sphincter function might be disturbed and, with cauda equina compression, a distended bladder might be palpable and anal tone will be lax.

Differential diagnosis

This will include intrinsic spinal cord tumours and paraneoplastic neuropathies. Transverse myelitis will give a similar clinical picture to cord compression and, in cancer patients, could be due to viral infection and rarely as a side-effect of chemotherapy or radiotherapy. Other unrelated causes include prolapsed intervertebral disc, subacute combined degeneration of the cord and a parasagittal intracranial tumour.

Acute onset of symptoms should raise suspicion of vertebral artery occlusion and cord infarction.

Investigations

Urgent investigations are required to confirm the diagnosis. Plain X-rays of the spine can demonstrate associated vertebral disease but urgent MRI of the spine will give the definitive diagnosis as shown in Figure 22.1. In the patient where MRI is contraindicated, e.g. those with a pacemaker or metal fragments, then a myelogram combined with CT scanning at the level of obstruction should be performed. Since multiple

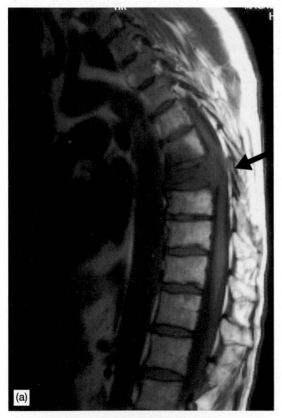

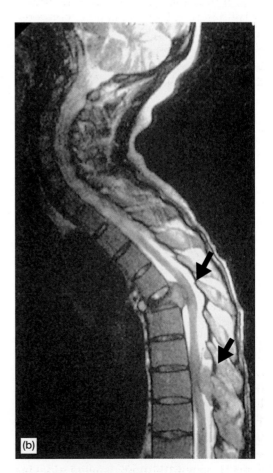

Figure 22.1 MRIs demonstrating (a) metastatic spinal canal compression owing to direct infiltration from a bone metastasis, (b) upper level: vertebral collapse and (b) lower level: an extradural metastasis.

levels of cord involvement will be found in a third of patients the entire spine should be imaged whenever possible.

Treatment

If spinal cord compression is the first manifestation of malignancy, then a primary site should be sought and cytology or histology obtained. If no primary site is apparent then a needle biopsy of the tumour at the site of spinal cord compression should be taken under CT guidance.

In the presence of a known histologically confirmed malignancy, treatment should proceed immediately as follows:

- All patients should start on high-dose steroids using dexamethasone 4 mg qds with, if necessary, prophylactic omeprazole or lansoprazole. Urine should be monitored for sugar, many patients having borderline glucose tolerance.
- Definitive treatment with surgery or radiotherapy should be given:
  - patients with spinal instability should all be reviewed by a spinal surgeon
  - those with localized cord compression, good performance status having primary breast cancer and no evidence of active metastases elsewhere have better outcomes with primary surgery and post-operative radiotherapy than with primary radiotherapy alone
  - most other patients should receive urgent local radiotherapy starting on the same day as the diagnosis is made. A course of 20–30 Gy over 1–2 weeks will usually be prescribed.
- Certain patients could be more appropriately treated with chemotherapy, in particular those with lymphoma, small cell lung cancer and germ cell tumours who have not been previously treated.
- In addition, appropriate general measures should continue. Patients with sphincter disturbance might require catheterization and analgesia should be given as necessary.
- Active physiotherapy and rehabilitation is a further important component of the management to optimize the chances of neurological recovery.

Prognosis

Survival following cord compression is defined by the underlying condition and the performance status of the patient. It is often a reflection of disseminated disease and average survivals are usually measured in only a few months from diagnosis.

The prognosis for neurological recovery is dependent almost entirely on the speed of diagnosis and instigation of treatment. Of patients who are mobile at the start of treatment, the majority (85 per cent) will walk after treatment. In contrast, fewer than 15 per cent of paraplegic patients will regain useful neurological function despite intensive treatment. For this reason there should be a high index of suspicion for this condition, particularly in patients known to have metastatic disease, with urgent referral to a specialist centre for treatment.

SUPERIOR VENA CAVA OBSTRUCTION

Superior vena cava obstruction (SVCO) is typically due to a large mediastinal tumour mass causing obstruction to venous return to the right side of the heart, and is often associated with other symptoms of mediastinal compression including dysphagia and stridor.

Aetiology

Any tumour involving the mediastinum could be the cause. The most common cause is carcinoma of the bronchus. In young patients in particular it is important to consider malignant lymphomas and germ cell tumours. Rarely a thymic tumour or retrosternal thyroid tumour can be the cause.

Post-mortem studies suggest that in most patients, although mechanical obstruction to venous flow may be the first event, thrombosis within the large veins inevitably follows although emboli are almost unknown.

Symptoms

Dyspnoea, stridor or dysphagia can be presenting symptoms. Intracranial venous congestion can cause headache or confusion. There might also be swelling of the face, neck and arms.

Signs

Oedema of the face, neck and arms can be apparent with fixed engorged jugular veins and dilatation of superficial skin veins over the chest, neck, face and upper limbs. Typical appearances are shown in Figure 22.2. There might be obvious respiratory distress or stridor. A tumour mass might be palpable arising out of the mediastinum in the supraclavicular fossae. Papilloedema can be present on fundoscopy.

Investigations

A chest X-ray will usually demonstrate a mediastinal mass, which will be better defined on CT scanning. Unless a diagnosis of malignancy has already been made, it is important to obtain a tissue diagnosis if at all possible. Other readily accessible disease sites should be sought such as a peripheral lymph node. If the mediastinum is the only site of disease, then a needle biopsy under CT control will usually be possible. More invasive approaches are usually avoided because of the theoretical risk of excessive haemorrhage from the area of raised venous pressure.

Treatment

Immediate treatment should take the form of high-dose steroids with dexamethasone 4 mg qds. Initial management should include consideration of vascular stenting, which is the most effective means of overcoming the venous obstruction in the early stages of SVCO and will result in immediate restoration of blood flow. An example is shown in Figure 22.3.

Definitive treatment will be either radiotherapy or chemotherapy. Where a diagnosis of lymphoma or germ cell tumour is made, further staging investigations should be completed as soon as possible followed by immediate

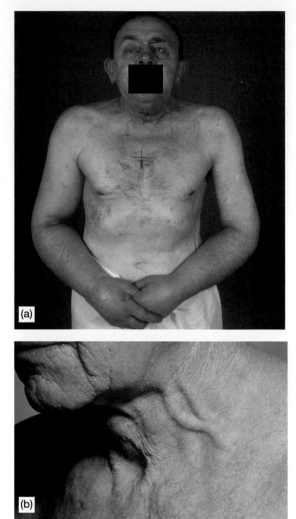

Figure 22.2 Superior vena cava obstruction characterized by arm and facial oedema, distended veins, plethora and (a) conjunctival suffusion and (b) distended, raised neck veins, which do not empty on lying flat ('fixed veins').

chemotherapy. In small cell lung cancer chemotherapy may also be the treatment of choice unless there has been previous exposure to chemotherapy or the patient is elderly or frail. All other patients should receive a course of radiotherapy to the mediastinum.

Prognosis

The prognosis of SVCO depends on the underlying condition and in itself this is not a poor

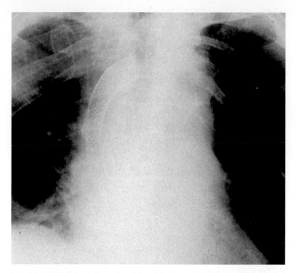

Figure 22.3 Vascular stent in situ in patient presenting with superior vena cava obstruction.

prognostic factor. For this reason it is important to identify those patients with lymphoma and germ cell tumour so that correct radical treatment can be given despite the acute nature of their presentation.

Most patients will benefit symptomatically from local treatment although recurrence of symptoms can occur at a later date.

NEUTROPENIC SEPSIS

Neutropenic sepsis is a major hazard and the principal cause of treatment-related death associated with the use of cancer chemotherapy. However, if promptly identified and aggressively treated, most episodes can be successfully controlled. Centres delivering chemotherapy will have a clearly defined neutropenic sepsis policy to ensure that all staff are familiar with the management of patients presenting with fever and neutropenia.

Aetiology

Neutropenia will occur after most chemotherapy and may also be a problem when radiotherapy encompasses large volumes of bone marrow, e.g. long spinal fields or large pelvic fields. Bone marrow infiltration by tumour is a further cause. Life-threatening infection is most likely to occur when the total neutrophil count falls below 1.0×10^9/L. The major cause of infection is from host organisms in the bowel or skin. The presence of a central venous line is a further risk factor. The common pathogens are Gram-negative bacteria such as *Escherichia coli*, *Klebsiella* and *Pseudomonas* and Gram-positive organisms including *Staphylococcus aureus*, *Staphylococcus epidermidis* and *Streptococcus faecalis*. Less often the organism may be an anaerobe, *Pneumocystis carinii*, cytomegalovirus or a fungal infection.

Symptoms

The patient might be initially asymptomatic or have non-specific symptoms such as malaise and anorexia. Specific symptoms related to a site of infection can include dysuria, cough or sore throat.

Signs

Any fever over 38.5°C in a patient with $<1.0 \times 10^9$/L neutrophils should be considered due to systemic infection even in the absence of any other positive findings. There might be specific signs of infection in the oropharynx or chest. Sites of intravenous catheters should be carefully inspected for erythema or discharge. In more severe cases there could be obvious septicaemic shock with hypotension and tachycardia.

Investigations

Any patient who is at risk of neutropenia and found to be febrile requires an urgent blood count. If a low white count is confirmed, blood cultures, a midstream urine, throat swab and chest X-ray are required together with swabs from other clinically relevent sites, such as a catheter or cannula site, and collection of sputum if produced.

Treatment

Intravenous antibiotics should be instigated as a matter of urgency. The results of cultures should not be awaited as life-threatening septi-caemia can develop if there is any delay. The precise antibiotic combination to be used will be guided by individual hospital antibiotic poli-cies but will take the form of broad-spectrum cover against both Gram-negative and -positive organisms. Typical combinations are an amino-glycoside with an extended spectrum penicillin, e.g. gentamicin or amikacin and carbenicillin, ticarcillin or piperacillin. Alternatively a single-agent cephalosporin can be used, such as cef-tazidime or cefotaxime. If the fever does not settle after 48 hours and there have been no positive results from culture, then it might be necessary to add metronidazole for anaerobic organisms or amphotericin for fungi. If there is clinical evidence for *Pneumocystis* then treat-ment with high-dose co-trimoxazole will be required.

Once the results of cultures become avail-able, then antibiotics can be adjusted appropri-ately. They should be continued for at least 5 days or for 48 hours after the fever has settled, whichever is the longer period.

Persistent fever in patients having a central intravenous line suggests colonization of the line and will require removal of that line to eradicate the source of infection.

In patients at high risk of infection then antibiotic prophylaxis is recommended. This includes those with leukaemia and lymphoma undergoing intensive chemotherapy. Co-trimoxazole, fluconazole and aciclovir are commonly used.

TUMOUR LYSIS SYNDROME

This is a syndrome arising as a result of rapid breakdown of large numbers of cells, usually at instigation of chemotherapy for a highly sensitive tumour such as lymphoma or leukaemia. This results in extensive metabolic disturbance charac-terized by hyperkalaemia, hyperuricaemia, hyperphosphataemia and hypocalcaemia.

If clinically significant, the syndrome presents as acute renal failure or acute cardiac arrhyth-mias with the risk of sudden death.

Treatment

Tumour lysis should be anticipated in any patient with a bulky lymphoma or leukaemia about to undergo chemotherapy. Preventative measures should be instigated prior to chemotherapy with 24 hours of prehydration ensuring good renal output and urine flow, and oral allopurinol should be started to prevent hyperuricaemia.

Rasburicase is an enzyme which oxidizes uric acid to allantoin, thereby resulting in rapid clearance of uric acid as it is formed. It is indi-cated in patients with a high risk of tumour lysis providing greater protection against tumour lysis syndrome than allopurinol. It is particu-larly indicated in those with acute leukaemias, Burkitt's lymphoma, chemosensitive paediatric tumours and other groups with renal impair-ment. It should be given prior to chemotherapy and daily for up to 7 days.

In patients who develop metabolic distur-bances after chemotherapy, intravenous hydra-tion should be continued. Alkalinization of urine with sodium bicarbonate can increase tubular excretion of potassium and phosphate. Specific measures to reduce very high levels of potassium might be required using insulin and glucose in order to prevent cardiac arrhythmias. In the most severe cases, particularly where renal function deteriorates, then dialysis may be required.

Prognosis

In most cases the metabolic sequelae of tumour lysis should be predictable and preventable. Where metabolic disturbance does occur, prompt treatment is usually successful and the effects are usually self-limiting with resolution within 5–7 days of chemotherapy.

FURTHER READING

Coffier B, Altman A, Pui CH, Younes A, Cairo MS. Guidelines for the management of pediatric and adult tumour lysis syndrome: an evidence-based review. *Journal of Clinical Oncology* 2008;**26**: 2767–78

SELF-ASSESSMENT QUESTIONS

1. Which of the following is true of malignant hypercalcaemia?
   a. It is a complication of lytic bone metastases
   b. It presents with diarrhoea
   c. The serum level of calcium should be corrected for the total protein
   d. Osteoclast-activating factors are important in its aetiology
   e. The serum phosphate is typically low

2. Which three of the following are true in the management of hypercalcaemia?
   a. Most patients will have fluid retention requiring diuretics
   b. Low calcium diet usually has little effect
   c. Bisphosphonates are the drug of choice
   d. If not repeated hypercalcaemia will recur after pamidronate
   e. Treatment of the underlying malignancy will be helpful
   f. Insulin and glucose will reduce the calcium rapidly in an emergency
   g. Phosphate supplements could also be required

3. Which of the following is true of spinal cord and cauda equina compression?
   a. It is usually due to extension of tumour from a vertebral metastasis
   b. Most cases have a sudden onset of neurological disability
   c. Hemiplegia is the most common motor deficit
   d. Typically back pain is absent
   e. Recovery is related to speed of initiation of treatment

4. Which three of the following are true in the management of cord compression?
   a. An urgent CT scan is essential for diagnosis
   b. High-dose steroids are started once the diagnosis is confirmed
   c. Treatment should be deferred where there is no known primary tumour
   d. Surgery is indicated for spinal collapse or instability
   e. Catheterization should be avoided to encourage bladder training
   f. Urgent radiotherapy is the treatment of choice for most cases
   g. Around 50 per cent of paraplegic patients will regain independent mobility

5. Which three of the following are true of superior vena cava obstruction?
   a. Lung cancer is the most common cause
   b. Widespread peripheral oedema will result
   c. Headache is a common presenting symptom
   d. Urgent embolectomy is indicated
   e. Most cases will resolve with heparin
   f. Superior vena cava stents are the treatment of choice
   g. Chemotherapy is contraindicated

6. Which of the following are common pathogens in neutropenic sepsis?
   a. *Streptococcus viridans*
   b. *Clostridium difficile*
   c. *Pseudomonas aeruginosa*
   d. *Helicobacter pylori*
   e. Herpes zoster

7. Which three of the following are true of the treatment of neutropenic sepsis?
   a. Intravenous antibiotics should be given despite no site of infection being found
   b. Urgent rehydration is required
   c. High-dose steroids should be started with antibiotics
   d. Inotropes may be required for hypotension
   e. Most patients can be managed as outpatients

SELF-ASSESSMENT QUESTIONS

f. Oral antibiotics are adequate once the neutrophils are $>1.0 \times 10^9/L$

g. All indwelling catheters must be removed

8. Which of the following is true of antibiotic use in neutropenic sepsis?
   a. Gentamicin alone is adequate for most patients
   b. If fever persists after 48 hours, metronidazole should be added
   c. The antibiotic of choice for initial use is cefuroxime
   d. Antibiotics should not be started until culture results are available
   e. If there is evidence of *Pneumocystis* infection, rifampicin should be added

9. In the treatment of which of the following does tumour lysis syndrome occur?
   a. Small cell lung cancer
   b. Follicular lymphoma
   c. Testicular seminoma
   d. Mycosis fungoides
   e. Burkitt's lymphoma

10. Which three of the following are seen in tumour lysis syndrome?
    a. Hypercalcaemia
    b. Hyperphosphataemia
    c. Renal failure
    d. Hyperkalaemia
    e. Hyponatraemia
    f. Hepatic failure
    g. Hypouricaemia

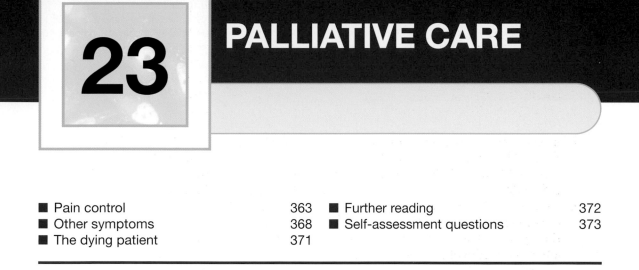

■ Pain control   363
■ Other symptoms   368
■ The dying patient   371

■ Further reading   372
■ Self-assessment questions   373

Medical care of a cancer patient does not stop when there is no curative treatment to offer and indeed over 50 per cent of cancer treatments are palliative. In this area lie many of the greatest challenges in patient care – controlling pain, dyspnoea, vomiting, haemorrhage and other tumour-related symptoms.

PAIN CONTROL

Cancer pain is a chronic pain distinct from that associated with acute events such as trauma, postoperative pain or a toothache. An important feature for its management is that it will often be associated with a significant emotional component alongside the physical cause of pain. Most cancer patients have associated anxiety, fear, depression and anger, which will modulate their perception of pain and attention to these features will be of equal importance to the use of analgesic drugs. Three components to the pain of advanced cancer have been described:

- physical
- emotional
- spiritual.

Careful evaluation of pain is important in this group of patients in order that treatment

can be directed to the principal underlying cause. Measurement of pain on an objective scale is of value, particularly in monitoring response to treatment. The use of a 10-point scale is common, sometimes in the form of a visual analogue scale, i.e. a 10 cm line on which the patient is asked to place a mark representing the severity of their pain. An example is shown in Figure 23.1.

Another important principle in the management of pain in this setting is that few patients will have a single cause of pain, the average will have three or four individual pains identified and in some circumstances several more. Such pains may be interrelated, and around one-quarter might not be directly due to the cancer but reflect pre-existing pathology, e.g. osteoarthritis, or be associated pains from the effects of treatment interventions. The overall picture for an individual patient can therefore be quite complex. Assessment and monitoring can be helped by the use of a 'pain diagram' alongside the use of pain scores as shown in Figure 23.1.

The incidence of pain in patients with advanced cancer is between 70 and 80 per cent. This can be effectively controlled in most cases by the application of simple rules governing the use of analgesics and related drugs:

PAIN CHART

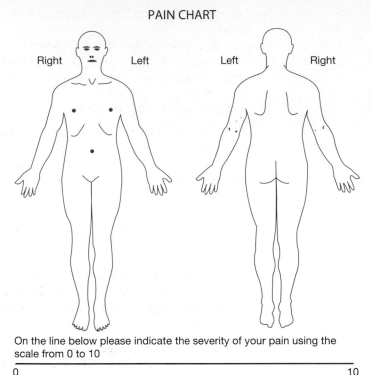

On the line below please indicate the severity of your pain using the scale from 0 to 10

0
No pain

10
Worst imaginable pain

Figure 23.1 Pain assessment chart showing pain diagram on which the patient is asked to mark sites of pain, and 10 cm visual analogue scale (VAS) on which the patient is asked to mark severity of pain (0 = no pain, 10 = worst imaginable pain).

1 Make a precise diagnosis of the cause of pain, e.g. whether a bone metastasis or nerve root pain.
2 Remember that many patients will have more than one pain and that pre-existing causes of pain such as arthritis will still be important.
3 Prescribe analgesics regularly, not as required, to prevent pain rather than wait for pain to return before the next dose.
4 Use and be familiar with a small number of drugs based on the analgesic ladder shown in Figure 23.2.
5 Consider specific cancer treatments, e.g. radiotherapy for bone pain whenever appropriate.
6 Establish realistic aims and expectations; not all patients will experience complete pain relief within a full range of activity and this should be made clear. Three levels of pain relief are described:
   ◾ pain free at night
   ◾ pain free sitting at rest
   ◾ pain free on movement.
Whilst the first two of these should be expected by most patients, pain control for movement-related pain is often much more difficult to achieve without limitation to movement.
7 Continually reassess the response to treatment and be prepared to modify regimens as the patient's condition evolves.

The use of analgesics in this situation should be based on a simple three-step analgesic ladder progressively escalating the potency of drug used. Alongside this it is important to consider more specific causes of pain that may respond to additional treatment, for example radiotherapy for bone metastases.

Level I analgesics

Although these are freely available non-prescription drugs, of patients who have not

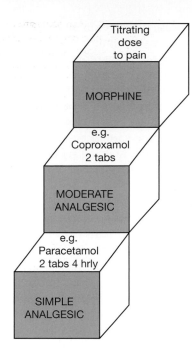

Figure 23.2 The analgesic ladder.

experienced regular analgesics around 20 per cent will achieve good pain control simply by starting regular level I analgesics. Paracetamol or ibuprofen are the drugs of choice, available 'over the counter' in many countries, but none the less highly effective drugs when given on a regular basis. Paracetamol has the advantage of a very low incidence of side-effects whilst ibuprofen or a similar non-steroidal anti-inflammatory drug (NSAID) might be better where an anti-inflammatory action is required, although it is associated with gastrointestinal side-effects, which occur particularly in the elderly.

Level II analgesics

When level I analgesics are no longer effective, the next step is to use regular level II analgesics. These drugs are weak opioids, i.e. they act by binding to the same opioid receptors as morphine but are less potent. Because of this, however, they tend to have a similar side-effect profile, in particular being associated with nausea and constipation. The drugs available in this group are:

- codeine, given as codeine phosphate 4 to 6 hourly
- dihydrocodeine, a derivative of codeine
- combination formulations of the above with paracetamol (co-codamol or co-dydramol)
- tramadol, a newer synthetic opioid.

There is no evidence to suggest that any one of the above is superior in the treatment of cancer pain; choice will be based upon availability, patient tolerance and physician preference.

Level III analgesics

Morphine

Morphine should be used when the pain is no longer responsive to a level II analgesic. The following principles apply to the use of morphine in this setting:

1 Start treatment with regular 4-hourly morphine solution or tablets. These are much more flexible for dose titration than controlled-release tablets.
2 Start a regular laxative with morphine, such as co-danthramer.
3 Start or be prepared to introduce a regular anti-emetic, such as haloperidol.
4 Slowly increase the dose from an initial 10 mg 4 hourly until pain control is achieved. Initially the dose can be doubled every 24–48 hours; beyond 60 mg, 4-hourly increments of 50 per cent might be better tolerated.
5 Warn the patient that during the introduction and dose titration, they could feel drowsy and that this will improve once they are on a stable dose.
6 Reassure the patient that addiction does not occur in this setting.

Parenteral opioids

Injection of opioid drugs such as morphine does not make them more potent when equivalent doses are given and should be considered only when oral or rectal administration is not possible. Remember, however, that because of its greater bioavailability when injected, the oral dose should be approximately halved to give an equivalent analgesic action.

Controlled-release morphine

Morphine tablets giving a 12- or 24-hourly release of morphine are generally preferred by patients once their dose requirements have been defined. Conversion from one morphine preparation to the other is simple as they are equivalent and a 12-hourly dose can therefore be given as a single controlled-release tablet or divided into three doses of immediate-release morphine at 4-hourly intervals.

If pain recurs then the cause should be investigated. Immediate-release morphine tablets or liquid should be available to be given in addition to controlled-release tablets for 'breakthrough pain'. It is important to remember that the breakthrough dose should reflect the 12-hourly dose, i.e. be equivalent to a further 4-hourly dose so that a patient on 30 mg 12 hourly will require 10 mg breakthrough doses, but another taking 120 mg 12 hourly will require 30 mg breakthrough doses.

Spinal opioids

Epidural or intrathecal administration, usually of diamorphine, can have a place in patients with very high morphine requirements or who are resistant to oral medication.

Alternatives to morphine

Whilst morphine is universally available and accepted as the level III analgesic of choice, some patients will have unacceptable side-effects, in particular drowsiness, hallucinations, confusion and constipation. In this setting, alternatives to morphine should be considered.

Fentanyl

This is a highly potent opioid drug with a short half-life. It is available in the form of skin patches allowing continuous transdermal absorption. This may have advantages over morphine in patients experiencing limiting side-effects or in those where oral administration is difficult. A single patch will provide analgesia for 72 hours at a time and a dose of 25 µg per hour gives equivalent analgesia to a 24-hour morphine dose of approximately 100 mg. There is, however, less flexibility with patches available in 25 µg/hour increments, up to 100 µg strength in a single patch. If necessary, breakthrough morphine doses can be combined with the use of fentanyl patches and, because of the delay in immediate absorption, the previous full dose of morphine should be continued for the first 24 hours after starting fentanyl patches to avoid withdrawal symptoms.

Hydromorphone

This is a synthetic strong opioid, similar to morphine but in some patients better tolerated. It is therefore a useful alternative to morphine when side-effects intrude. It is available in the same oral formulations as morphine but, because it is more potent, a dose reduction is needed, with 1.5 mg hydromorphone giving equivalent analgesia to 10 mg morphine.

Oxycodone

This is another alternative strong opioid. It has for many years been available as a suppository, but is now also produced as an oral drug in both immediate-release and controlled-release formulations. With hydromorphone it represents a suitable alternative to morphine for patients who cannot tolerate morphine because of limiting side-effects, although since it is also a strong opioid a similar spectrum of unwanted effects are to be expected with both these drugs, in particular nausea and constipation. The use of these drugs should therefore follow similar guidelines to those for morphine with the accompanying use of regular prophylactic laxatives and anti-emetics.

Diamorphine (diacetyl morphine)

This is preferred for injections because of its greater solubility. Otherwise it has no advantages and is converted to morphine rapidly on passing through the liver.

Morphine-resistant pain

Whilst the above approach will work well for most patients, there is undoubtedly a group of patients whose pain is not sensitive to morphine or other opioid drugs. It is important to recognize these patients and not submit them to ever-increasing doses of morphine for no benefit. In particular musculoskeletal pains and neurogenic pains can fall into this category. A further group of patients has been identified whose pain has been described as 'morphine irrelevant pain'. This refers to those where the overriding aetiology of their pain is due to an affective or spiritual component.

Therefore, in patients who, after dose titration to 40 or 60 mg morphine 4 hourly, are reporting no pain reduction with medication, it is important to reconsider the further use of morphine and explore alternative approaches with adjuvant analgesics, non-drug teatments or specific treatment such as local radiotherapy. A small group of patients can be identified who have true 'morphine resistance'. This has been attributed to an adaptive central response resulting in 'wind up', with altered perception of painful and non-painful stimuli (hyperalgesia and allodynia). This is thought to be mediated by a specific neurotransmitter, N-methyl-D-aspartate (NMDA). Specific NMDA inhibitor drugs are available including methadone and ketamine. Methadone dosage is often difficult to titrate and ketamine can be associated with significant psychotomimetic side-effects. Such measures should be considered only under careful supervision in a specialist pain unit.

Adjuvant analgesics

This includes all drugs that do not have intrinsic analgesic activity but in specific situations will help in pain relief.

Non-steroidal anti-inflammatory drugs (NSAIDs)

These are useful in bone pain and soft tissue infiltration by tumour. They include drugs such as aspirin, ibuprofen or naproxen and can be adequate used alone as step I analgesics in some patients. Their main disadvantage is their association with gastritis and gastrointestinal haemorrhage. The risk is least with ibuprofen and greatest with ketorolac. Where there is a previous history of dyspepsia or proven peptic ulceration, then particular care is required and concomitant use of a protective drug such as omeprazole, lansoprazole or misoprostol is rec-ommended. They are also contraindicated in patients with renal impairment and significant asthma.

Steroids

These are of value in nerve root pain, raised intracranial pressure, hepatomegaly and soft tissue infiltration. Dexamethasone might be more convenient than prednisolone but both are effective in moderate doses, e.g. dexamethasone 4 mg twice daily or prednisolone 20–40 mg daily. There may be the added advantage of increased wellbeing experienced by many patients on taking steroids, but care should be taken not to induce steroid-related side-effects in particular fluid retention, restlessness and insomnia. The latter can be avoided by taking single early morning doses.

Bisphosphonates

Both pamidronate and clodronate can be effective in metastatic bone pain even in the absence of hypercalcaemia. Oral absorption is variable and oral formulations are often not well tolerated; many patients are therefore better served by intermittent intravenous infusions. Hypocalcaemia and transient fevers during administration can occur and serum calcium requires occasional monitoring. A rare complication of prolonged use is mandibular necrosis.

Anxiolytic drugs

Small doses of drugs such as diazepam might be required where anxiety is either a major component of pain or a debilitating condition in its own right. In the terminal phase patients often become restless and agitated and then midazolam given by subcutaneous infusion is effective.

Antidepressants

These could be required for some patients who are significantly depressed and can also be of value for neuropathic pain. Evidence for a role in neuropathic pain is greatest for amitriptyline, whereas, where a true antidepressant effect is sought, newer drugs with selective serotonin uptake inhibitor activity such as fluoxetine, paroxetine and sertroline may be preferable.

Muscle relaxants

Baclofen can be of value where muscle spasm is a significant component of pain, for example in paraplegia or associated with underlying bone or soft tissue metastases.

Anticonvulsants

Pain owing to peripheral nerve damage, either from tumour infiltration or other associated conditions, for example herpes zoster, can be particularly difficult to control and is often not very responsive to pure analgesics. It is typically a burning or stabbing pain within the affected dermatome. Alongside amitriptyline, gabapentin and pregabalin have emerged as the most useful in neuropathic pain largely replacing older drugs such as carbamazepine, sodium valproate or clonazepam, although objectively they each appear effective.

Specific cancer treatments for pain control

For local pain from a growing and infiltrating tumour, specific therapy aimed at a reduction in tumour bulk and growth arrest is often the most effective approach.

Radiotherapy

This is highly effective for metastatic bone pain and also of value in relieving headache owing to raised intracranial pressure from primary or metastatic intracranial tumours. In this setting it is, however, important to select those patients with good performance status whose symptoms cannot otherwise be controlled with medication or those in whom medication such as morphine and steroids causes troublesome side-effects.

In other situations where tumour is invading nerve roots or plexuses, as with an apical lung tumour invading the brachial plexus or presacral rectal tumour invading the lumbosacral plexus, radiotherapy is indicated for pain control.

Chemotherapy

In sensitive tumours, such as small cell lung cancer, breast cancer and myeloma, chemotherapy can be of value for both bone and soft tissue pain where tumour infiltration is the main cause of pain. Despite only modest objective activity, chemotherapy is often associated with improvements in quality of life including pain and mobility scores. Examples include cisplatin and gemcitabine in non-small cell lung cancer, taxotere in hormone-resistant prostate cancer and gemcitabine in pancreatic cancer. Again careful patient selection is required to optimize benefits and avoid unnecessary treatment in the face of disease that will inexorably progress.

Other pain treatments

Pain can have many components. The pain associated with malignant disease can have a major affective (emotional) component, and neuropathic pain and incident movement-related pain can present major challenges. In such pain analgesics and adjuvant drugs are often not successful alone. Alternative non-drug treatments can be very effective in selected patients. These include:

- transcutaneous electrical nerve stimulation (TENS) – sometimes particularly valuable for neuropathic pains
- specific nerve blocks – sometimes dramatically successful in selected cases
- neurosurgical procedures such as cordotomy, rhizotomy or thalotomy
- massage – including the use of heat and cold to painful and tender areas
- acupuncture – can be particularly successful for difficult neuropathic pains
- relaxation and techniques such as aromatherapy – may also have a place in alleviating distress related to advanced malignancy.

OTHER SYMPTOMS

Many symptoms other than pain can affect the patient with advanced cancer. These include anorexia, nausea and vomiting, constipation, sore mouth, confusion, cough and dyspnoea.

TABLE 23.1 Anti-emetic drugs in advanced cancer

Site of action	Drugs	Indication
Vomiting centre	Cyclizine	Can be useful in all causes as this is the final common pathway for vomiting reflex
Chemoreceptor trigger	Prochlorperazine	Drug-induced
	Chlorpromazine	Metabolic, e.g. hypercalcaemia, uraemia, hepatic
	Haloperidol	Metastases
	Metoclopramide	
	Domperidone	
	Ondansetron	
Peripheral	Metoclopramide	Gastric stasis
	Domperidone	
	Ondansetron	

Management of these symptoms should focus on the basic principle of diagnosing the precise cause for each symptom on the basis of which the most effective treatment can be devised.

Anorexia

This may have many causes, often inter-related, including:

- anxiety
- nausea
- pain
- liver metastases
- sore mouth
- uraemia.

Specific treatment for each of these could be required, alongside which appetite can be stimulated by the use of low-dose steroids such as dexamethasone 4 mg daily or prednisolone 10–20 mg daily. An alternative is a progestogen such as medroxyprogesterone or megestrol which has the advantage of fewer steroid side-effects.

It is important to have clear goals and realistic expectations. Patients with advanced cancer do not typically regain the weight lost prior to diagnosis and there is no evidence that specific dietary approaches will prolong life at this stage. Often considerable anxiety and tension develop between patients and those caring for them who, with the best possible motives, wish to see them eating heartily. Small, perhaps more frequent, meals with the emphasis on patient enjoyment and avoiding dehydration rather than high calorie intake is a preferable approach.

Nausea and vomiting

This can be a side-effect of many drugs used in advanced cancer, in particular morphine. Other potential causes include:

- mechanical bowel obstruction
- hepatic metastases
- uraemia
- hypercalcaemia
- cerebral metastases.

A simple biochemical test should be made as the initial step in management with correction, where possible, of any biochemical disturbance. In addition anti-emetic drugs will be required. Many drugs are available; choice for any individual should be based on the cause of nausea and the drug's site of action, as shown in Table 23.1.

Where there is no clear individual cause, then treatment should be started with metoclopramide 10 mg 4–6 hourly, haloperidol 1.5–3 mg nocte or cyclizine 50 mg 8 hourly. A similar principle of regular medication to prevent symptoms rather than 'as required' medication applies to the use of anti-emetics as to analgesics. Often patients end up on a cocktail of three or four drugs and it is important to evaluate carefully the response to each and discontinue them if there is no clear benefit.

Patients with nausea and particularly those who are already vomiting might have difficulty taking oral medication which may, if anything, simply provide an additional stimulus to emesis. In this situation rectal administration using domperidone or prochlorperazine suppositories or buccal prochlorperazine can be helpful. Alternatively, subcutaneous administration, the infusion often also incorporating analgesics, can be used; metoclopramide, cyclizine and haloperidol are all compatible in this setting.

Constipation

Constipation and fear of constipation is often a major concern to patients and should be actively managed to avoid the situation where effective medication such as opioid analgesia is refused because of this. Constipation can be a side-effect of drugs, in particular morphine and other opioids, or related to dehydration, hypercalcaemia or mechanical restriction of the bowel from intra-abdominal or pelvic tumour. Good hydration and, where appropriate, a diet containing fruit and other fibre should be encouraged. Fruit juices are often welcome when solid food is no longer taken.

Laxatives should be given regularly to all patients receiving opioid medication. Co-danthramer, which has a combination of a bowel stimulant and faecal softener, is useful for opioid-related constipation and the dose can be titrated to the patient's requirements. Alternatives such as senna formulations, bisacodyl, docusate, osmotic salts, and lubricants, such as liquid paraffin, are also effective. Whilst oral agents are in general preferable in stubborn constipation, glycerine suppositories or phosphate enemas might be necessary to break a difficult cycle, particularly when preventive measures have not been used.

Sore mouth

This may be due to dryness of the oral cavity as a side-effect of drugs, including morphine and phenothiazine anti-emetics, radiotherapy to the mouth, mucositis related to chemotherapy or candidiasis.

Oropharyngeal candidiasis can cause severe symptoms in these patients and should be treated actively with topical nystatin or amphotericin and, for persistant cases, oral ketoconazole. Regular mouthwashes, sucking ice cubes, carbonated drinks or ascorbic acid are also recommended.

Confusion

This can be one of the most difficult symptoms to deal with. There is often an identifiable precipitating cause which may include:

- medication, e.g. morphine
- hepatic failure
- renal failure
- hypercalcaemia
- hypoxia
- infection
- cerebral metastases.

Specific attention to the above can be supplemented with mild sedation using low doses of a benzodiazepine or, in more severe disturbance with hallucinations, haloperidol might be required in the acute phase. However, drugs should not take the place of sympathetic psychological support and reassurance counteracting the cycle of misinterpretation and overreaction which builds up.

Cough and dyspnoea

This is commonly the result of progressive intrathoracic tumour causing bronchial irritation or obstruction, lung collapse, lung metastases or pleural effusion. Chest infections are also common in this group of patients.

Alongside specific management of these problems, for example aspiration of effusion and antibiotics for overt infection, cough sedatives based on codeine linctus could be tried. When this is unsuccessful, morphine in doses of 10–20 mg 4 hourly can be effective. Steroids can be of value in diffuse lung infiltration with metastases or lymphangitis carcinomatosa.

Common patterns are seen to emerge when the above symptoms are considered. In particular many symptoms can be attributable to biochemical disturbance, and simple investigations including blood urea, creatinine and electrolytes, liver function tests and serum calcium may provide the cause for specific problems. It is always important to take a full and detailed drug history, since many of the problems encountered will be related to medication. Renal and hepatic dysfunction will also influence drug handling, and a change in these can suddenly destabilize a previously satisfactory drug schedule. In particular remember that active metabolites of morphine are excreted through the kidney and in impaired renal function morphine toxicity can quickly develop owing to their accumulation if appropriate dose adjustments are not made.

THE DYING PATIENT

Inevitably there will come a time when death is imminent. This may require changes in medication to minimize the physical distress for both the patient and relatives. The following points should be considered.

Place of death

Only a small minority of patients die in a specialist palliative care setting such as a hospice. The majority die in a general hospital ward or at home. When it is clear that the terminal course of the disease is approaching, the patient and their carers should have the opportunity to discuss the anticipated course of events and the place they would choose to die. The extent to which this is possible will depend upon the individual patient, their wish to freely discuss such issues and to take part in such decisions. It is often a greater burden for the family of the patient who may worry about their ability to care for them at home, whilst having misgivings about the care available in local institutions. This is a particular concern where the patient expresses a strong wish to die at home but may live with only one elderly spouse whose physical capacity to provide the care required is limited.

It is therefore important to identify the level of support that may be required for each individual, to have realistic plans for their care and to enable them to die in the surroundings in which they and their family are most comfortable.

Medication for the dying patient

Diminishing levels of consciousness will require a switch from oral medication. It is rarely necessary to give drugs intravenously or intramuscularly and the subcutaneous route should be chosen. If the patient is expected to succumb within a day or so, intermittent injections can be acceptable, but it is often easier and less traumatic to set up a continuous infusion pump. Diamorphine or morphine can be given by this route (remembering to reduce the oral dose by 50 per cent) and, if anti-emetics are required, haloperidol or metoclopramide can be added to the infusion. Alternatively these can be given in suppository form.

Agitation and restlessness

Terminal agitation and restlessness can develop. This is best treated by haloperidol, levopromazine or midazolam in the subcutaneous infusion.

Respiration

Pooling of secretions can make respiration unpleasantly noisy and uncomfortable. This is best controlled with subcutaneous hyoscine in doses of 0.2–0.4 mg. Levopromazine is also a useful drug in this setting, compatible with subcutaneous infusions and, as a phenothiazine, it also has anti-emetic actions if required.

Reassessment of medication

Many patients continue to be left on large numbers of oral medications, most of which are irrelevant in these final hours. It is important therefore to review carefully all medication and in general most routine oral medical treatments such as antihypertensives, anti-inflammatory drugs and laxatives can be discontinued without causing distress to the patient or hastening death.

Acute haemorrhage

Acute deaths are unusual in oncology but rarely a tumour can erode a large enough blood vessel to cause acute haemorrhage. The typical sites for this are the carotid artery in the neck, femoral artery in the groin or an intrapulmonary vessel. These are inevitably terminal events and can cause considerable distress. Sedation with parenteral diamorphine and local pressure to control blood loss should be administered. A dark-coloured blanket is also of great value in masking the dramatic loss of blood.

Resuscitation

It is always distressing following a chronic illness with inevitable death for the final moments to be submitted to inappropriate resuscitation procedures. It is important therefore that clear policies regarding resuscitation are given to those caring for the patient, arrived at only after full discussion with the patient and their family.

FURTHER READING

Hanks GW, Cherney N, Christakis N, Fallon MT, Kassa S, Portenoy RK (eds). *Oxford Textbook of Palliative Medicine*. Fourth Edition. Oxford University Press, Oxford, 2009

Forbes K (ed.). *Opioids in Cancer Pain*. Oxford University Press, Oxford, 2007

Rice A, Howard R, Justins D, Miaskowski C (eds). *Clinical Pain Management*. Second Edition. Volume 3: *Cancer Pain*. Arnold, London, 2008

Twycross RG, Wilcock A. *Symptom Control in Advanced Cancer*. Third Edition. Blackwell, Oxford, 2007

SELF-ASSESSMENT QUESTIONS

1. Which of the following is true of cancer pain?
   a. It is usually traced to a single physical cause
   b. It is affected by emotional responses to cancer
   c. It is constant day and night
   d. Treatment is based on similar principles to postoperative pain
   e. It is difficult to assess accurately

2. Which three of the following apply to managing cancer pain?
   a. Analgesics should be given 'as required'
   b. Radiotherapy can play an important role
   c. A wide range of analgesics should be available
   d. Treatment might need to change regularly
   e. Different treatments may be required for individual pains
   f. Relief of daytime pain is the first goal
   g. Once pain is controlled, medication should be reduced

3. Which three of the following apply to the analgesic ladder?
   a. Non-steroidal anti-inflammatory drugs may be used as step 1
   b. Tramadol is a useful level 2 analgesic
   c. Paracetamol is avoided as chronic use causes hepatic damage
   d. Severe pain will require level 3 analgesics
   e. Codeine is the most effective level 1 analgesic
   f. Morphine should be given only in the last weeks of life
   g. Level 2 analgesics should be discontinued when morphine is started

4. Which of the following is true of morphine use in cancer pain?
   a. Controlled-release formulations are best avoided
   b. Laxatives should be routinely prescribed with morphine
   c. Initially it can be introduced 'as required'
   d. Regular administration every 6 hours is most effective
   e. Regular anti-emetics are rarely required

5. Which of the following is a useful alternative to oral morphine in cancer pain?
   a. Sublingual buprenorphine
   b. Oral pethidine
   c. Oral tramadol
   d. Transcutaneous fentanyl
   e. Oral diamorphine

6. Which three of the following are useful adjuvant analgesics in cancer pain?
   a. Paracetamol
   b. Salbutamol
   c. Flucloxacillin
   d. Vitamin E
   e. Gabapentin
   f. Tamsulosin
   g. Methotrimeprazine

7. Which of the following is used in the treatment of anorexia?
   a. Acupuncture
   b. Diazepam
   c. Oravite
   d. Megestrol
   e. Methtrimeprazine

8. Which three of the following causes nausea and vomiting in advanced cancer?
   a. Hypercalcaemia
   b. Hyperuricaemia
   c. Cisplatin
   d. Renal failure
   e. Candidiasis
   f. Ascites
   g. Acoustic neuroma

SELF-ASSESSMENT QUESTIONS

9. Which of the following is true in constipation in advanced cancer?
   a. It may be due to renal failure
   b. Most patients respond to dietary changes
   c. Hyperuricaemia should be actively treated
   d. It will often respond to diuresis
   e. Patients on opioids will require daily laxatives

10. Which of the following is true in the dying patient?
    a. Regular meals should be maintained for as long as possible
    b. Sedation should be avoided
    c. Drugs and fluids are best given intravenously
    d. Analgesia can often be reduced
    e. Subcutaneous midazolam is used for terminal agitation

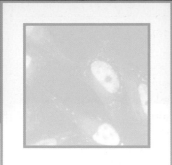

APPENDIX 1

Number of new cancers and deaths annually in the UK by site – males and females* (ranked by incidence)

Rank	Site	No. cases	(%)**	No. deaths
1	Breast	44 659	15.7	12 400
2	Lung	38 313	13.5	34 150
3	Colorectal	36 109	12.7	16 000
4	Prostate	34 986	12.3	10 000
5	Bladder	10 093	3.5	4800
6	Non-Hodgkin's lymphoma	10 003	3.5	4500
7	Malignant melanoma	8939	3.1	1900
8	Stomach	8178	2.9	5300
9	Oesophagus	8000	3.0	7405
10	Pancreas	7398	2.6	7300
11	Kidney	7044	2.5	3800
12	Leukaemia	6998	2.5	4300
13	Ovary	6615	2.3	4400
14	Uterus	6438	2.3	1700
15	Oral	4769	1.7	1700
16	Central nervous system	4413	1.6	3600
17	Multiple myeloma	3788	1.3	2600
18	Liver	2867	1.0	3100
19	Cervix	2726	1.0	900
20	Mesothelioma	2167	0.8	2000
21	Larynx	2166	0.8	800
22	Testis	1958	0.7	80
23	Bone/connective tissue	1853	0.7	1000
24	Thyroid	1641	0.6	300
25	Hodgkin's disease	1519	0.5	300

* Adapted from Cancer Research UK 2004 incidence data and 2006 mortality data.

** Excluding non-melanomatous skin cancer.

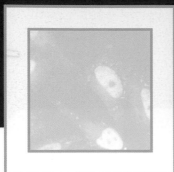

APPENDIX 2

Number of new cancers and deaths annually in the UK by site – males* (ranked by incidence)

Rank	Site	No. cases	(%)**	No. deaths
1	Prostate	34 986	24.4	10 000
2	Lung	22 495	15.7	19 600
3	Colorectal	19 657	13.7	8500
4	Bladder	7168	5.0	3200
5	Non-Hodgkin's lymphoma	5288	3.7	2400
6	Stomach	5157	3.6	3300
7	Oesophagus	4943	3.5	4900
8	Kidney	4348	3.0	2400
9	Leukaemia	4035	2.8	2500
10	Malignant melanoma	4015	2.8	1000
11	Pancreas	3603	2.5	3600
12	Oral	3149	2.2	1100
13	Central nervous system	2587	1.8	2100
14	Multiple myeloma	2065	1.4	1400
15	Testis	1958	1.4	80
16	Mesothelioma	1826	1.3	1700
17	Larynx	1789	1.2	600
18	Liver	1713	1.2	1900
19	Bone/connective tissue	1060	0.7	600
20	Hodgkin's disease	844	0.6	200
21	Small intestine	450	0.3	200
22	Thyroid	455	0.3	150
23	Penis	418	0.3	100
24	Breast	324	0.2	70
25	Salivary glands	307	0.2	100

* Adapted from Cancer Research UK 2004 incidence data and 2006 mortality data.

** Excluding non-melanomatous skin cancer.

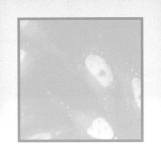

APPENDIX 3

Number of new cancers and deaths annually in the UK by site – females* (ranked by incidence)

Rank	Site	No. cases	(%)**	No. deaths
1	Breast	44 335	31.3	12 300
2	Colorectal	16 452	11.6	7400
3	Lung	15 818	11.2	14 600
4	Ovary	6615	4.7	4400
5	Uterus	6438	4.6	1700
6	Malignant melanoma	4924	3.5	800
7	Non-Hodgkin's lymphoma	4715	3.3	2100
8	Pancreas	3795	2.7	3700
9	Stomach	3021	2.1	2000
10	Leukaemia	2963	2.1	1800
11	Bladder	2925	2.1	1600
12	Cervix	2726	1.9	900
13	Oesophagus	2711	1.9	2500
14	Kidney	2696	1.9	1400
15	Central nervous system	1826	1.3	1500
16	Multiple myeloma	1723	1.2	1200
17	Oral	1620	1.1	600
18	Thyroid	1196	0.8	200
19	Liver	1154	0.8	1200
20	Vulva	1022	0.7	400
21	Bone/connective tissue	793	0.6	500
22	Hodgkin's disease	675	0.5	200
23	Gallbladder	412	0.3	300
24	Larynx	377	0.3	200
25	Small intestine	361	0.3	200

* Adapted from Cancer Research UK 2004 incidence data and 2006 mortality data.

** Excluding non-melanomatous skin cancer.

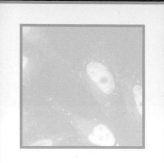

APPENDIX 4

ANSWERS TO SELF-ASSESSMENT QUESTIONS

Chapter 1

1. a, c, g
2. b
3. b, e, g
4. e

Chapter 2

1. b, d, e
2. d
3. b, d, f
4. c, e. g

Chapter 4

1. b, c, g
2. b

Chapter 5

1. c
2. d
3. b, d, e
4. d
5. d
6. c, e, f
7. b, c, f
8. e

Chapter 6

1. a, d, g
2. c

3. b
4. b
5. b, c, f
6. b, c, d
7. c, e, f
8. c
9. d
10. a, c, g

Chapter 7

1. a, c, g
2. e
3. d, e, g
4. d
5. b, c, g
6. c
7. a, b, f

Chapter 8

1. d, e, f
2. b
3. a, c, f
4. d
5. e, f, g
6. d
7. b, c, g
8. c

Chapter 9

1. c, d, g

2. b
3. b, c, e
4. a, d, e
5. d
6. c, e, g
7. a
8. a, b, g
9. c
10. b, e, f
11. a, d, g
12. e
13. b, c, e
14. c

Chapter 10

1. c
2. b
3. b, d, g
4. d
5. a, d, e
6. c, f, g
7. e
8. b
9. d
10. e
11. d
12. a, d, g
13. b
14. a

Chapter 11

1. e
2. c
3. a, e, g
4. d
5. e
6. b
7. d
8. a
9. b, d, f
10. c
11. a
12. b
13. c
14. a, b, f

Chapter 12

1. b, c, d
2. d
3. b, e, f
4. b
5. b. d. f
6. b

Chapter 13

1. b, e, g
2. d
3. c, d, f
4. e
5. a, b, c

6. a
7. a, c, e
8. b

Chapter 14

1. c, d, f
2. c
3. a, d, g
4. d

Chapter 15

1. c
2. b
3. b, c, e
4. b
5. e
6. c
7. e, f, g
8. b, d, g

Chapter 16

1. c
2. b
3. a, e, f
4. d
5. e

6. a, b, c
7. c
8. b
9. c, e, g
10. a, b, g

Chapter 17

1. b
2. a, c, f
3. b
4. e
5. b
6. b
7. a, b, g
8. e
9. b
10. d
11. a, d, e
12. b, d, g

Chapter 18

1. a
2. a, b, g
3. d
4. d
5. a, b, d

6. c
7. c
8. a, f, g
9. c
10. d

Chapter 19

1. c
2. a, c, d
3. c, f, g
4. b, e, g
5. a, c, d
6. b, d, f
7. b
8. b, c, d

Chapter 20

1. c, e, f
2. c
3. a, c, e
4. b, c, e

Chapter 21

1. c, e, g
2. a, b, d

Chapter 22

1. d
2. c, d, e
3. e
4. b, d, f
5. a, c, f
6. c
7. a, d, f
8. b
9. e
10. b, c, d

Chapter 23

1. b
2. b, d, e
3. a, b, g
4. b
5. d
6. c, e, g
7. d
8. a, c, d
9. e
10. e

INDEX

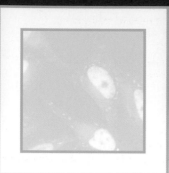

ABL see BCR-ABL
ABVD regimen, Hodgkin's lymphoma 271, 272, 273
AC regimen, breast cancer 106
acquired immune deficiency syndrome *see* HIV disease and AIDS
ACTH-secreting pituitary tumours 214, 215
active surveillance *see* surveillance
acute lymphoblastic leukaemia 288–92
acute myeloid/myeloblastic leukaemia 292–4
adenocarcinoma
  bladder 177
  cervical 191
  lung 68
  ovarian 194
  of unknown primary, likely sites 348
adenoid cystic carcinoma
  oesophageal 124
  salivary 236
adenolymphoma, salivary 236
adenoma
  parathyroid 246
  pituitary 214–16
  salivary 236
adenomatous polyposis, familial (FAP) 143
adjuvant (postoperative) treatment 24–5
  chemoradiotherapy
    pancreatic cancer 133
    stomach cancer 127–8
  chemotherapy
    cervical cancer 190
    endometrial cancer 193
    pancreatic cancer 133
    soft tissue sarcoma 258
    Wilms' tumour 320
  hormone therapy, prostate cancer 169
  radiotherapy 37
    breast cancer 24–5, 104–5
    cervical cancer 176–8
    colorectal carcinoma 148
    endometrial cancer 193
    medulloblastoma 312
    neuroblastoma 318
    Wilms' tumour 320
Adjuvant prognostic model of breast cancer 113–14
adrenal gland tumours 246–8
aetiology 1–9
aflatoxin 4, 136
afterloading brachytherapy 43–4
age
  and breast cancer 89
  and prostate cancer 163
aggressive (intermediate/high-grade) non-Hodgkin's lymphoma
  classification 276
  treatment 280–4
agitation, dying 371
AIDS *see* HIV disease
AJCC staging, lung cancer 76
alanine dye industry 3
alentuzumab 64
alkylating agents 53
  carcinogenicity 4
all-trans-retinoic acid, promyelocytic leukaemia 294
alpha-fetoprotein (AFP; α-fetoprotein)
  hepatocellular carcinoma and 137
  testicular cancer and 19, 178, 180
amelanotic melanoma 333
American Joint Committee on Cancer (AJCC) staging, lung cancer 76
amputation
  osteosarcoma 261, 262
  soft tissue sarcoma 258
anal carcinoma 152–6
analgesic drugs 363–8

anaplastic/undifferentiated tumours
    thyroid carcinoma 239, 240
    of unknown primary, differential diagnosis
        347
anastrozole 25, 61, 62, 106, 109, 113
    preventive use 115
androgens
    antagonism *see* antiandrogens
    breast cancer therapy 62
angiogenesis inhibitors *see* antiangiogenic drugs
angiography
    hepatic
        carcinoids 250
        hepatocellular carcinoma 137
    magnetic resonance, CNS tumours 210
angiosarcoma, hepatic 139
    see also lymphangiosarcoma
Ann Arbor classification
    Hodgkin's lymphoma 270–1
    non-Hodgkin's lymphoma 279
anorexia 369
antiandrogens/androgen antagonism, prostate
        cancer 62–3, 169, 172
    prostate cancer 171
antiangiogenic drugs 54, 65
    colorectal carcinoma 150
    hepatocellular carcinoma 138
    multiple myeloma 304
    renal cancer 162
    renal cell carcinoma 162
antibiotics, neutropenic sepsis 359–60
anticonvulsants 368
antidepressants 367
antiemetics 59–60, 369–70
antiepileptics (anticonvulsants) 368
antimetabolites 52–3
antimitotic agents 53
antioestrogens
    breast cancer 61, 62, 105
        adverse effects 113
        metastatic disease 108–9
        prophylactic use 115
    melanoma 336
anus, carcinoma 152–6
anxiolytic drugs 367
APC 143
apoptosis, drugs inducing 53
aromatase inhibitors 61, 62, 106, 113
    adverse effects 113
    metastatic disease 109
    prophylactic use 115
arsenic 4
    and skin cancer 4, 325–6
asbestos 3, 67–8, 84–5
    preventing exposure 87
Askin's tumour 258

aspiration
    bone marrow *see* bone marrow sampling
    fine needle *see* fine needle aspiration
    pleuropericardial 80
astrocytoma 211–13
axillary node metastases 93
    management 103–4, 105
azo dyes 3

B-cell lymphoma
    classification 276
    monoclonal antibody therapy 64
Bacillus Calmette–Guérin (BCG), bladder cancer
        175
baclofen 368
bacterial infections causing neutropenic sepsis,
        antibiotics 359–60
barium studies
    colorectal carcinoma 145
    gastric carcinoma 126
    oesophageal cancer 120
Barrett's oesophagus 118, 119, 124
'basal' breast cancer 92
basal cell carcinoma
    skin 325–31
    vagina 202
basophil adenomas 214
BCG, bladder cancer 175
BCR-ABL 2, 294–5, 296
    agents targeting 8, 296
betel nut 225, 226
bevacizumab 54, 64
    breast cancer 109–10
    colorectal carcinoma 150
    lung cancer 80
    multiple myeloma 304
    renal cancer 162
    renal cell carcinoma 162
biliary cancer 139–41
Binet classification, chronic lymphocytic
        leukaemia 298
biochemical tests *see* laboratory tests
biological therapy 63–4
    breast cancer metastases 109–10
    colorectal carcinoma 150
    hepatocellular carcinoma 138
    lung cancer 80
    melanoma 336
    pancreatic cancer 133
    renal cell carcinoma 162–3
    see also specific types of therapy
biopsy 11
    bone marrow 16
    breast 99
    cervical 187
    chronic lymphocytic leukaemia 298

biopsy – (*contd*)
  CNS tumours 210
  endometrial 192
  hepatocellular carcinoma 137
  Hodgkin's lymphoma 270
  lung cancer metastases 75
  oral 227
  penile 181
  pleural 86
  prostate 167
  renal cell carcinoma 161
  sarcoma
    Ewing's 264
    soft tissue 257, 314
  skin
    basal and squamous cell carcinoma
      329
    melanoma 335
  thyroid 231
  unknown primary carcinoma metastases
    348
  see also histology
bisphosphonates 367
  in hypercalcaemia 355
  metastatic bone pain 367
    in breast cancer 110
  multiple myeloma 304
bitumen 4, 325
bladder cancer 172–80
blast crisis, chronic granulocytic leukaemia 294,
  295, 296
bleomycin 53
blood
  faecal occult 152
  tumour markers in 18
  see also peripheral blood progenitor cells
blood count (blood cell count)
  Ewing's sarcoma 263
  leukaemia
    acute lymphoblastic 290
    acute myeloid 293
    chronic granulocytic 295
    chronic lymphocytic 297–8
  lymphoma
    Hodgkin's 270
    non-Hodgkin's 277
  multiple myeloma 301
blood tests *see* laboratory tests
blood vessel formation, new, drugs targeting *see*
  antiangiogenic drugs
bone
  destruction by multiple myeloma 300
  lymphoma 284
  metastases *see* bone metastases
  sarcoma 259–65
    oral cavity 232

bone marrow
  ablative chemotherapy *see* high-dose marrow
    ablative chemotherapy
  infiltration by multiple myeloma 300, 301
  suppression (myelosuppression), and AIDS-
    related tumour treatment 342
  transplantation
    acute lymphoblastic leukaemia 291
    neuroblastoma 318
bone marrow sampling (aspiration and trephine)
  and examination 16
  embryonal rhabdomyosarcoma 314
  leukaemia
    acute lymphoblastic 290
    acute myeloid 293
    chronic granulocytic 295
    chronic lymphocytic 298
  lymphoma
    Hodgkin's 270
    non-Hodgkin's 278
  multiple myeloma 301
  neuroblastoma 317
bone metastases (skeletal metastases)
  breast cancer 93–6
    bisphosphonate therapy 110
  multiple myeloma vs 300
  radionuclide scan for *see* bone scan
bone scan
  for metastases 14
    bladder cancer 174
    osteosarcoma 261
    prostate cancer 167
    renal cell carcinoma 161
  multiple myeloma 301
bortezomib 304, 306
bowel
  large, cancer *see* colorectal carcinoma
  small, radiation damage 45
bowel habit change 144–5
brachytherapy 43
  oral carcinoma 229
  prostate cancer 168–9
    complications 171
  thyroid cancer 242–4
    complications 245
brain tumours *see* central nervous system;
  metastases
BRCA genes 90–1
  ovarian cancer and 194
breast cancer 89–117
  aetiology 90–1
  bilateral 92
  case histories 101, 110
    metastastic disease with unknown primary
      351–2
  differential diagnosis 96–7

epidemiology 89–90
investigations 97–100
    in exclusion with unknown primary 349
natural history 92–5
pathology 91–2
prevention 115
prognosis 113–14
screening 114–15
staging 100
symptoms and signs 95–6
therapy 8, 24–5, 61–2, 100–13
    complications 112–13
breathlessness *see* dyspnoea
Brenner tumours 197
Breslow thickness 335, 336–7
bronchial carcinoid 83
bronchoalveolar carcinoma 83
bronchoscopy
    lung cancer 72–3
    oesophageal cancer 120
Burkitt's lymphoma 281
Butchart staging classification, modified 86

CA 19-9 assay 131
CA 125 assay 195, 196, 197
Calvert formula 57
candidiasis, oropharyngeal 370
capecitabine, colorectal carcinoma 148, 159
carcinoembryonic antigen (CEA) 18, 127, 130,
    140, 144
carcinogens 1–9
    bladder cancer 172–3
    oral cancer 225–6
    skin cancer 4, 325–6
    see also specific (types of) carcinogens
carcinoid 248–51
    bronchial 83
    gastroenteropancreatic 135, 248–51
        stomach 130
    oesophageal 124
carcinoid syndrome 249, 250
carcinoma, of unknown primary 347–52
    *see also specific histological types and tissue/organ
        sites*
carcinoma in situ of breast *see* ductal carcinoma
    in situ; lobular carcinoma in situ
carcinomatous meningitis 221–3
case–control studies 34
Castleman's disease 285
catecholamines
    neuroblastoma 317
    phaeochromocytoma 247
cauda equina compression 209, 355–7
causation 1–9
cell cycle-specific antiangiogenic drugs 54
central nervous system, radiation damage 45

central nervous system tumours 207–24
    childhood 310–13
    general principles 207–11
        aetiology 207
        epidemiology 207
        investigations 210
        natural history 208–9
        pathology and classification 207–8
        symptoms and signs 209
        treatment 210–11
    leukaemia
        acute lymphoblastic 289, 290, 291
        acute myeloid 292, 293
    lymphomas 218, 278, 282
        AIDS-related 343–4
    MRI 14
    secondary *see* metastases
    see also spinal tumours
central venous access for chemotherapy 58–9
cerebral tumours *see* central nervous system;
        metastases
cervical cancer 185–91
cervical node metastases 226
    dissection 229
cetuximab
    colorectal carcinoma 150
    lung cancer 80
    oral cancer 230, 231
CHART *see* continuous hyperfractionated
        accelerated radiotherapy
chemical carcinogens 3–4
    bladder cancer 172–3
    oral cancer 225–6
    skin cancer 325–6
chemoradiotherapy
    anal carcinoma 155
    cervical cancer
        complications 190
        for extra-cervical disease 189
        for local disease 187–9
    lung cancer 78
    non-Hodgkin's lymphoma (aggressive/high-
        grade forms) 281
    pancreatic cancer 133
    stomach cancer 127–8
chemotherapy (cytotoxic drug) 54–7
    acute lymphoblastic leukaemia 290–1
    acute myeloid leukaemia 293
        complications 294
    administration 57–61
        routes 57, 58–9
        scheduling 60–1
    anal carcinoma, complications 156
    bladder cancer 176
        intravesical 176
        palliative 176

chemotherapy (cytotoxic drug) – (*contd*)
  breast cancer 105
    adjuvant 25
    complications 113
  cervical cancer 190
    palliative 190
  cholangiocarcinoma, palliative 141
  choriocarcinoma 203–4
    complications 204
  chronic granulocytic leukaemia 296
  chronic lymphocytic leukaemia 298
    complications 299
  clinical use (in general) 56
    palliative (pain control) 368
  CNS tumours 211
    astrocytoma 213
    lymphoma 218, 344
  colorectal carcinoma 148
    palliative 149–50
  combination 56
  complications/side-effects/toxicity (general
    aspects) 54–6, 56
    avoidance 59–60
    carcinogenicity 4, 292
    tumour lysis syndrome *see* tumour lysis
      syndrome
    see also specific cancer in subheadings
      above/below
  efficacy 54–6
  embryonal rhabdomyosarcoma 314–15
    palliative 315
  endometrial cancer 193
    palliative 193
  Ewing's sarcoma 264
    complications 264
    palliative 264
  hepatocellular carcinoma, palliative 138
  Hodgkin's lymphoma 271, 273
    case history 272
    complications 274
  Kaposi's sarcoma 343
  lung cancer 77, 78, 79, 84
    adverse effects 81
    palliative 79–80
  lymph node enlargement treated with 38
  multiple myeloma 303–4
    complications 304
  myeloablative *see* high-dose chemotherapy
  neuroblastoma 318
    complications 318
  non-Hodgkin's lymphoma 56
    aggressive/high-grade forms 280–1, 282
    AIDS patients 344, 344–5
    case history 293
    CNS 218, 344
    complications 284

    indolent/low-grade forms 279, 280
  oesophageal cancer 122
    complications 124
    neoadjuvant 121–2
    palliative 122
  oral cancer 230
    palliative 231
  osteosarcoma 261
    complications 262
  ovarian cancer 196
    complications 196
    palliative 196
    rare tumours 197, 198
  pancreatic cancer
    adjuvant 133
    palliative 133
  penile cancer, palliative 182
  prostate cancer 169–70
  resistance to 56–7
  skin cancer
    basal and squamous cell carcinoma 330
    melanoma 336
  soft tissue sarcoma 258
    embryonal rhabdomyosarcoma *see*
      subheading above
  stomach cancer 128
    palliative 128
  superior vena cava-obstructing tumours 358
  testicular cancer 179–80
    complications 180
  thyroid cancer, palliative 244
  types of agents 52–4
  unknown primary carcinoma 350–1
  vulval cancer, palliative 201
  Wilms' tumour
    complications 321
    palliative 320
    postoperative 320
chest (thorax)
  complications in lung cancer 80–1
  infections, recurrent 70
  pain 70
chest X-rays
  leukaemia
    acute lymphoblastic 290
    acute myeloid 293
  lung cancer 72
  lung metastases
    anal cancer 153
    bladder cancer 174
    hepatocellular carcinoma 137
    oral cancer 228
    ovarian cancer 195
    pancreatic carcinoma 131
    renal cell carcinoma 161
    soft tissue sarcoma 255, 314

thyroid cancer 241
vulval cancer 201
Wilms' tumour 320
lymphoma
Hodgkin's 270
non-Hodgkin's 278
mesothelioma 85–6
children 310–24
chloroma 294
cholangiocarcinoma 139–41
cholangiography *see* percutaneous transhepatic cholangiography
cholangiopancreatography *see* endoscopic retrograde cholangiopancreatography
cholecystectomy 142
chondrosarcoma 265
chordoma 218
choriocarcinoma 202–4
chromates 4
chromogranin A 250
chromophobe adenomas 214
chromosome (cytogenetic) abnormalities
acute lymphoblastic leukaemia 288, 289
chronic lymphocytic leukaemia 297
chronic myeloid leukaemia 2, 294–5
embryonal rhabdomyosarcoma 313
multiple myeloma 300
neuroblastoma 316
unknown primary carcinoma 349
chronic lymphocytic leukaemia 64, 297–9
chronic myeloid (granulocytic) leukaemia 2, 294–7
therapy 8, 296
complications 296
chronic trauma/inflammation/irritation 5
bladder cancer and 173
oral cancer and 226
soft tissue sarcoma and 254
Clark's levels 335
clinical evidence 28–9
clinical trials *see* trials
clotting profile
acute myeloid leukaemia 293
hepatocellular carcinoma 136
pancreatic cancer 131
CMF regimen, breast cancer 106
alternative drugs with failure of 109
coagulation profile *see* clotting profile
cohort studies 34–5
colonoscopy 145
colorectal carcinoma 142–52
aetiology 142–3
case history 151
epidemiology 142
hereditary non-polyposis *see* hereditary non-polyposis colon cancer

investigations 145–6
management 146–50
natural history 144
pathology 143–4
prevention 152
prognosis 150–1
screening 151–2
staging 146
symptoms and signs 144–5
combination chemotherapy, general aspects 56
see also references under chemotherapy *and specific acronyms/abbreviations for regimens*
combined modality therapy *see* chemoradiotherapy
communication 26–8
complete response (CR) 30
chemotherapy 55
compression, spinal tumours 209, 355–7
computed tomography (CT) 14
acute lymphoblastic leukaemia 290
bladder cancer 174
carcinoid 250
CNS tumours 210
pituitary tumours 215
gastrointestinal/digestive tract cancer
anal carcinoma 154
cholangiocarcinoma 140
colorectal carcinoma 145–6
hepatocellular carcinoma 137
oesophageal cancer 120
pancreatic cancer 131
stomach carcinoma 126
stomach carcinoma, for metastases 127
testicular cancer 178
gynaecological cancer
cervical cancer 187
choriocarcinoma 203
endometrial cancer 192
ovarian cancer 195
vulval cancer 201
lung cancer 73–4
lymphoma
Hodgkin's 270
non-Hodgkin's 278
medulloblastoma 311
mesothelioma 86
neuroblastoma 317
oral cancer 228
penile cancer 182
prostate cancer 166
renal cell carcinoma 161
sarcoma
Ewing's 263–4
osteogenic 261
soft tissue 256, 314
skin cancer 329

computed tomography (CT) – (*contd*)
  thyroid cancer 241
  unknown primary carcinoma 349
conformal radiotherapy 46
confusion 370
consolidation (intensification) chemotherapy
  acute lymphoblastic leukaemia 290
  acute myeloid leukaemia 293
  neuroblastoma 318
  see also high-dose marrow ablative
      chemotherapy
constipation 370
continuous hyperfractionated accelerated
      radiotherapy (CHART)
  lung cancer 78
  oral cancer 230
contrast studies, gastrointestinal *see* barium
      studies
controlled trials, randomized 29–34
corticosteroids (steroids) 367
cough 70, 370–1
Cowden's syndrome 91, 143, 239
CPT11 149
cranial/craniospinal (CNS) irradiation
  medulloblastoma 312
    complications 312–13, 313
  prophylactic
    acute lymphoblastic leukaemia 290
    lung cancer 78–9
craniopharyngiomas 216
creatinine clearance, ovarian cancer 195
cryotherapy, basal and squamous cell carcinoma
      of skin 330
culture and communication 26
curettage, basal and squamous cell carcinoma
      330
Cushing's syndrome 248
cutaneous problems/tumours etc. *see* skin
cyberknife 47
cystectomy 176
  complications 176
cystic ovarian cancer 194
cystoscopy 174
cytogenetic abnormalities *see* chromosome
      abnormalities
cytology 10–11
  breast cancer 99
  cervical cancer 187
  fine needle aspiration *see* fine needle aspiration
  lung cancer 72
  skin cancer 328–9
cytotoxic drug therapy *see* chemotherapy

data monitoring committee 33
death
  place of 371

as trial end-point 31
UK, by site 375–7
  see also dying
decision-making, treatment 23–8
denosumab 172
dermatofibroma 259
dermatological lesions *see* skin
desmoid tumour 259
diacetyl morphine 366
diagnosis, tissue *see* tissue diagnosis
diamorphine 366
diet
  carcinoid management 250
  colorectal carcinoma aetiology 142
digestive system cancer 118–59
digital examination
  rectum 145, 152
  vagina 145
disease-free survival 30
DNA
  anticancer drugs acting on structure 52–3
  ionizing radiation-induced damage 44–5
dopamine agonists, pituitary tumours 216
dose, radiotherapy 47–8
Down syndrome, acute lymphoblastic leukaemia
      288
drug-induced immunosuppression 7
drug therapy (non-anticancer medication)
  carcinoids 251
  dying patient 371
    reassessment 371–2
  pituitary tumours 216
  tumour lysis syndrome 360
  see also specific (types of) drugs
dry mouth 370
  radiotherapy-induced 231
ductal carcinoma in situ (DCIS) 90, 91
  treatment 100–2
Dukes staging system 146
duration of radiotherapy 47–8
Durie–Salmon staging system 302
dying
  discussing 27
  management 371–2
dysgerminomas
  brain 216–17
  ovary 197
dysphagia
  lung cancer 70
  oesophageal cancer 119
dyspnoea 70, 370–1
  lung cancer 70

EBV *see* Epstein–Barr virus
ECF regimen, oesophageal cancer 122
E/CMF regimen, breast cancer 107

economic assessments in trials 31–2
EDTA clearance, ovarian cancer 195
education *see* health education
EGFR *see* epidermal growth factor receptor
embolization, hepatic artery 138, 139
embryonal rhabdomyosarcoma 313–15
emergencies 354–62
emesis and its prevention 59–60, 369–70
endobronchial laser therapy 80
endobronchial stent 80
endocrine factors predisposing to cancer 8
endocrine therapy *see* hormone therapy
endocrine tumours 239–53
    see also hormone-secreting tumours; multiple
        endocrine neoplasia
endocrinologist referral for pituitary adenoma
    214
endometrial cancer 191–3
endometrial cancer therapy 63
endoscopic retrograde cholangiopancreatography
    cholangiocarcinoma 140
    pancreatic carcinoma 132
endoscopy, gastrointestinal
    anal carcinoma 153
    colorectal carcinoma 145
    gastric carcinoma 126
        palliative procedures using 128
    oesophageal cancer 120
    see also bronchoscopy; cystoscopy; laparoscopy;
        laryngoscopy; mediastinoscopy
end-points 29–32
environment
    communication and 26
    excess background radiation in *see* ionizing
        radiation
eosinophilic granuloma 321
ependymomas 217, 313
epidermal growth factor receptor (EGFR)
        inhibitor
    colorectal carcinoma 150
    lung cancer 150
    oral cancer 230
epidural opioids 366
Epstein–Barr virus (EBV) 6
    Hodgkin's lymphoma and 6, 268
    non-Hodgkin's lymphoma and 275, 281
erlotinib
    lung cancer 80
    pancreatic cancer 133
error, type I and II 33
erythrocyte sedimentation rate
    acute lymphoblastic leukaemia 290
    lymphoma
        Hodgkin's 270
        non-Hodgkin's 277
erythroderma 338

ethanol injection, percutaneous, hepatocellular
        carcinoma 138
ethics in trials 33–4
evidence, clinical 28–9
Ewing's tumour/sarcoma 263–5
    extraosseous 258
examination 12
    carcinoma of unknown primary 347
    under anaesthetic
        anal carcinoma 153
        oral cancer 227
excision biopsy 11
    breast cancer 99
    skin
        basal and squamous cell carcinoma 329
        melanoma 335
external beam radiotherapy
    basic principles 42–3
    conformal 46
extravasation of chemotherapy 59
eye
    radiation damage to lens 45
    tumours 237
        children 321–2
        secondary 221

faecal occult blood 152
FAM regimen, pancreatic cancer 133
familial adenomatous polyposis (FAP) 143
familial history/familial occurrence
    bladder cancer 173
    breast cancer 90–1
    prostate cancer 163
    soft tissue sarcoma 254
    see also genetic factors
family conflict 28
FEC regimen, breast cancer 106
females
    gynaecological cancer 185–206
    new cancers and deaths by site 376–7
fentanyl 366
fertility, male, chemotherapy affecting 180
α-fetoprotein *see* alpha-fetoprotein
FIGO staging
    cervical cancer 187
    endometrial cancer 192
    ovarian cancer 196
    vaginal cancer 199
fine needle aspiration (FNA) 11
    anal cancer, nodal 153
    breast cancer 97, 99
    cutaneous tumours, nodal
        basal and squamous cell carcinoma 329
        melanoma 335
    lung cancer, metastases 75
    oral cancer, nodes 228

fine needle aspiration (FNA) – (*contd*)
   penile cancer, nodal 182
   renal cell carcinoma 161
   thyroid cancer 241
   unknown primary carcinoma 348
   vaginal cancer, nodal 199
   vulval cancer, nodal 201
fluid cytology 10
   nipple discharge 99
   pleural 86
5-fluorouracil (5-FU)
   colorectal carcinoma 148, 149, 150
   cutaneous basal and squamous cell carcinomas
      330
   folinic acid and *see* folinic acid
   oesophageal cancer 122
   stomach cancer 128
   see also CMF; E/CMF; FAM; FEC
folic acid, drugs inhibiting reduction 53
folinic acid (leucovorin) + 5-fluorouracil 56
   colorectal carcinoma 148, 149, 150
follicular lymphoma
   classification 276
   therapy 279
follicular thyroid carcinoma 239, 240
fractionation of radiotherapy 48
fracture reduction and fixation 39
fungation
   breast cancer 94, 111
   surgical management 39

gallbladder carcinoma 141–2
Gammaknife® 47
Gardener's syndrome 143, 239
gastric cancer *see* stomach cancer
gastrinoma 135
gastrointestinal cancer 118–59
gastrointestinal stromal tumor (GIST) 8, 129
G-CSF 64
gefitinib 80
genetic (inherited) diseases, cancer predisposition
   2, 3
   basal cell carcinoma 326
   CNS tumours 207
   colorectal cancer 143
   leukaemia
      acute lymphoblastic 288
      acute myeloid 292
   Wilms' tumour 319
genetic factors 1–2
   bladder cancer 172–3, 173
   breast cancer 90–1
   ovarian cancer 194
   prostate cancer 163
genital tract/reproductive organ cancer
   females 185–206

   males 177–82
germ cell tumours
   brain 216–17
   childhood 322
   ovarian 194, 197
   testicular 178, 180
giant cell tumour of bone 265
Gleason score 164, 167
glial tumours *see* ependymoma; glioblastoma
   multiforme; oligodendroglioma
glioblastoma multiforme 209, 211, 213
glottic carcinoma 233
glucagonoma 135
gonadotrophin-releasing hormone analogues,
   prostate cancer 169
Gorlin's syndrome 326
granulocyte colony-stimulating factor 64
granulocytic leukaemia *see* myeloid leukaemia
granulocytic sarcoma 294
granuloma, eosinophilic 321
granulosa cell tumour 194, 198
Gray 48
growth factors 64–5
growth hormone-producing pituitary tumours
   214, 215
gynaecological cancer 185–206

haemangioblastoma, brain 218
haematological disorders 288–309
   in lung cancer 71
   neoplastic 288–309
haemoptysis 70
haemorrhage
   acute 372
   surgical management 39
hairy cell leukaemia 299
Halstead mastectomy 102
Hand–Schüller–Christian syndrome 321
head and neck cancer 225–34
health care professionals, HIV infection risk
   342
health economic assessments in trials 31–2
health education 8
   breast self-examination 180
   melanoma 337
   oral cancer 232
   smoking and lung cancer and smoking 83
heat, cancer risk 5
Helicobacter pylori and MALToma 125, 129, 275,
   282
hepatic angiography *see* angiography
hepatic artery embolization 138, 139
hepatitis, viral
   HBV 6, 135
   HCV 135
   serological tests 136

hepatocellular carcinoma (hepatoma) 135–9
  causes 4, 6, 135–6
HER2-targeting drugs
  metastatic breast cancer 109
  monoclonal antibody *see* trastuzumab
hereditary non-polyposis colon cancer 143
  bladder cancer in 173
  endometrial cancer in 191
  ovarian cancer in 194
HHV 8 (human herpes virus type 8) 7, 345
hidradenocarcinoma 339
high-dose marrow ablative chemotherapy
  acute lymphoblastic leukaemia 291
  multiple myeloma 303–4
  neuroblastoma 318
  non-Hodgkin's lymphoma 281
histiocytosis
  Langerhans' cell 321
  malignant 285
histology, choriocarcinoma 203
  see also biopsy
history-taking 12
  carcinoma of unknown primary 347
HIV disease and AIDS 7, 341–5
  non-Hodgkin's lymphoma 275, 343–5
Hodgkin's lymphoma 268–75, 315–16
  aetiology 268–9
    EBV 6, 268
  AIDS-related 345
  childhood 315–16
  nodular lymphocyte-predominant 285
homosexual activity and anal cancer 152, 156
hormone replacement therapy (oestrogens)
  breast cancer risk and 109
  in cervical cancer, post-treatment 190
hormone therapy (endocrine therapy) 61–3
  breast cancer 61–2, 105–7
    complications 113
    metastatic disease 108–9
  endometrial cancer 193
  melanoma 336
  pancreatic cancer 133
  prostate cancer 62–3, 169
    complications 171
    palliative 169
  thyroid cancer 244
    complications 245
hormone-secreting tumours
  ectopic, lung 71, 81
  gastroenterohepatic 135
  pituitary 214, 216
  see also endocrine tumours
Horner's syndrome 71
HPV *see* human papilloma virus
HTLV-1 *see* human T-cell lymphotrophic virus
  type 1

human chorionic gonadotrophin (HCG) levels
  choriocarcinoma 203, 204
  testicular cancer 19, 178, 180
human herpes virus type 8 (HHV-8) 7, 345
human immunodeficiency virus *see* HIV
  disease
human papilloma virus (HPV) 6
  anal cancer and 153–4
  cervical cancer and 185
  vaginal cancer and 198
  vulval cancer and 200
human T-cell lymphotrophic virus type 1
  (HTLV-1) 7
  chronic lymphocytic leukaemia (CLL; T-cell
    leukaemia/lymphoma) and 275, 297,
    298, 299
Hutchinson's melanotic freckle 334
hydatidiform mole 202, 203
hydromorphone 366
5-hydroxyindoleacetic acid, urinary 250
5-hydroxytryptamine (5-HT), carcinoid
  syndrome 249, 250
hypercalcaemia 354–5
  multiple myeloma 300
hypopharyngeal carcinoma 233–4
hysterectomy 193
  complications 193
  ovarian cancer 196

ibritumomab 64, 285
imaging *see* radiology
imatinib 8
  acute lymphoblastic leukaemia 290
  adverse effects 296
  chordoma 218
  chronic granulocytic leukaemia 296
  gastrointestinal stromal tumour 8, 129
immunocytochemistry, unknown primary
  carcinoma 349
immunosuppressed/immunodeficient states,
  cancer predisposition 7
  non-Hodgkin's lymphoma 275
  see also HIV disease
immunotherapy, Kaposi's sarcoma 342–3
  see also monoclonal antibodies
incision biopsy 11
  basal and squamous cell carcinoma 329
indolent (low-grade) non-Hodgkin's lymphoma
  classification 276
  treatment 279–80
induction chemotherapy
  acute lymphoblastic leukaemia 290
  acute myeloid leukaemia 293
  multiple myeloma 303–4
industrial carcinogens *see* occupational (incl.
  industrial) carcinogens

infections
  chest, recurrent 70
  neutropenic 359–60
  viral, in aetiology *see* viruses *and specific viruses*
infertility, male, chemotherapy causing 180
inflammation, chronic *see* chronic
      trauma/inflammation
inflammatory carcinoma of breast 91–2
information, communicating to patient 26–8
infusion of chemotherapy 58
inherited diseases *see* genetic diseases
insulinoma 135
intensification chemotherapy *see* consolidation
      chemotherapy
intensity-modulated radiotherapy (IMRT) 47
  oral cancer 230
interferon (IFN-α) 63
  complications 336
  melanoma 336
  renal cell carcinoma 162–3
interleukin-2 (IL-2)
  complications 336
  melanoma 336
  renal cell carcinoma 162
internal isotope therapy 44
interstitial treatment 43
intestine *see* bowel
intracavitary treatment 43
intraepithelial neoplasia
  cervical (CIN) 185
  prostate (PIN) 164
  vaginal (VAIN) 198, 200
intramedullary spinal tumours 208
  secondary (metastases) 221
intrathecal administration
  chemotherapy 58
  opioids 366
intravenous administration
  chemotherapy 58–9
  opioids 365–6
intravenous urography
  bladder cancer 174
  cervical cancer 187
  prostate cancer 166
intravesical chemotherapy, bladder cancer 176
investigations 12–20
iodine-131 in thyroid cancer 242–4
  complications 245
ionizing radiation
  biological actions 44–5
  carcinogenicity 5, 49
    acute lymphoblastic leukaemia 289
    acute myeloid leukaemia 292
    non-Hodgkin's lymphoma 275
    soft tissue sarcoma 254
    thyroid cancers 239

excessive background (environmental) 5
  lung cancer 68
  protection 49–50
irinotecan 149
irradiation *see* ionizing radiation
irritation, chronic *see* chronic
      trauma/inflammation/irritation
isotope(s), radioactive
  implants *see* brachytherapy
  safety considerations (patients and staff) 50
  systemic (internal) administration 44
  see also specific isotopes
isotope scan
  bone *see* bone scan
  thyroid 241
  see also meta-iodobenzyl guanidine scan

Jackson stage, penile cancer 182

Kaposi's sarcoma 338, 342–3
  oral cavity 232
Karnofsky performance scale and chemotherapy
      55
keratoacanthoma 328
keratosis, solar 328
kidney *see entries under* renal
knowledge, lack of 28
Krukenberg tumours 95, 125, 194, 198

laboratory tests (incl. blood/biochemistry) 12
  acute myeloid leukaemia 293
  choriocarcinoma 203
  Ewing's sarcoma 263
  lymphoma
    Hodgkin's 270
    non-Hodgkin's 277–8
  multiple myeloma 301
  prostate cancer 165–6
  renal cell carcinoma 161
  in trials 31
  unknown primary carcinoma 349
  Wilms' tumour 319
Langerhans' cell histiocytosis 321
laparoscopy
  diagnostic
    hepatocellular carcinoma, for biopsy 137
    stomach cancer 127
  therapeutic (surgical), phaeochromocytoma
      247
laparotomy, pancreatic carcinoma 132
lapatinib 109
large bowel cancer *see* colorectal carcinoma
laryngeal carcinoma 232–3
laryngoscopy, indirect 75
laser therapy, endobronchial 80
laxatives 370

leiomyoma, gastric 129–30
leiomyosarcoma
    endometrial 193
    oesophageal 124
lenalidomide (lenolidamide) 54, 304
lens, radiation damage 45
lentigo maligna 334
letrozole 61, 62, 109, 113
Letterer–Siwe disease 321
leucophoresis (leukophoresis), chronic
        granulocytic leukaemia 296
leucovorin see folinic acid
leukaemia 288–99
    acute lymphoblastic 288–92
    childhood 310–13
    chronic lymphocytic 64, 297–9
    myeloid/granulocytic see myeloid/
        myelogenous/granulocytic leukaemia
    rare forms 299
leukophoresis, chronic granulocytic leukaemia
        296
Li–Fraumeni syndrome 2, 91, 207, 254, 260
lip carcinoma, aetiology 226
live source implants 43
liver cancer 135–9
    angiosarcoma 139
    hepatoma see hepatocellular carcinoma
    secondary, from carcinoid 249
        symptoms 249
        treatment 250, 251
liver function tests
    acute lymphoblastic leukaemia 290
    hepatocellular carcinoma 136
    pancreatic cancer 131
lobectomy, lung cancer 76
lobular carcinoma in situ (LCIS) 90, 91
local radiation effects 48
local treatment vs systemic 24
localization of tumour for radiotherapy 46
lumbar puncture 16, 210
lumpectomy 102
lung
    function tests 75
    radiation damage 45
lung cancer 67–84
    aetiology 67–8
    case histories 77, 84
    differential diagnosis 72
    epidemiology 67
        screening 83
    investigations 72–5
    natural history 68–9
    pathology 68
    prevention 83
    secondary see metastases
    staging 75–6

symptoms and signs 69–72
treatment 76–80
    complications 81
    prognosis 81–3
    tumour-related complications 80–1
lymph node involvement
    chronic lymphocytic leukaemia, biopsy 298
    Hodgkin's lymphoma 269–70
        assessment (for staging) 270–1
    non-Hodgkin's lymphoma 277
        treatment 280
lymph node metastases
    anal cancer 153
    breast cancer 93, 103, 105
        assessment and treatment 103–4
    cervical cancer 186
    cutaneous basal and squamous cell carcinoma
        329
    cutaneous melanoma
        assessment for 335
        dissection 335
    fine needle aspiration for see fine needle
        aspiration
    oral cancer 226
        assessment 228
        dissection 229
    penile cancer, assessment 182
    principles concerning
        assessment 11
        surgery 37–8
    prostate cancer 164–5
    testicular cancer, dissection 180
    thyroid cancer 231
    see also TNM staging system
lymphangiosarcoma 255, 259
lymphoblastic leukaemia, acute 288–92
lymphoblastic lymphoma 281
lymphocyte-depleted Hodgkin's disease 269
lymphocyte-predominant Hodgkin's disease 269
    nodular 285
lymphocytic leukaemia, chronic 64, 297–9
lymphoedema of the arm 112, 113
lymphomas, Hodgkin's see Hodgkin's lymphoma
lymphomas, non-Hodgkin's (and unspecified)
        275–85, 315
    aetiology 275
    AIDS-related 275, 343–5
    childhood 315
    differential diagnosis 278–9, 300
    epidemiology 275
    extranodal 281–4, 284
        CNS see central nervous system tumours
        cutaneous 282, 338
        gastrointestinal 130, 275, 276, 282
        ovarian 198
        salivary 237

lymphomas, non-Hodgkin's (and unspecified) –
(*contd*)
  extranodal – (*contd*)
    testicular 180
    thyroid 246
  investigations 277–8
  natural history 277
  pathology 275–7
  prognosis 284–5
  rare forms 285
  staging 279
  symptoms and signs 277–8
  treatment 56, 64, 279–84, 315, 344, 344–5
    aggressive (high-grade) forms 280–4
    complications 284
    indolent (low-grade) forms 279–80
    tumour-related complications 284
Lynch syndrome 143

M band in protein electrophoresis 301
β_2-macroglobulin in multiple myeloma 301
macroglobulinaemia, Waldenström's 285,
  300
magnetic resonance angiography, CNS tumours
  210
magnetic resonance imaging (MRI) 14–15
  bladder cancer 174
  breast cancer 99
  carcinoids 250
  CNS tumours 210
    pituitary tumours 215
    spinal cord compression 356
  gastrointestinal/digestive tract cancer
    anal carcinoma 154
    colorectal carcinoma 146
    hepatocellular carcinoma 137
    oesophageal cancer 120
    pancreatic carcinoma 131
  gynaecological cancer
    cervical cancer 187
    choriocarcinoma 203
    endometrial cancer 192
    vaginal cancer 199
  Hodgkin's lymphoma 270
  lung cancer 74
  medulloblastoma 311
  neuroblastoma 317
  oral cancer 228
  prostate cancer 166
  sarcoma
    Ewing's sarcoma 263–4
    osteogenic 261
    soft tissue 256, 314
maintenance chemotherapy
  acute lymphoblastic leukaemia 290
  acute myeloid leukaemia 293

males/men
  breast cancer 92
  genital cancers 177–82
  new cancers and deaths by site 375–6
MALTomas 130, 275, 276, 282
mammography 97
  screening 114–15
manual afterloading brachytherapy 43
mastectomy 102
  pre-invasive disease 100
  risk factors for recurrence 105
MDR1 57
mediastinoscopy 75
mediastinotomy 75
medication *see* drug therapy
medullary spinal tumours *see* intramedullary
  spinal tumours
medullary thyroid carcinoma 239, 240
  screening in MEN-2 245–6
medulloblastoma 217–18, 311–13
megavoltage machines 42
melanoma 331–8
  cutaneous 331–8
  oesophageal 124
  vaginal 202
men *see* males
meningioma 213–14
meningitis, carcinomatous 221–3
menopausal status and breast cancer
  chemotherapy 106
menopausal symptoms with hormone therapy in
  breast cancer 113
Merkel cell carcinoma 339
mesodermal tumours of ovary, mixed 194
mesothelioma 84–7
  peritoneal 157
  pleural 84–7
meta-analysis 34
meta-iodobenzyl guanidine (mIBG) scan
  neuroblastoma 317
  phaeochromocytoma 247
metastases
  biopsy in lung cancer for 75
  lymph node *see* lymph node metastases
metastases, distant (secondaries)
  assessment (in staging) 11
  from bone 261, 262
  in bone *see* bone metastases; bone scan
  from breast 94–6
    case history with unknown primary 351–2
    exclusion 100
    treatment 107–12
  from carcinoma of unknown primary 347–52
  from choriocarcinoma 202, 204
  from CNS 209
  in CNS/brain/cerebral 219–23

choriocarcinoma 204
MRI 14
prophylactic cranial irradiation *see*
cranial/craniospinal irradiation
from kidney 161
from liver 136
in liver *see* liver cancer
from lung, prophylactic cranial irradiation 78–9
in lung
chest X-ray *see* X-ray
osteosarcoma, resection 261
from neuroblastoma 316
in staging 317
in oral cavity 226
in orbit 237
from ovaries 194
in ovaries (incl. Krukenberg tumours) 95, 125, 194, 198
from prostate 165
in skin 338
from skin melanoma 333–4
exclusion 335
from soft tissue sarcoma 255, 258
from stomach, exclusion 127
from thyroid 240
in TNM system *see* TNM staging system
mIBG scan *see* meta-iodobenzyl guanidine scan
mineral oils 4
mitosis, drugs acting on 53
mixed mesodermal tumours of ovary 194
mixed multiple endocrine neoplasia 252
molar pregnancy 202, 203, 204
monitoring, radiation 50
monoclonal antibodies 8, 63–4
antiangiogenic 54
breast cancer 8, 107
adverse effects 113
metastatic disease 109
chronic lymphocytic leukaemia 297
colorectal carcinoma 150
gastrointestinal stromal tumour 8, 129
lung cancer 80
lymphomas 64, 280, 285
oral cancer 230
prostate cancer 172
MOPP regimen, Hodgkin's lymphoma 273
morphine 365
alternatives to 366
controlled-release 366
pain resistant to 366–7
mortality *see* death
mould treatment 43
mouth *see* oral cavity
multidrug resistance 57
multiple endocrine neoplasia (MEN) 251–2

gastrinoma 135
MEN-1 135, 239, 251
MEN-2 135, 239, 252
screening for medullary carcinoma 245–6
mixed 252
thyroid cancer in 239
multiple myeloma *see* myeloma
muscle relaxants 368
mycosis fungoides 282, 338
myeloablative chemotherapy *see* high-dose
marrow ablative chemotherapy
myelography 210
myeloid/myelogenous/granulocytic leukaemia
acute 292–4
chronic *see* chronic myeloid leukaemia
myeloma (plasma cell) 299–306
multiple 299–306
treatment 54, 303–4
solitary (plasmacytoma) 299, 301, 302, 303, 304–6
myelosuppression and AIDS-related tumour
treatment 342

nasopharyngeal carcinoma 234
nausea and vomiting and their prevention 59–60, 369–70
neck and head cancer 225–34
needle biopsy 11
breast cancer 99
CNS tumours 210
neoadjuvant (preoperative) treatment
chemotherapy
bladder cancer 176
cervical cancer 188–9
oesophageal cancer 121–2
stomach cancer 128
hormone therapy, prostate cancer 169
radiotherapy 37
colorectal carcinoma 147–8
nephrectomy 162
nephroblastoma 318–21
neuroblastoma 316–18
neuroendocrine tumours, gastroenteropancreatic
135
neurofibromatosis 217
type 1 (von Recklinghausen's disease) 3, 254, 316
neurological syndromes, neuroblastoma 317
neuromuscular manifestations of lung cancer 71
neurosurgery 210–11
neutron beam therapy 44
neutropenic sepsis 359–60
nickel 4
nipple
discharge cytology 99
Paget's disease 92

nitrosamines 4
NMDA inhibitors 367
nodular lymphocyte-predominant Hodgkin's
  lymphoma 285
nodular sclerosing Hodgkin's lymphoma 268,
  269
non-Hodgkin's lymphoma *see* lymphoma
non-small cell lung cancer (NSCLC) 68
  management 76–8, 79, 80
  prognosis 83
non-steroidal anti-inflammatory drugs (NSAIDs)
  365, 367

obstructive symptoms, palliation 39
occupational (incl. industrial) carcinogens 3–4
  basal and squamous cell carcinoma and 325
octreotide (somatostatin analogue) 135, 251
ocular tumours and problems *see* eye
oesophageal cancer 118–24
oestrogen(s), endometrial cancer aetiology 191
  see also hormone replacement therapy
oestrogen receptor status in breast cancer 61–2,
  105
  metastatic disease treatment and 108–9
oligodendroglioma 213
oncogenes 2
ophthalmological tumours and problems *see* eye
opioids 365–7
  weak 365
optic nerve metastases 221
oral cavity (mouth) 225–32
  carcinoma 225–32
  other tumours 232
  soreness 370
oral route, chemotherapy 58
orbital tumours 237
orchidectomy 179
  complications 180
  prostate cancer 169
oropharyngeal candidiasis 370
oropharyngeal carcinoma 232
orthovoltage machines 42
osteoclastoma 265
osteosarcoma 259–62
ovarian cancer 194–8
  metastases (incl. Krukenberg tumours) 95,
    125, 194, 198
oxaliplatin, colorectal carcinoma 148, 150
oxycodone 366
oxygenation, tumour, radiosensitivity related to
  45

p53 (*TP53*) 2
  breast cancer and 90
paediatric tumours 310–24
Paget's disease of bone 260, 261, 262

Paget's disease of breast 92
pain 363–8
  chest 70
  control 363–8
palliative treatment 363–74
  bladder cancer 176
  breast cancer 107, 109
  gastrointestinal/digestive tract cancer
    anal carcinoma 155
    cholangiocarcinoma 141
    colorectal carcinoma 148–50
    hepatocellular carcinoma 138
    oesophageal cancer 122
    pancreatic cancer 133
    stomach cancer 128
  gynaecological cancer
    cervical cancer 190
    endometrial cancer 193
    ovarian cancer 196
    vaginal cancer 199
  lung cancer 79–80
  neuroblastoma 318
  non-Hodgkin's lymphoma 280
  oral cancer 230–1
  penile cancer 182
  prostate cancer 169–71
  radical vs 23–4
  radiotherapy in *see* radiotherapy
  renal cell carcinoma 162
  sarcoma
    embryonal rhabdomyosarcoma 315
    Ewing's 264
    osteogenic 261–2
  surgery in 38–9
  thyroid cancer 244
  Wilms' tumour 320
Pancoast tumour 73
pancreas 130–5
  carcinoma 130–5
  rare tumours 135
pantogram, oral 228
Pap (cervical) smear 190–1
papillary thyroid carcinoma 239, 240
paracetamol 364
paranasal sinus carcinoma 235
paraneoplastic conditions
  in neuroblastoma, neurological 317
  renal cell carcinoma 161
paraproteins 299, 301
  electrophoresis 301
parathyroid tumours 236
parenteral opioids 365–6
parosteal sarcoma 262
parotid gland tumours 235–7
partial response (PR) 30
  chemotherapy 55

Patey mastectomy 102
pathogenesis 1–9
pathological information, use 20
Patterson–Brown-Kelly (Plummer–Vinson)
        syndrome 118, 119
pelvic surgery, testicular cancer 180
Pendred's syndrome 239
penile cancer 180–2
percutaneous ethanol injection, hepatocellular
        carcinoma 138
percutaneous transhepatic cholangiography
    cholangiocarcinoma 140
    pancreatic carcinoma 132
performance status
    AIDS patients, poor 342
    chemotherapy and 55
peripheral blood progenitor cells following
        myeloblative therapy in non-Hodgkin's
        lymphoma 281
peritoneal tumours 156–7
Peutz–Jeghers syndrome 143
phaeochromocytoma 246–8
pharyngeal carcinoma 232, 233–5
phase 1/2/3 studies of chemotherapeutic drugs
        65
Philadelphia chromosome 2, 8, 288, 291, 294,
        295
physical carcinogens 4–5
physical examination see examination
pineal tumours 216
pituitary tumours 214–16
placebo-controlled trials 32
placenta-derived tumours 202–4
plain X-rays see X-rays
planning of radiotherapy 46–7
plasma cell neoplasms 299–306
    myeloma see myeloma
    other 299
pleomorphic adenoma, salivary 236
pleural biopsy 86
pleural fluid cytology 86
pleural tumours 84–7
pleurectomy 86–7
pleuropericardial aspiration 80
pleuropneumonectomy 86, 87
Plummer–Vinson syndrome 118, 119
pneumonectomy 76
    see also pleuropneumonectomy
polymerase chain reaction, unknown primary
        carcinoma 349
polyposis, familial adenomatous (FAP) 143
positioning of patient for radiotherapy
        45–6
positron emission tomography 15–16
    CNS tumours 210
    lung cancer 74–5

lymphoma
    Hodgkin's 270
    non-Hodgkin's 278
oesophageal cancer 121
pancreatic carcinoma 131–2
soft tissue sarcoma 256
unknown primary carcinoma, whole body 349
post-marketing surveillance of new drugs 65
postoperative therapy see adjuvant treatment
precursors of breast cancer see ductal carcinoma
        in situ; lobular carcinoma in situ
pregnancy, molar 202, 203, 204
preoperative therapy see neoadjuvant treatment
prevention see screening and specific cancers
primary tumour
    management 36–7
    unknown, carcinoma of 347–52
primitive neuroectodermal tumour (PNET)
        263
    childhood 310–11
    extraosseous 258
proctoscopy
    anal carcinoma 153
    colorectal carcinoma 145
progestogens, breast cancer therapy 62, 109
prognosis, communicating 27
progressive disease (PD) 30
    chemotherapy 55
prolactin-producing pituitary tumours 214, 215,
        216
prolymphocytic leukaemia 299
promyelocytic leukaemia 294
prophylaxis see screening and specific cancers
prostate cancer 163–72
    therapy 62–3, 167–72
        complications 171
prostate-specific antigen (PSA) 165–6, 167, 168,
        170
protection, radiation 49–50
protein electrophoresis, multiple myeloma 301
proteosome inhibitor 304
proton beam therapy 44
pseudomyxoma peritoneii 157
PTEN 91, 143, 191

quality of life (and its measurement) 25
    chemotherapy 55–6
    in trials 30, 31

radiation
    ionizing see ionizing radiation
    solar see solar radiation
radical treatment
    bladder cancer 174–6
    breast cancer 102
    carcinoids 250–1

radical treatment – (*contd*)
   gastrointestinal/digestive tract cancer
      anal carcinoma 155
      cholangiocarcinoma 140–1
      colorectal carcinoma 146–8
      gastric carcinoma 127
      hepatocellular carcinoma 138
      oesophageal cancer 121–2
      pancreatic carcinoma 132–3
      peritoneal tumours 157
   gynaecological cancer
      cervical cancer 187–90
      choriocarcinoma 203–4
      endometrial cancer 192
      ovarian cancer 196
      vaginal cancer 199
      vulval cancer 201
   lung cancer 76–9
   mesothelioma (pleural) 86–7
   oral cancer 228–30
   palliative vs 23–4
   penile cancer 182
   prostate cancer 167, 168–9
   with radiation 48
   renal cell carcinoma 162
   sarcoma
      Ewing's 264
      osteogenic 261
   sarcoma, soft tissue 258
      embryonal rhabdomyosarcoma 314–15
   skin cancer
      basal and squamous cell carcinoma 329–30
      melanoma 335–6
   testicular cancer 179–80
   thyroid cancer 242–4
radiofrequency ablation, hepatocellular
   carcinoma 138
radiography *see* X-rays
radioisotopes *see* isotope; isotope scan *and specific*
   elements
radiology (imaging) 12–20
   bladder cancer 174
   breast cancer 97–9
   carcinoids 250
   cholangiocarcinoma 140
   CNS tumours 210
      pituitary tumours 215
      spinal cord compression 356–7
   cutaneous basal and squamous cell carcinoma
      329
   gastrointestinal/digestive tract cancer
      anal carcinoma 153–4
      colorectal carcinoma 145–6
      hepatocellular carcinoma 137
      oesophageal cancer 120, 120–1
      pancreatic carcinoma 131–2

stomach carcinoma 126
gynaecological cancer
   cervical cancer 187
   choriocarcinoma 203
   endometrial cancer 192
   ovarian cancer 195
   vaginal cancer 199
   vulval cancer 201
leukaemia
   acute lymphoblastic 290
   acute myeloid 293
   chronic granulocytic 295
lung cancer 72, 73–5
lymphoma
   Hodgkin's 270
   non-Hodgkin's 278
medulloblastoma 311
mesothelioma 85–6, 86
multiple myeloma 301
neuroblastoma 317
oral cancer 228
   palliative 231
penile cancer 182
phaeochromocytoma 247
prostate cancer 166–7
for radiotherapy guidance 47
renal cell carcinoma 161
risk of cancer with radiation exposure 5, 49
sarcoma
   Ewing's 263–4
   osteogenic 261
sarcoma, soft tissue 255–6
   children 314
testicular cancer 178
in trials 31
unknown primary carcinoma 349
Wilms' tumour 320
radiosensitivity, factors affecting 45
radiotherapy 36–7, 42–51
   anal carcinoma
      complications 156
      palliative 155
   bladder cancer 176
      complications 176
      palliative 176
   breast cancer 104–5
      adjuvant 24–5, 104–5
      complications 112
      metastatic disease 108
   carcinoids 251
   causing cancer 5, 49
   cervical cancer 187–9
      complications 190
      palliative 190
   cholangiocarcinoma 141
      complications 140

palliative 141
chronic granulocytic leukaemia 296
clinical use (principles) 45–7
CNS tumours 211
    meningioma 214
    metastases 219–20, 221
    pituitary tumours 215–16
    spinal cord compression 357
    see also cranial/craniospinal irradiation
colorectal carcinoma 147–8
    palliative 149
complications/side-effects (general aspects)
    48–9
    *see also specific cancers in subheadings
        above/below*
cutaneous basal and squamous cell carcinoma
    330
    complications 330
cutaneous melanoma 335–6
embryonal rhabdomyosarcoma 315
    complications 315
endometrial cancer 193
    complications 193
    palliative 193
hepatocellular carcinoma 138
    palliative 138
Hodgkin's lymphoma 271
    complications 273
Kaposi's sarcoma 342
lung cancer 76–7, 78–9
    complications 81
    palliative 79
lymph node 38
medulloblastoma 312
    complications 312–13, 313
neuroblastoma 318
    complications 318
    palliative 318
non-Hodgkin's lymphoma 282, 283
    complications 284
oesophageal cancer 121–2
    complications 123
    palliative 122
oral carcinoma 229–30
    palliative 231
ovarian cancer
    palliative 196
    rare forms 197, 198
in pain control (general aspects) 368
palliative (general aspects) 48, 368
    *see also specific cancers in subheadings
        above/below*
pancreatic cancer 132–3
    complications 134–5
    palliative 133
penile cancer 182

complications 182
    palliative 182
prostate cancer 168–9
    complications 171
protection from radiation 49–50
sarcoma
    Ewing's 264, 265
    osteogenic 261
sarcoma, soft tissue 258
    embryonal rhabdomyosarcoma *see
        subheading above*
stomach cancer 127–8
    complications 128–9
    palliative 128
superior vena cava-obstructing tumours 358
surgery combined with *see* adjuvant treatment;
        neoadjuvant treatment
testicular cancer 179
    complications 180
thyroid cancer 242–4
    palliative 244
types and forms 42–4
vaginal cancer 199
    palliative 199
vulval cancer 201
Wilms' tumour
    complications 321
    palliative 320
    postoperative 320
    see also chemoradiotherapy
Rai classification, chronic lymphocytic leukaemia
    298
randomization 32
randomized controlled trials 29–34
rasburicase 260
RCHOP regimen 56, 57, 280, 282, 283
RCVP regimen, non-Hodgkin's lymphoma 279
RECIST response criteria 30
    chemotherapy and 55
rectum
    carcinoma *see* colorectal carcinoma
    digital examination 145, 152
    endorectal ultrasound 146
redistribution phenomenon 45
Reed–Sternberg cells 269
regional vs systemic treatment 24
relapse treatment
    acute lymphoblastic leukaemia 291
    acute myeloid leukaemia 293
    multiple myeloma 304
remote afterloading brachytherapy 43–4
renal failure, multiple myeloma 300, 302
renal tumours
    childhood 318–21
    renal cell carcinoma 160–3
repair of ionizing radiation-related damage 45

repopulation, tumour and normal cell 45
reproductive tract *see* genital tract
resistance
    chemotherapy 56–7
    hormone, breast cancer 62
respiratory (chest) infections, recurrent 70
respiratory symptoms, palliation 370–1
    dying patient 371
response to treatment 30
    chemotherapy 55
restlessness, dying 371
resuscitation 372
retinoblastoma 45
retinoid (all-trans-retinoic acid) therapy,
        promyelocytic leukaemia 294
rhabdoid tumour of kidney 321
rhabdomyosarcoma, embryonal 313–15
rituximab
    chronic lymphocytic leukaemia, combined
            with chemotherapy 298
    lymphomas 64, 280
        combined with chemotherapy 279, 280,
            283
Royal Marsden Stage, testicular cancer 179
rubber industry 3

salivary gland tumours 235–7
salpingo-oophorectomy, bilateral, hysterectomy
        and 193, 196
sarcoma 254–67
    bone *see* bone
    granulocytic 294
    Kaposi's *see* Kaposi's sarcoma
    soft tissue 254–9, 313–15
        childhood 313–15
        cutaneous 339
        endometrial 193
        oral cavity 232
        ovarian 198
        subtypes 255
        vaginal 202
scintigraphy *see* isotope scan
scrapings 10–11
    skin cancer 328–9
screening
    acute myeloid leukaemia 294
    bladder cancer 177
    breast cancer 114–15
    gastrointestinal/digestive tract cancer
        anal carcinoma 156
        colorectal carcinoma 151–2
        hepatocellular carcinoma 139
        oesophageal cancer 124
        stomach cancer 129
    gynaecological cancer
        cervical cancer 190–1

    choriocarcinoma 204
    ovarian cancer 197
    vaginal cancer 200
lung cancer 83
mesothelioma 87
oral cancer 231–2
prostate cancer 172
renal cell carcinoma 163
skin cancer
    basal and squamous cell carcinoma 331
    melanoma 337
testicular cancer 180
thyroid cancer 245–6
second cancers (treatment-related)
    in Hodgkin's lymphoma 274
    in non-Hodgkin's lymphoma 284
    with radiotherapy 5, 49
self-examination, breast 114
seminoma 177
    treatment 179, 180
sentinel lymph node mapping 37
    breast cancer 103
    melanoma 335
sepsis, neutropenic 359–60
serotonin (5-HT), carcinoid syndrome 249, 250
Sertoli cell tumour 194
Sertoli-Leydig cell tumours 198
sexual activity
    and anal cancer 152–3, 156
    and cervical cancer 185
Sézary syndrome 338
sigmoidoscopy, colorectal carcinoma 145
signal transduction inhibitors 53
sinuses (paranasal), cancer 235
skeletal metastases *see* bone metastases
skin 325–40
    lung cancer effects 71
    tumours 325–40
        causes 4, 325–6, 332
        dermatofibroma 259
        non-Hodgkin's lymphoma 282, 338
        T-cell lymphoma 228, 338
small bowel, radiation damage 45
small cell carcinoma
    lung (SCLC) 68
        management 78–9, 79, 80
        prognosis 83
        staging 76
    oesophagus 124
smear, cervical 190–1
smoking 3, 67
    bladder cancer and 172–3
    lung cancer and 67, 83
    oesophageal cancer and 118
    reduction/cessation and avoidance of passive
        exposure 83

soft tissue sarcoma *see* sarcoma
solar keratosis 328
solar radiation (incl. UV) 4
    basal and squamous cell carcinoma and 325
    melanoma 332
somatostatin analogue (octreotide) 135, 251
soot 3, 325
sorafenib/sorafinib 53, 54
    hepatocellular carcinoma 138, 139
    renal cancer 162
    renal cell carcinoma 162
sore mouth 370
spinal opioids 366
spinal tumours 209
    classification 208
    secondary (metastases) 221
    symptoms and signs 209
        compression 209, 355–7
spindle cell sarcoma 265
spindle poisons 53
splenic irradiation in chronic granulocytic
        leukaemia 296
sputum cytology, lung cancer 72
squamous cell carcinoma
    bladder 177
    lung 68
    skin 325–31
stable disease (SD) 30
    chemotherapy 55
staging 11–20
    bladder cancer 174
    breast cancer 100
    carcinoids 250
    gastrointestinal/digestive tract cancer
        anal carcinoma 154–5
        cholangiocarcinoma 140
        colorectal carcinoma 146
        gastric carcinoma 127
        hepatocellular carcinoma 137
        oesophageal cancer 121
        pancreatic carcinoma 132
    gynaecological cancer
        cervical cancer 187
        choriocarcinoma 203
        endometrial cancer 192
        ovarian cancer 196
        vaginal cancer 199
        vulval cancer 201
    head and neck cancer
        laryngeal carcinoma 233
        nasopharyngeal carcinoma 234–5
        oral cancer 228
    leukaemia
        acute lymphoblastic 290
        chronic lymphocytic 298
    lung cancer 75–6

lymphoma
    Hodgkin's 270–1
    non-Hodgkin's 279
medulloblastoma 311–12
mesothelioma 86
multiple myeloma 301–3
neuroblastoma 317–18
penile cancer 182
prostate cancer 167
renal cell carcinoma 161–2
sarcoma
    Ewing's 264
    osteogenic 261
    soft tissue 257, 314
skin cancer
    basal and squamous cell carcinoma 329
    melanoma 335
testicular cancer 178–9
thyroid cancer 241–2
Wilms' tumour 320
statistics, trial 32–3
stem cell transplantation, autologous, multiple
        myeloma 303–4
stent, endobronchial stent 80
stereotactic techniques
    needle biopsy with CNS tumours 210
    radiotherapy 47
        with CNS tumours 221
steroids 367
Stewart–Treves tumour 259
stomach cancer 124–30
    lymphomas (incl. MALTomas) 130, 275, 276,
        282
    rare tumours 129–30
        lymphomas (incl. MALTomas) 130, 275,
            276, 282
stratification 32
subglottic carcinoma 233
sumatinib 162
sunitinib 163
superficial voltage 42
superior vena cava obstruction 357–9
supportive therapy
    CNS tumours 211
    multiple myeloma 304
supraglottic carcinoma 233
surgery 36
    anal carcinoma 155
        complications 156
        palliative 155
    bladder cancer 176
        complications 176
    breast cancer 102–4
        metastatic disease 107–8
        pre-invasive disease 100–2
        risk factors for recurrence 105

surgery – (*contd*)
  carcinoids 250
    palliative 250
  cervical cancer 187
    complications 190
  cholangiocarcinoma 141
    complications 140
    palliative 141
  choriocarcinoma 203
  CNS tumours 210–11
    astrocytoma 211–12
    metastases 220–1
    pituitary tumours 215
    in spinal cord compression 357
  colorectal carcinoma 146–7
    palliative 149
  embryonal rhabdomyosarcoma 315
    complications 315
  endometrial cancer 193
    complications 193
  gallbladder carcinoma 142
  hepatocellular carcinoma 138
    complications 139
    palliative 138
  lung cancer 76, 78
    complications 81
  lymph node 37–8
  medulloblastoma 312
  oesophageal cancer 121
    complications 123
  oral carcinoma 228–9
    complications 231
    palliative 230
  other therapies before or after *see* adjuvant treatment; neoadjuvant treatment
  ovarian cancer 196
    palliative 38–9
  pancreatic carcinoma 132
    complications 134
    palliative 133
  penile cancer 182
  peritoneal tumours 157
  phaeochromocytoma 247
  pleural mesothelioma 86–7
  prostate cancer 168
    complications 171
  renal cell carcinoma 162
  sarcoma
    Ewing's 264
    osteogenic 261
  sarcoma, soft tissue 258
    embryonal rhabdomyosarcoma *see subheading above*
  skin cancer
    basal and squamous cell carcinoma 329
    melanoma 335
  stomach cancer 127
    complications 128
    palliative 128
  systemic treatment vs 24
  testicular cancer 179, 180
    complications 180
  thyroid cancer 242
    complications 244–5
    palliative 244
  vaginal cancer 199
  vulval cancer 201
    complications 202
  Wilms' tumour 320
surveillance
  prostate cancer 167–8
  testicular cancer 179
survival
  communication about 27
  as end-point 29–30
swallowing difficulty *see* dysphagia
symptoms
  measurement in trials 31
  palliation *see* palliative treatment
systemic isotope therapy 44
systemic treatment (in general) 52–6
  breast cancer, adjuvant 25–6
  local or regional treatment vs 24
  renal cell carcinoma 162–3

T-cell lymphoma
  adult (adult T cell leukaemia/lymphoma), HTLV-1 and 275, 297, 298, 299
  classification 276
  cutaneous 282, 338
TAC regimen, breast cancer 107
tamoxifen
  breast cancer 61, 62, 105
    adverse effects 113
    metastatic disease 108–9
    prophylactic 115
  melanoma 336
tar 4, 325
taxanes, metastatic breast cancer 109
temozolomide
  astrocytoma 213
  melanoma 336
teratoma
  brain 216–17
  childhood 322
  ovarian 194, 197
  testicular 177
    treatment 179
terminal care *see* dying
testicular cancer 177–80
  markers 18, 19, 178
thalidomide 54, 304, 305

thoracotomy 75
thorax *see* chest
thymoma 83–4
thyroid cancer 239–46
tissue diagnosis 10–11, 16
   unknown primary carcinoma 348
   see also specific methods
TNM staging system 19–20
   bladder cancer 174
   embryonal rhabdomyosarcoma 314
   gastrointestinal/digestive tract cancer
      anal carcinoma 154–5
      cholangiocarcinoma 140
      colorectal carcinoma 146
      gastric cancer 127
      hepatocellular carcinoma 137
      oesophageal cancer 121
      pancreatic carcinoma 132
   head and neck cancer
      laryngeal carcinoma 233
      nasopharyngeal carcinoma 234–5
      oral cancer 228
   lung cancer 75–6
   osteosarcoma 261
   penile cancer 182
   prostate cancer 167
   renal cell carcinoma 161–2
   testicular cancer 178–9
   thyroid cancer 241–2
   vulval cancer 201
tobacco
   chewing 225
   smoking *see* smoking
tomotherapy 47
topoisomerase inhibitors 53
toxicity in trials 30
TP53 see p53
transitional cell tumours
   bladder 173
   prostate 172
translocations, chromosome
   acute lymphoblastic leukaemia 288, 289
   chronic myeloid/granulocytic leukaemia 2,
      294–5
transurethral resection
   bladder 174–5
   prostate (TURP) 167
trastuzumab (Herceptin) in breast cancer 8, 64,
   107
   adverse effects 113
   metastatic disease 109
trauma, chronic *see* chronic trauma
treatment (general aspects)
   choices and decision-making 23–8
   clinical evidence 28–9
   clinical trials *see* trials

   communication about 26–8
   primary tumour 36–7
   see also specific modes of treatments and specific
      sites or origin of tumours
trephine, bone marrow *see* bone marrow sampling
trials, clinical 28–35
   chemotherapy 65
trisomy 21 (Down syndrome), acute
   lymphoblastic leukaemia 288
Troisier's sign 125, 145
trophoblastic disease 202–4
tubulin polymerization 53
tumour lysis syndrome 360
   in acute lymphoblastic leukaemia 291
   in acute myeloid leukaemia 294
   in chronic granulocytic Hodgkin's lymphoma
      296
   in chronic lymphocytic leukaemia 299
   in Hodgkin's lymphoma 271
   treatment 360
tumour markers 16–19
   ovarian cancer 195
   testicular cancer 18, 19, 178
   thyroid cancer 241
   unknown primary carcinoma 349
   in urine *see* urine tests
tumour suppressor genes 2
Turcot's syndrome 143
type I and II error 33
tyrosine kinase inhibitors 53
   chronic granulocytic/myeloid leukaemia 8,
      296
   lung cancer 80

UK, new cancers and deaths by site 375–7
ultrasound 13
   anal carcinoma 154
   breast cancer 97
   choriocarcinoma 203
   chronic granulocytic leukaemia 295
   hepatocellular carcinoma 137
   mesothelioma 86
   ovarian cancer 195
   prostate cancer 166
   rectal carcinoma 146
   testicular cancer 178
   thyroid cancer 241
ultraviolet radiation *see* solar radiation
United Kingdom, new cancers and deaths by site
   375–7
unknown primary, carcinoma of 347–52
urine tests (incl. tumour markers) 18–19
   bladder cancer 174
   carcinoid 250
   multiple myeloma 301
   neuroblastoma 317

urine tests (incl. tumour markers) – (*contd*)
   phaeochromocytoma 247
   Wilms' tumour 319
urography, intravenous *see* intravenous
    urography
urological cancer 160–77
UV radiation *see* solar radiation

VAC regimen
   complications 315
   embryonal rhabdomyosarcoma 314, 315
   Ewing's sarcoma 264
vaccine
   HPV 191
   prostate cancer therapy 172
vagina
   cancer 198–200
   digital examination 145
vanillylmandelic acid, urinary 247
vascular endothelial growth factor-targeting drugs
    54, 64, 162
   breast cancer 109–10
   lung cancer 80
   renal cell carcinoma 162, 163
vasculature, tumour, drug targeting *see*
    antiangiogenic drugs
VEGF *see* vascular endothelial growth factor
vena cava obstruction, superior 357–9
venous access for chemotherapy 58–9
verification of radiotherapy planning 47
vesicant properties of cytotoxic drugs 59
vinyl chloride monomer 4

VIPoma 135
viruses 5–7
   see also specific viruses
visual field perimetry 215
vocal cord apposition 80
voltage levels in radiotherapy 42
vomiting and its prevention 59–60, 369–70
von Recklinghausen's disease 3, 254, 316
vulval cancer 200–2

Waldenström's macroglobulinaemia 285
Waldeyer's ring lymphoma 282
WHO performance scale and chemotherapy 55
WHO-REAL classification of non-Hodgkin's
    lymphoma 268, 276
Wilms' tumour 318–21
women *see* females
wood dust 3
World Health Organization *see* WHO
WT1 319

X-rays, plain 12–13
   chest *see* chest X-rays
   Ewing's sarcoma 263
   multiple myeloma 301
   neuroblastoma 317
   osteosarcoma 271
   pituitary tumours 215
   skin cancer 329
   see also mammography
xeroderma pigmentosum 4
xerostomia *see* dry mouth